VIKING

MEDICINE
The Self-help Guide

General editors
Professor Michael Orme
Dr. Susanna Graham-Jones

VIKING

VIKING

Published by the Penguin Group
27 Wrights Lane, London W8 5TZ, England
Viking Penguin Inc., 40 West 23rd Street, New York, New York 10010, USA
Penguin Books Australia Ltd, Ringwood, Victoria, Australia
Penguin Books Canada Ltd, 2801 John Street, Markham, Ontario, Canada L3R 1B4
Penguin Books (NZ) Ltd, 182-190 Wairau Road, Auckland 10, New Zealand

Penguin Books Ltd, Registered Offices: Harmondsworth, Middlesex, England

First published 1988

Filmset in Britain by Modern Reprographics Ltd, Hull, North Humberside

Made and printed in Hong Kong by Regent Publishing Services

British Library Cataloguing in Publication Data

Orme, Michael
    Medicine: the self-help guide.
    1. Chemotherapy
    I. Title
    615.5'8   RM262

ISBN 0-670-81705-8

The ideas, procedures and suggestions in this
book are not intended to replace the services of
doctors; they are intended to enable patients to
collaborate more effectively with health professionals in combatting illness and disease. All matters regarding health require some degree of
medical supervision, and any applications of
treatments set forth in this book are made at the
reader's own risk.

THE CONTRIBUTORS

The consultant editors and publishers are grateful to the many doctors who have contributed to *Medicine – The Self-help Guide:* all are listed on page 303.

Many are colleagues of Professor Orme and Dr. Graham-Jones at Liverpool University, and at the Royal Liverpool and other local hospitals. Just as many are in hospital posts and general practice all round Britain.

Besides Michael Orme and Susanna Graham-Jones, Dr. Mary Belshaw, Dr. Peter Campion, Dr. P.Carey, Dr. J.M. Carey, Dr. Peter Elliot, Dr. R.M. Graham and Dr. Denise Kitchener made particularly extensive contributions.

CONTENTS

Medicine – The Self-help Guide has 12 sections, corresponding to the main branches of medicine. For a detailed breakdown of illnesses covered, plus their page numbers, see the section opener pages listed below.

Introduction 8

Gastro-intestinal problems 20

Cardio-vascular 44

Respiratory and associated diseases 66

Problems of the central nervous system 82

Infections 132

Metabolic and endocryn disorders 152

Obstetrics, gynaecology, urinary and children 170

Malignant disease and the immune system 200

Blood and nutritional 218

Skeletal, joint and muscular disorders 232

Ear, nose, throat and eye 252

Skin and hair 272

Index 294

Contributors 303

Acknowledgements 304

INTRODUCTION

Michael Orme

The ultimate purpose of this book is to increase understanding of medicine. All the doctors who have contributed believe that a suitably informed patient is generally happier with the treatment and perhaps more able to cope with illness. Certainly the medications in question are more likely to give a beneficial result. But medicine is, of course, a complex subject; it is difficult, if not impossible, to understand about the treatment for an illness unless one first understands the illness itself. For this reason, *Medicine – The Self-help Guide* is organized by illnesses, rather than the daunting chemical classifications of modern medicine.

Each of the 90-odd sections are devoted to an illness, or group of similar illnesses or diseases. Each begins with a clear definition of what the illness or disease actually is; then moves on to describe to drugs used and how they work. This approach involves some repetition, but this is worth it for the sake of easy reference.

Of course, treatment of illness or disease does not always involve drugs. In many cases non-drug treatment is highly effective. Dietary treatment of, for example, diabetes or disorders of fat metabolism is often at least as important as the use of drugs. In some cases treatment requires the removal of some insult to your system. So, working alongside the mainstream drug information are sections on how to lose weight; how to relax more effectively and thus give up tranquillizers; how to cope with fatigue and stress in general.

Not all drug treatment involves the use of prescribed medicines. For many conditions there are treatments that can be bought at pharmacists; thus every section contains advice on over-the-counter treatments. It is, however, important to realize that such medicines can occasionally have disagreeable side-effects, and that they may interact with the medicines a doctor is prescribing. Make a habit of discussing with your doctor whether an over-the-counter treatment is appropriate for you.

Another aim of this book is to help the patient work with the doctor to achieve the best result possible from the treatment given. Each section suggests certain questions to ask a doctor during consultation. These cannot, of course, be comprehensive; but they are intended to be a useful starting point. They are in no way a substitute for questions that concern you particularly. You are not challenging a doctor's competence when you ask such questions: in fact, you will be showing that you are interested in the treatment and want to achieve the best possible result.

These features are of course entirely appropriate to a modern drug handbook; but to them we have added others which, we hope, will give the book added value. Many of the sections go into considerable detail about self-management during illness. This typically includes advice on maximizing the effectiveness of the medicines taken – or of cutting them down so as to achieve results with minimum intake. But they also include many practical suggestions for coping with illness, and indeed preventing it. The aim is to involve the patient as far as possible in *actively* fighting the illness rather than being the passive recipient of medicines. Obviously this is far more relevant to some illnesses than others; but there is usually something the patient can do. Thus *Medicine – The Self-help Guide* is an all-round approach to drugs and to illness: it sees illness, medicines, doctor, and patient as equally important parts of a whole.

Adverse drug effects

Although all drugs are tested exhaustively before being released on to the market, absolute safety can never be guaranteed. Indeed, practically no drug is without some side-effect(s) which basically need to be taken in the patient's stride. These are listed in each section; the patient is not bound to have them; often they are minimal. By contrast, there will always be the occasional individual who responds adversely to a medicine, and these grave, or potentially grave side-effects are also mentioned. In general they are uncommon; don't assume that, because they are mentioned, they are likely to happen. If you are unlucky enough to suffer an adverse effect from any medicine, discuss it with your doctor as soon as possible: in most cases he or she will want to change the treatment. If you feel really awful on your medicine and cannot see a doctor, it *may* be sensible to stop taking the medicines straight away. However this is not always the best course because sometimes it is harmful to stop a medicine before the course is finished. Therefore, make every effort to get in touch with a doctor to ask if it is alright to stop a medicine. Doctors should be interested in adverse effects and may want to report these to the appropriate drug watchdog body.

Drugs today

The words 'drug' or 'drugs' have acquired a tarnished reputation over the last decade and this is primarily because of the problems of drug abuse and addiction. In this context 'drugs' means heroin, cocaine or amphetamine in its various forms. In medical practice the word 'drug' is used interchangeably with 'medicine' and only a tiny fraction of the medicines in use today produce addiction. There are currently some 2,500 different drugs available for prescription in the UK alone and when the various combination preparations are included this number increases substantially.

Modern medicines are, in large part, the end result of years of patient research. The original idea for a drug has to undergo extensive laboratory testing before being tried out in humans. If all goes well, the government's watchdog committee on drugs (in the UK, the C.S.M.) will grant a clinical trials certificate, or give an exemption to that certificate. Then, extensive trials will take place in humans before the drug is given a product licence – only then may the new drug be prescribed by doctors.

The majority of new drugs are developed by the pharmaceutical companies and it is estimated that it takes at least 12 years and costs £70 million to develop a new drug. To allow the company to recoup some of their development costs the new drug is initially protected by a patent which lasts for about 20 years. When the product licence is finally granted, the drug will be sold under a trade name, although it will also have a chemical or generic name. The generic name, for example cimetidine, tells doctors and other professionals what type of drug it is. The trade name (in this case Tagamet) is chosen as a catchy label and may also tell the doctor something about the type of drug it is. In this book, the **NAMES YOU WILL HEAR** section gives a selection of both generic names and trade names of most of the drugs likely to be prescribed.

Once a patent has expired, companies other than the original developer may decide to sell the drug and thus it may acquire more than one trade name. However, much prescribing today is done using the generic name only.

We hope that by giving a range of names, including the main variants in English-speaking markets worldwide (excluding the USA), you will usually find the one that is applicable to your case. But with the vast array of drugs and different drug names that are now used it is not possible to provide a complete listing.

The future
Research goes on continuously into all areas of drug treatment to find substances that are more effective or have fewer side effects. In certain areas where drugs are not as yet very useful (for example drugs to prevent premature aging, drugs to treat obesity, drugs to treat AIDS) there is real promise of better treatments to come. Against this must be balanced the fact that medicine will probably never provide a drug which can be guaranteed 100 per cent safe and 100 per cent effective.

Healthy diet
The source of daily energy supply

Carbohydrates 50%
Proteins 10-15%
Fats 35-40%

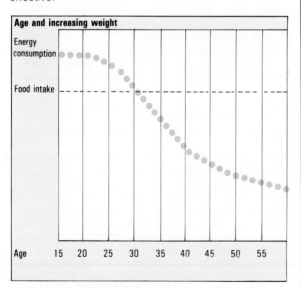

Age and increasing weight

Energy consumption

Food intake

Age   15   20   25   30   35   40   45   50   55

Prevention of illness and disease
The main focus of modern medicine is still on correcting the disease process once disaster has struck; the shortcomings of this approach are well-illustrated in the

Effects of alcohol

12 pints
(¾ bottle whiskey)
Loss of consciousness

5 pints
(10 whiskies)

Chances of road accident
are 25 times greater than
normal.

2½ pints
(5 whiskies)

The risk of having
an accident
is increased × 4

1 pint of beer
(2 single whiskies)

Judgement becomes
slightly impaired, and
reactions slower

patient who suffers a major stroke: once brain cells have died, the only recourse is to retrain other parts of the brain to take over from the damaged parts. Much more effective would be to try to prevent the stroke in the first place and increasingly people in the health care professions are directing their attention to the prevention of illness.

In some cases, the causes of disease are in the environment and the ability of the individual to control these factors is limited. Central government, or local authorities have here a clear responsibility: pollutants in the air, radioactivity and indeed noise are, or should be, controlled by a public body in every country. However, there are ways in which the individual can take action, and they tend to boil down to awareness, and respect for, the risk factors for certain diseases. Thus for heart attack (*myocardial infarction* – see page 52) the main risk factors are cigarette smoking, obesity, high blood pressure and high serum cholesterol. The first two factors are for the individual to control; the second two are, strictly speaking, the concern of the doctor, but attending a clinic for health checks regularly is the only certain way to alert the professional to the need for action.

Primary and second prevention
These terms have recently crept into the medical vocabulary. In the case of a heart attack, primary prevention means taking steps to prevent a heart attack ever happening. If an individual has already had one heart attack, secondary prevention aims to prevent a further one happening. Between primary and secondary prevention, methods may widely differ.

Diet
The average Western diet is not healthy. Generally, we all eat too much salt, too much animal fat and too much sugar as sucrose (the ordinary sugar bought as granulated or castor sugar). Fat, in particular, supplies 40 per cent of the average person's energy needs and this should be reduced to 30 per cent. Protein intake is about right and this is usually the expensive part of our diet. We generally need to increase the amount of fibre we eat and the amount of fruit and vegetables. Convenience foods like fish and chips, hamburgers and so on often contain much animal fat and salt. They are not necessarily bad foods; but in excess they do not provide a healthy diet. Adjusting diet in this way will help to prevent obesity and heart disease.

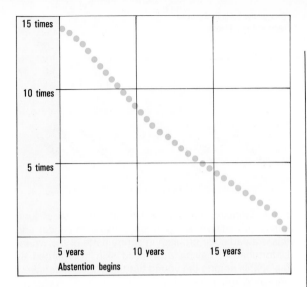

Chances of smokers'
dying from lung cancer
compared to non-smokers

15 times
10 times
5 times

5 years   10 years   15 years
Abstention begins

Alcoholic content of drinks

Beer
5% by
volume

Wine
10% by
volume

Fortified
wine
20% by
volume

Spirits
40% by
volume

Smoking

This is probably the biggest single cause of preventable disease. Smoking is strongly linked with chest disease, heart disease, arterial disease, stomach disease and cancer to name but a few. Unfortunately, many people who smoke feel that disasters only happen to other people and it is always possible to point to an individual who has smoked all his life and who is fit and well in his eighties. He is the exception that proves the rule. The fewer cigarettes you smoke (preferably none), the more likely you are to remain healthy.

Alcohol

People in most Western countries drink alcohol to excess. Alcohol is strongly linked with liver disease, heart disease and intestinal disease – amongst others. However it is not necessary to stop consuming alcohol completely. Small amounts of alcohol seem to be actually beneficial to long-term health. Women should not exceed 10 units of alcohol per week and men should not exceed 15 units per week (a unit is half a pint of beer, a glass of wine or a single standard measure of spirits).

Cancer

There is no doubt that many cancers are preventable. For some, this depends on central control to reduce radioactivity or chemical contamination of the environ-

Type of exercise: Walking Housework Gardening/Weeding Golf Brisk walk Badminton Horse riding Gymnastics

ment. Stopping smoking will reduce the risk of lung cancer. Excessive sunlight can cause skin cancer and this is a particular problem in sunny parts of the world. Unfortunately, having a bronzed skin is regarded as fahionable among the young but this vogue is definitely unhealthy in the long run.

Cancer in women is a particular problem, particularly cancers of the breast, the neck of the womb (cervical cancer) and of the body of the womb itself. Screening systems now exist to look at all these problem areas. Women should be encouraged to examine their own breasts for unusual lumps and should have a cervical smear every three to five years. Many centres are setting up 'well women' clinics for just these purposes. It is hoped that mammography, a simple X-ray examination of the breasts, will improve matters further.

Exercise
In general we all take too little exercise and this contributes to being overweight. This does not mean compulsory jogging for life, but everyone should try to take *some* exercise *each* day. Choose the form of exercise you enjoy most: it should be sufficiently strenuous to increase the heart rate.

Infectious diseases
The big improvement in community health has come from the reduction in infectious diseases following the provision of clean water. It follows that general habits of cleanliness are important to health and everyone should, for example, wash their hands before preparing food before eating.

Immunization has done much to reduce the problems of infectious disease in childhood. Children should cer-

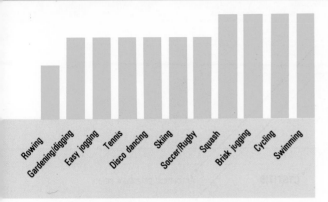

Rowing · Gardening/digging · Easy jogging · Tennis · Disco dancing · Skiing · Soccer/Rugby · Squash · Brisk jogging · Cycling · Swimming

tainly be immunized against diptheria, tetanus and poliomyelitis and girls against rubella (German measles) if they have not had the natural disease by the age of 12. The whooping cough vaccine has brought immunization into poor repute, but there is little doubt that the risks of this vaccine have been over-stated and the benefits outweigh the risks in the large majority of children. Whooping cough in children can be fatal, even with modern drugs.

If you are going abroad, particularly to the tropics, you will need to take special advice on preventing illness. It is, for example, essential to take drugs to prevent malaria, which probably kills more people throughout the world than any other disease. The problem of AIDS is now a real one: the AIDS virus is not easily spread, but is present in the vaginal secretions of women and the semen of men. The contraceptive sheath seems to give considerable protection against infection during sexual intercourse.

All this amounts to only a brief summary of the possibilities of preventitive medicine. One of the best ways to discover more is to contact one of the many local or national self-help groups. There is one for almost every disease though the more common, long-term disabling conditions such as diabetes and multiple sclerosis are represented by especially active groups. The chance to discuss problems with someone who has faced them too is reassuring and often prevents those same problems arising. Ask a doctor, community nurse, social worker or community health council about the existence of such organizations in your area.

Michael Orme
Liverpool, August 1987

USING THE BOOK

Principal drug 'families' relevant to the illness/disease.

Definition of illness/disease, including selective list of symptoms.

The book's scope is essentially drug treatment of illness. Medical problems never tackled with drugs are generally not included.

A selection (not an exhaustive list) of the common chemical (generic) names of drugs plus some of their most familiar trade names. The list begins with UK names, then moves on to give some of the commoner overseas names in English-speaking countries such as Australia, New Zealand, Canada and South Africa, but excluding the USA.

Prescription drugs for the illness/disease; how they are given, and, in simple terms, how they work.

A selection of remedies generally available from chemists, with comments on their usefulness.

Usual (generally tolerated) and adverse side effects. These are not exhaustive lists, and reactions in individuals vary widely.

CYSTITIS

Antibiotics, potassium citrate

NAMES YOU WILL HEAR

Antibiotics
Chemical name: sulphamethizole; trade names: Urolucosil, Urolex, Uroz, Thiosulfil, S-Methizole, Thiosulfil. Chemical name: ampicillin; trade names: Ampifen, Penbritin, Pentrexyl, Vidopen, Austrapen, Bristin, Amcill, Ampicin, Ampilean, Biosan, Ampil, Famicilin, Pentrex, Petercilin, Synthecillin. Chemical name: co-trimoxazole; trade names: Bactrim, Fectrim, Nodilon, Septrin. Chemical name: nalidixic acid; trade names: Mictral, Negram, Uriben. Chemical name: nitrofurantoin; trade names: Furadantin, Macrodantin. Chemical name: nolidixic acid; trade names: Mictral, NeGram, Uriben. Chemical name: nitro furantoin; trade names: Furadantin, Macrodantin.

Potassium citrate
Chemical name: potassium citrate; trade name: Effercitrate.

RISKS WITH POTASSIUM CITRATE
Recent studies have indicated that potassium citrate may under some circumstances cause kidney damage. Raise this issue with your doctor before taking the drug.

WHAT IS CYSTITIS?
– Painful passing of urine, commonly in women. Passing urine becomes frequent, uncontrollable, and sometimes the urine contains blood. These symptoms are due to inflammation of the urethra, the tube leading from the bladder to outside the body. A pain in the lower abdomen means that the bladder is also inflamed. If the kidneys are involved, a dull backache develops, often accompanied by a fever – a condition known as pyelitis.

CAUSES The root cause is either infection or bruising. The infection may be present in the kidneys or bloodstream and descend to the bladder, but more commonly it ascends from the urethra.

PRESCRIPTION DRUGS
Antibiotics: the common remedy. Many types are available; those listed here are particularly suited to treating cystitis; typically taken as tablets.
How they work: By killing bacteria responsible for infection. However, some bacteria can become resistant to some antibiotics; the antibiotic becomes ineffective, and a different one has to be prescribed. Antibiotics also have a tendency to kill not only the 'target' bacteria, but others as well; as some bacteria are naturally helpful in fighting harmful bacteria, a course of antibiotics can leave you without natural defences.
Potassium citrate helps relieve discomfort of cystitis.
How it works: by neutralizing acid in the urine.

OVER-THE-COUNTER TREATMENTS
Potassium citrate is available under several brand names; sometimes it is referred to simply as 'pot. cit.' (pronounced ''pot sit''). A good pharmacist will recommend a dosage and trial treatment period. If this fails, see a doctor straightaway.

QUESTIONS TO ASK THE DOCTOR
■ How long should I take the antibiotics?
■ How soon will the symptoms go?
■ How will I know whether they are working?
■ What happens if I am allergic to the antibiotics?

SIDE EFFECTS
Antibiotics are usually prescribed for less than one week, but for recurrent cystitis, a course may last several weeks. Antibiotics can make you feel under-the-weather and lethargic; some people are allergic to

142

16

The self-management/self-help sub-sections are, where appropriate, sub-divided to include measures for chronic (on-going) illness and acute episodes (sudden attacks).

them, and may develop a rash. Report this to a doctor immediately.

Potassium citrate: A helpful treatment, but it tastes awful, and this may make you vomit.

SELF-MANAGEMENT

If you have had cystitis once, work against future infection – and the need to take antibiotics:

■ After using lavatory paper in the usual way, soap hands and gently cleanse anus; rinse hands, then pour a bottle of warm water over anus away from vagina.

■ Wear cotton underpants and change them daily. Avoid wearing tights. Rinse underwear well and do not use strong soap powders or bleach.

■ Always pass urine within 15 minutes of sexual intercourse and then wash the uro-genital area with cool water. Rest – if possible.

■ Drink as little alcohol as possible, and if you do, try to have long drinks, and some bland liquid afterwards.

■ Drink 3-4 pints of bland liquid or water daily.

SELF-HELP IN AN ATTACK

As soon as the attack begins:

1 Put the kettle on for two hot water bottles. **2** Drink one pint of cold water and let your stomach settle. **3** When the kettle has boiled and the hot water bottles are filled, take one teaspoon of bicarbonate of soda mixed in water or jam. **4** Take two strong painkillers. **5** Fill a jug and glass with bland liquid; keep them by you and drink often. **6** Once each hour drink strong, coffee. **7** Try to put your feet up, or go to bed. Take your jug and glass, but before resting, drink another half pint of fluid. **8** Put one hot water bottle on your back and the other high up between your legs, resting against the urethral opening. **9** Every time you pass water, wash the surrounding area and gently dab it dry. **10** CONTINUE TO DRINK HALF A PINT OF LIQUID EVERY 20 MINUTES.

The kidneys produce, and excrete urine. Waste materials in the blood are extracted in the kidneys and transformed into urine. This passes via the ureter tubes to the bladder where it is stored until the bladder fills up. It then passes through a valve to the urethra, down which it passes to be expelled from the body.

PATIENT'S EXPERIENCE
"My first treatment for cystitis was a month's course of antibiotics which made me really sick. A few weeks later, back came the cystitis, and more antibiotics were prescribed. Over the next few months I had to take 14 different types of pills. After a variety of investigations, including cauterizing of my urethra, I was prescribed yet more antibiotics. In the end, it was my doctor who said 'try passing water after intercourse'. After all that fruitless medication, it was this simple advice which worked."

The case histories do not relate to actual individuals; they are amalgamations of the typical accounts of illness and disease heard by doctors during consultation. Similarity to any individual's circumstances is purely coincidental. No confidential patient information is disclosed.

143

1

Keep medicines out of the reach of children.

2

Keep medicines in the containers in which you receive them – never transfer medicines from one container to another.

3

Your medicines have been prescribed especially for you. Never allow other people to take them. Do not accept medicines which have been prescribed for anyone else.

4

If you have difficulty in opening your medicine container please ask your pharmacist for alternative packaging.

5

If you find the instructions on the label difficult to read, please tell your pharmacist.

6

Always follow the instructions carefully when taking or using medicines. If you have not been given instructions, or if you do not understand them, ask your pharmacist for advice.

The contributors to *Medicine – The Self-help Guide* are not the only people to believe that a better understanding of medicines allows them to be used to better effect. In Britain, and other countries throughout the world, government health departments, pharmaceutical companies and medical faculties of univer-

7

Keep medicines in a cool, dry place unless otherwise directed: some medicines may need to be kept in a refrigerator.

8

Some medicines have an expiry or 'use before' date. Do not use them after this date.

9

Dispose of unwanted medicines carefully. If in doubt, return them to your pharmacist who will dispose of them for you.

10

When buying medicines, please tell the pharmacist about any medicines your doctor has prescribed for you.

11

Some medicines take several days to achieve their intended benefit.

12

If you experience side effects with a medicine, please tell your doctor or pharmacist.

sities are starting to tackle the task of ensuring that patients receive information about their medicines in an easily understandable form.

In the UK, for instance, drugs manufacturers are including (from mid-1988) descriptive leaflets with most medicines.

Gastro-intestinal problems

The gastro-intestinal system includes the oesophagus (or gullet), the stomach, and the intestines – both small and large bowel. Food is partly digested in the stomach and then, in the small intestine, further digestion and absorption of nutrients takes place. In the large bowel (or colon) water is removed from the contents to form faeces (stools) which are discharged through the anus via the rectum. The liver, with the gall bladder, is included in the gastro-intestinal system because this is primarily where all the nutrients absorbed into the body are put to use and 'metabolised'

INDIGESTION AND HIATUS HERNIA — 22-23

NAUSEA AND VOMITING — 24-25
including motion sickness

PEPTIC ULCER, — 26-27
including gastric and duodenal

DIARRHOEA, — 28-29
including dysentery

CONSTIPATION — 30-31

IRRITABLE BOWEL SYNDROME — 32-33

HAEMORRHOIDS (PILES) — 34-35

MALABSORPTION, — 36-37
including coeliac disease

ULCERRATIVE COLITIS — 38-39

JAUNDICE, — 40-41
including hepatitis

CIRRHOSIS — 42-43

See also: *Obesity, page 154; organ transplants, page 216; blood and nutritional, pages 218-231; food intolerance, page 230.*

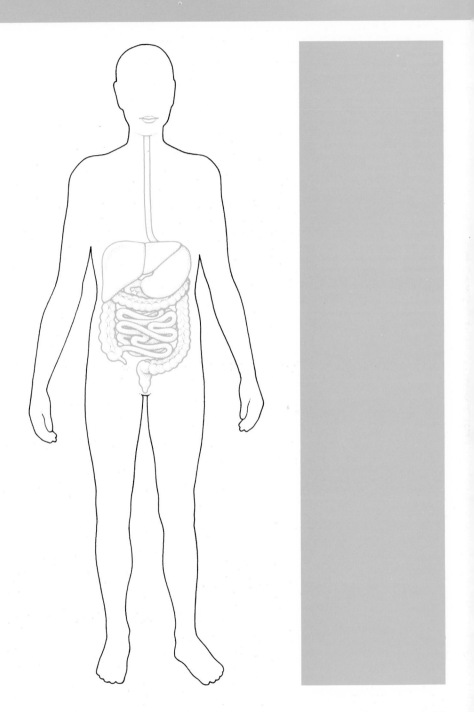

WHAT IS INDIGESTION?

Pain – typically the aching variety – in the upper abdomen, just under the ribs, in the mid line. It can be associated with heartburn, a burning pain in the centre of the chest, sometimes extending up to the throat, with an acid taste in the mouth; also with waterbrash, when saliva floods into the mouth, often accompanied by nausea. Another meaning of indigestion, used by some people, is belching or burping wind.

"Hiatus hernia" is a condition in which the stomach bulges up through the diaphragm into the chest, and is often, but not always, accompanied by the symptoms described above.

Oesophagitis is inflammation of the gullet, and this causes similar pain, especially after drinking hot liquids. It is caused by stomach acid leaking up into the gullet, particularly when there is a hiatus hernia.

CAUSES Anything which irritates or inflames the stomach can cause these symptoms: too much food or drink, especially alcohol, stress, or spicy foods, and smoking. These all cause inflammation of the stomach lining, or gastritis. Ulcers, either gastric, in the stomach, or duodenal, in the duodenum, represent a more severe form of inflammation, when lining is completely lost over a small area – *see **peptic ulcer**, page 26.*

PRESCRIPTION DRUGS

Antacids: available either as tablets to be chewed or as white mixture.
How they work: by mopping up, or neutralizing acid normally produced by the stomach. It is a common misconception that stomach acid actually causes the condition. In fact its role is to aggravate already existing inflammation. Some preparations also contain alginic acid, which helps the antacid to coat the lining of the stomach or gullet.
Anti-emetics lessen the symptoms of indigestion, nausea and heartburn.
How they work: by reducing the time food and acid remain in the stomach by stimulating stomach emptying. They also act on the brain to cut down nausea.
H2 antagonists are expensive, but are highly effective for ulcer healing, both gastric and duodenal, and also for oesophagitis, for which higher doses are used. They are less useful for other forms of indigestion and are not normally used unless the diagnosis has been proved by tests.
How they work: The output of acid by the stomach is

almost completely stopped by these drugs. *See **peptic ulcer**, page 26*.

QUESTIONS TO ASK THE DOCTOR
■ When should I take the antacids?
■ Should I change my diet?
■ Will smoking or drinking affect my symptoms?
■ Have I got an ulcer?

SIDE EFFECTS
Antacids are relatively free from serious side effects, unless taken in gross excess. Bicarbonate of soda, which is often used as a home remedy, will cause serious disturbance to the body's fluid balance if taken regularly. Aluminium-based antacids tend to cause constipation, while magnesium leads to diarrhoea: this is why most are a mixture of the two.

Anti-emetics may, rarely, cause unpleasant involuntary movements of the limbs, especially in the young and the old. They stop as soon as the drug wears off.

H2 antagonists have no serious side effects, although cimetidine may interfere with other prescribed drugs, and occasionally causes diarrhoea. *See **peptic ulcer**, page 26*.

OVER-THE-COUNTER TREATMENTS
A wide range of antacids is available without prescription, such as Rennies, Settlers, Bisodol, Gelusil or Milk of Magnesia, but if you need to take them continually you should consult your doctor. Expensive preparations are unlikely to be any more effective than simple magnesium trisilicate mixture, magnesium trisilicate compound tablets, or aluminium hydroxide (either tablets or mixture).

SELF-MANAGEMENT
A number of basic changes to your lifestyle may help to reduce the amount of indigestion or heartburn you suffer – but not to eliminate it:
■ If you smoke, give up. All forms of tobacco stimulate the stomach to produce acid, the main cause of pain and ulcers.
■ If you are overweight, lose weight. Fat in and around the abdomen presses on the stomach, leading to acid regurgitation and heartburn.
■ Avoid large meals late at night. Avoid fatty food, as fat delays stomach emptying, encouraging acid regurgitation.
■ Avoid foods you know will provoke trouble.

ALCOHOL
If you drink more than 15 units of alcohol per week, cut down. This amount represents the lower safe limit for men; for women the limit is less – *see **alcoholism**, page 94*.

SELF-HELP IN AN ATTACK
Once pain starts, a proprietary antacid will probably help; bicarbonate of soda can be used in an emergency, but not regularly. If food relieves your pain, and the symptoms occur frequently, it is quite likely you have an ulcer: see your doctor.

NAMES YOU WILL HEAR
General anti-emetics
Chemical name: prochlorperazine;
trade names: Stemetil, Compazine,
Anti-Naus, Mitil, Vertigon **Chemical name:** trifluoperazine; **trade name:** Stelazine. **Chemical name:** cyclizine;
trade names: Marzine, Valoid.
Chemical name: cinnarizine; **trade name:** Stugeron. **Chemical name:** metoclopranide; **trade names:** Maxolon, Metox, Metramid, Parmin, Primperan, Gastrobid. **Chemical name:** domperidone; **trade names:** Evoxin, Motilium. **Chemical name:** promethazine; **trade names:** Phenergan, Avomine, Progan, Prothazine, Histantil, Lenazine, Prohist, Profan. **Chemical name:** meclozine;
trade names: Ancoloxin, Ancolan, Bonamine, Navicalm.

Meniére's Disease
Chemical name: betahistine; **trade name:** Serc.

Glucose-salt solutions
Chemical name: sodium chloride:
trade names: Dioralyte, Rehidrat.

CAUSES
Gastroenteritis or general infection (for example tonsillitis, ear infection, meningitis, kidney infection, appendicitis); obstructions in the bowel, scars from previous operations, or tumours; hormonal changes as in pregnancy and diabetes; disorders of balance, including motion sickness, Meniére's Disease and certain viral infections of the ear; brain disease causing pressure on the brain or migraine; certain drugs (digitalis, opiate analgesics, some drugs used in the treatment of cancer and the oestrogen component of the contraceptive pill); poisons (iron, lead), alcohol, radiotherapy; psychogenic factors such as anxiety or bulimia (see pages 84 and 220).

WHAT ARE NAUSEA AND VOMITING?
Vomiting is a reflex action caused by a stimulus from the vomiting centre in the base of the brain. It is usually preceded by nausea – the inclination to vomit – accompanied by sweating, pallor, excessive salivation and dizziness (see page 96). Profuse or prolonged vomiting can result in dehydration.

CAUSES See list in margin. All those listed can stimulate the vomiting centre in the brain, either via substances in the bloodstream, or by stimulation of nerves.

PRESCRIPTION DRUGS
The choice of drug depends partly on the cause:
Anti-emetic drugs can be used to treat vomiting generally, but the side effects are significant. They should not be used if the cause can be rapidly treated and they are only appropriate for cases of persistent vomiting, not for nausea. This applies especially to children and old people, in whom side effects are commonest. They can be given by mouth, or by injection or suppository if the patient is vomiting continuously.
How they work: by acting on the brain, suppressing the stimulus to vomit.
After vomiting, one should drink clear fluid to replace what has been lost. A glucose-salt solution may be a useful alternative to clear fluid, particularly in young children. See **diarrhoea,** page 28.
Cinnarizine can be very effective against motion sickness, and it is less sedative than others of its kind; however, no single drug should be regarded as outstanding. Duration of action and the degree of drowsiness caused vary widely. Test different varieties to find which suits you best.
Promethazine and **meclozine** have been used for many years to treat vomiting in early pregnancy, with no reports of adverse effects. However, drugs should only be used if vomiting is really severe, not for nausea: there is always the potential for drug-induced abnormalities in the foetus. See **pregnancy,** page 184.
Severe nausea and vomiting associated with Meniére's Disease and vertigo can be difficult to treat. See **dizziness,** page 96. **Betahistine** is said to have a specific effect; if it does not work, any of the general anti-emetics could be tried.
How it works: not fully understood, but it is thought to improve circulation to the brain. Metoclopramide antagonises dopamine in the brain and thus calms the vomiting centre (see **migraine,** page 100).

OVER-THE-COUNTER TREATMENTS

Oral rehydration fluids (Dextrolyte, Rehydrat) are useful for maintaining adequate hydration in children; they may be used as soon as vomiting starts. Some motion sickness drugs can be bought without a prescription; self-treatment is appropriate, but it is worth experimenting to find the one that suits best.

QUESTIONS TO ASK THE DOCTOR

■ When can I start on solid foods again?
■ Should I avoid any foods?
■ How long is the vomiting likely to last?
■ Are drugs necessary?
■ How often can I take the treatment?

SIDE EFFECTS

Anti-emetics are often antihistamines and tend to have similar side effects. However, the frequency and severity vary as much between people as between drugs. They all cause drowsiness and should not be taken while driving or working in a potentially dangerous environment. This drowsiness is made worse by alcohol. Other side effects include dry mouth, headache and irritability. Muscle stiffness and spasms can occur, usually associated with high doses, but children and some individuals are more sensitive. The effect is reversible with an appropriate drug.

These drugs should not be used in children under $1\frac{1}{2}$ stones (10 kg), in people who are dehydrated, nor in people with glaucoma.

Betahistine (not an antihistamine) causes headache and must not be used in people with asthma or peptic ulcer.

SELF-MANAGEMENT

■ Some normal babies regurgitate their feeds. This is no cause for worry if the baby is gaining weight, and it can be at least partially improved by frequent winding, thickening feeds and propping up after feeds. It usually resolves once the baby is on a mixed diet. ■ Any patient who has vomited should be given clear fluids to drink. The most suitable are sugar-salt solution, water, diluted pure apple juice or soda water. ■ Milk and other dairy products should be avoided, as should all fatty foods. Digesting fat causes extra strain on an already irritated stomach. ■ Small amounts of fluid, taken frequently, are easiest to absorb. ■ Fever can cause or aggravate vomiting, particularly in young children, so get the patient's temperature down: *see **common cold**, page 134.* ■ Do not take aspirin .

TREATMENT OF MOTION SICKNESS

■ Take the pills about half an hour before starting the journey. ■ Avoid heavy, fatty meals before or during the journey. ■ If in a car or train, face forwards and look out of the window. ■ If on a boat, lie flat, or if you wish to be up and about, try to keep your gaze on the horizon. ■ Have small frequent meals. ■ Don't read or write while in motion.

TREATMENT OF VOMITING DURING PREGNANCY

■ Have something to eat BEFORE getting up in the morning. ■ Eat small, frequent meals during the day – but remember, weight gained now is not easily lost.

WHEN TO SEE A DOCTOR

■ If vomiting persists for more than 24 hours. ■ If a child under six years has diarrhoea or fever as well as vomiting: there is a danger of dehydration. ■ If there is vomiting after a head injury. ■ If the patient is not only vomiting but generally ill.

PEPTIC ULCER

Antacids, H₂ antagonists, muscosal strengtheners, anticholinergics

WHAT IS A PEPTIC ULCER?

A defect, or a hole, in the lining of the gut – the mucosa. Peptic ulcers can occur in the gullet (oesophageal ulcer), stomach (gastric ulcer), duodenum (duodenal ulcer) or rarely in other parts of the gut. Pain in the upper abdomen, or sometimes the chest and back, is the most common symptom. The pain is related to meals, often being relieved by food or milk, and may wake the patient from sleep. Most cases of peptic ulcer are treated with drugs, but surgery may be needed for complications such as bleeding.

CAUSES Although this is a common disease, the mechanism of ulcer formation is not understood. Smoking and heavy alcohol consumption are thought to increase the risk; drugs such as aspirin and indeed various drugs used to treat arthritis can cause ulcers.

PRESCRIPTION DRUGS

Antacids: taken as liquid, or tablets; often taste 'chalky' or 'minty'. (Also widely available over the counter.)
How they work: as the name suggests, antacids work by neutralizing the acid secreted by the stomach.
H₂ Antagonists: powerful, ulcer-healing drugs, given as tablets, but can be injected into the bloodstream in hospital. They are typically used to relieve the symptoms of indigestion.
How they work: by blocking the H₂ receptors in the stomach. The H₂ receptors of the stomach cause the production of acid to help digest food. It is this acid which causes the pain, and enlarges the ulcer.
Mucosal strengtheners: These are also powerful ulcer-healing drugs. Depending on type, they may be taken in liquid form or as capsules or tablets.
How they work: normally, the gut lining (mucosa) defends itself against the acid within the stomach by covering itself with thick slime (mucus). Some of the mucosal strengtheners work by increasing the rate of production of the protective mucus. Others bind to the ulcer itself, protecting it against further erosion by acid.
Anticholinergics: also ulcer-healing drugs.
How they work: by blocking nervous impulses which produce stomach acid.

OVER-THE-COUNTER TREATMENTS

There are many antacids available without prescription, even if the antacid helps with the pain, still see your doctor.
ULCERS CAN BE HAZARDOUS.

QUESTIONS TO ASK THE DOCTOR
■ For how long should I take the medication?
■ Are there any foods or drinks I should avoid?

SIDE EFFECTS
Antacids: It is important to tell the doctor about other drugs that you may be taking because antacids can stop them working. Some antacids (those containing calcium or aluminium) tend to constipate, while others (containing magnesium) may cause diarrhoea; otherwise side effects are uncommon.

H$_2$ antagonists: may be given as a course (for example, lasting two months) until the ulcer heals; but sometimes continued indefinitely to prevent recurrence. Side effects are unusual, but in men, impotence and enlargement of the breasts have been occasionally reported, and these drugs can cause confusion in the elderly. H$_2$ antagonists can interfere with other drugs taken simultaneously; discuss with your doctor.

Mucosal strengtheners: Bismuth salts (such as De-Nol) taste unpleasant, and cause the faeces to turn black. Liquorice derivatives (such as carbenoxolone) are not used in elderly patients because they cause salt and water retention; for the same reason, people with high blood pressure should not take mucosal strengtheners.

Anticholinergics: In the past, before the development of better ulcer-healing drugs, several anticholinergics were used which often produced adverse effects, including dry mouth, constipation, blurred vision and difficulty passing urine. With pirenzipine, a modern compound, adverse effects are less common. Patients with glaucoma should not take anticholinergics.

SELF-MANAGEMENT
Four steps towards helping an ulcer heal quickly:
■ If you smoke, stop. This will speed healing.
■ Avoid drinking large amounts of alcohol.
■ Eat regular meals. Obviously you should avoid foods which upset you, but there are no hard rules about diet.
■ Don't take aspirin or other painkillers without consulting your doctor.

SELF-HELP IN AN ATTACK
1 You can relieve the ulcer pain quickly by drinking milk, or taking an antacid.
2 If you have ulcer-healing drugs left from a previous attack, **don't take them without consulting a doctor.**
3 See a doctor, soon. If you vomit blood, pass a black motion, or pass out, call your doctor or go to hospital.

Oesophagus
Stomach
Duodenum

Ulcer
Debris in base of ulcer
Stomach wall
Muscle

27

WHAT IS DIARRHOEA?
– The frequent passage of loose or liquid faeces. Normally the large bowel absorbs most of the water in the digestive system, leaving a semi-solid residue – the faeces. When surplus fluid passes down the bowel, or when the bowel is unable to absorb fluid, the normally solid faeces become liquid, and are passed more frequently. Excessive loss of fluid causes dehydration, which can be fatal.

CAUSES The infection known as gastroenteritis is responsible for most attacks of diarrhoea in babies and youngchildren, but can affect people of any age. It is usual-ly caused by rotaviruses, but many other organisms can be involved. All are infectious.

In adults the commonest cause is food poisoning. One type, caused by poisons produced by bacteria in food, starts two to four hours after eating. The other is caused by bacteria (often *salmonella*) themselves multiplying in food; it starts 1 2-24 hours after eating. Both types may be accompanied by vomiting; the first is less prolonged than the second and is not contagious.

Travellers' diarrhoea is a form of gastroenteritis suffered by people newly arrived in a foreign, usually hot, country. It is caused by various bacteria or viruses, such as *E.coli*, against which the body has no immunity.

In old people 'false diarrhoea' can result from constipation: an overflow of liquid faeces passes along with the hard constipated stool, giving the appearance of diarrhoea. Medical advice is needed here.

PRESCRIPTION DRUGS
Glucose-salt solution: for infants and young children, or whenever diarrhoea is severe, this solution, containing glucose and various salts in the correct proportions, is by far the most important form of treatment, and will prevent dehyration if started early.
How it works: The addition of glucose in the correct amount increases twenty-fold the intake of water and salts into the bowel to replace the sodium, potassium and bicarbonate lost with water in the faeces.
Anti-diarrhoeal drugs: These relieve the painful spasms, and reduce the frequency of diarrhoea. They DO NOT prevent dehydration, as fluid continues to be lost into the bowel.
How they work: By paralyzing the bowel muscle. They cause severe constipation if used for too long. They

should never be used in children under our, and only with caution in older children and the elderly.

Antibiotics are only used in certain forms of diarrhoea. **How they work:** by killing the bacteria responsible.

OVER-THE-COUNTER TREATMENT

Both glucose-salt solutions and anti-diarrhoeal drugs are available from chemists. If you feel confident in using them, and take care to follow the guidelines on the packets, you will save unnecessary visits to the doctor. BUT for babies under two years, or anyone with severe pain or vomiting, medical advice is essential.

QUESTIONS TO ASK THE DOCTOR

■ How can I prevent it spreading to other people?
■ Should I drink milk, or avoid it?
■ When should I start solid food again?

SIDE EFFECTS

Glucose-salt solution may cause nausea: try one of the flavoured varieties, or add a little fruit squash. **Anti-diarrhoeal drugs** readily cause constiption if continued too long. Some, including Lomotil, can cause drowsiness.

SELF-MANAGEMENT

■ Prevention: Food poisoning results from unhygienic food preparation, and inadequate cooking or re-heating. Always wash your hands before preparing food, use clean utensils, refrigerate food quickly and re-heat thoroughly. ■ Travel abroad: Avoid eating un-washed, unpeeled fruit, or drinking tap water unless you are sure it has been boiled, or chemically purified. Avoid ice cubes in drinks, unless prepared from clean water. ■ For short trips abroad (less than one week), when an attack of diarrhoea would be a disaster, an an-tibiotic such as co-trimoxazole may be taken as a preventive measure.

SELF-HELP IN AN ATTACK

■ Children with diarrhoea require immediate fluid replacement. Use glucose-salt solution if possible, but any fluid will help. ■ For adults, the discomfort and em-barrassment of diarrhoea can be reduced by taking anti-diarrhoeal drugs, but remember also to take plenty of fluids. ■ Solid food should be stopped for 24 hours, but as soon as you feel able, start again with dry bread or toast and small amounts of vegetables. Avoid fatty food and milk, which can aggravate the symptoms.

HOME-MADE GLUCOSE-SALT SOLUTION

A safe substitute for commercial glucose-salt solution can be made up from 1/10 oz (3.5 grams) of salt and $1\frac{1}{2}$ oz (40 grams) of sugar (or half the amount of glucose) in 1 3/4 pints (1 litre) of water. Too much salt is dangerous: 3.5 grams is slightly less than one small level teaspoon. The solution should not be more salty than tears. Fruit juice or squash can be added for taste.

SIGNS OF DEHYDRATION

Dehyrdration results in thirst, dry mouth, fast breathing, and sometimes fever. An early sign is reduction in the amount and frequency of urine passed. Drink enough to keep up normal output.

Bulking agents
Chemical name: methylcellulose;
trade names: Celevac, Cellucon,
Cologel, BFL, Cellulon, Nilstim.
Chemical name: ispaghula husk;
trade names: Agiolax, Fybogel,
Isogel,Regulan. **Chemical name:**
sterculia; **trade names:** Normacol,
Inotaxine, Karagum, Prefil. **Chemical
name:** bran; **trade names:** Fybranta,
Proctofibre, Trifyba.

Osmotic laxatives
Chemical name: lactulose; **trade
names:** Duphalac, Cephulac,
Chronulac, Lactalose Solution.
Chemical name: magnesium
hydroxide; **trade name:** Milk of
Magnesia.

Lubricant
Chemical name: liquid paraffin; **trade
name:** Petrolagar.

Stimulant laxatives
Chemical name: bisacodyl; **trade
names:** Dulcolax, Dulcodos, Toilex,
Bisacolax, Laco, Perilax. **Chemical
name:** senna; **trade names:** Senna
Tablets, Senokot. **Chemical name:**
docusate sodium; **trade names:**
Dioctyl-Medo, Normax, Constiban,
Regulex.

WHAT IS CONSTIPATION?
– Failure to pass normal faeces ("stools"). What constitutes 'normal' is open to a wide range of interpretations, but constipation implies the infrequent passage of hard faeces, which may be accompanied by pain or discomfort. By contrast, the normal faeces passed by people living in rural Africa are semi-liquid, due to their high-fibre diet of unrefined grain, fruit, and vegetables.

CAUSES By far the commonest cause of constipation is a diet lacking sufficient fibre or roughage. This is a hazard of modern life, with its convenience foods, which are highly processed, removing most of the natural fibre.

Many drugs and medicines can interfere with the normal working of the bowel, causing constipation. The most significant of these are antidepressants and painkillers such as codeine. Lack of thyroid hormone (myxoedema) is a rare but important cause of severe constipation, as are many diseases of the nervous system, especially dementia and depression in the elderly. Irritable bowel syndrome *(page 32)* is another cause of constipation.

Constipation in young children is often a result of anxiety about emptying the bowel (fear of pain, embarrassment); or part of a more complex psychological disturbance. This can become a severe problem; treatment often involves the whole family, and is directed at behaviour and feelings rather than at the constipation itself. *See also* **haemorrhoids,** *page 34,* which may result from constipation.

PRESCRIPTION DRUGS
Bulking agents: When prescribed, these are supplements to the diet, and should only be necessary if the patient really finds a high-fibre diet – at least 1 oz (30 grams) – of coarse bran per day too unpleasant (see SIDE EFFECTS).

All bulking agents should be taken with plenty of fluid: at least $2\frac{1}{2}$ pints (1.5 litres) per day.
How they work: by increasing the water in the faeces.
Osmotic laxatives also increase the water content of the stool, leading to a larger, softer stool.
How they work: The laxative contains sugars and/or salts which the body happens not to absorb and these attract (by osmosis) water into the bowel.
Stimulant laxatives may be necessary in the initial treatment of constipation, provided an obstructing cause has been excluded.

How they work: by acting on the muscle wall of the large bowel, making it propel the contents forward. In excess, they readily cause diarrhoea.

Suppositories: Glycerine suppositories stimulate defecation without any risk of side effects. They are best avoided in young children, who find them frightening or painful.

How they work: uncertain, but lubrication plays a part. Enemas, usually administered by a nurse, are sometimes necessary in the initial management of severe constipation, especially in the elderly.

How they work: by softening hard, dry faeces; they also stimulate the bowel muscle by increasing the volume of the faeces.

QUESTIONS TO ASK THE DOCTOR
- Why am I constipated?
- How can I improve my diet?
- How long should I use the medicines?
- Have I got piles?

SIDE EFFECTS
Bulking agents (including bran) can lead to bloating, increased wind (flatus), and to discomfort. Reducing the quantity, and then building it up gradually, with plenty of fluids, should solve this. **Stimulant laxatives** cause colicky pains as a direct result of their action on the bowel. This is probably inevitable, and acceptable, if the laxative is used for a short period only. **Osmotic laxatives** and **suppositories** have no significant side effects.

OVER-THE-COUNTER TREATMENTS
All the preparations discussed here are available without prescription. Buy them from a pharmacist who is prepared to advise on their use.

SELF-MANAGEMENT
- In addition to bran, many foods are high in fibre, and prevent constipation: wholemeal bread, whole grain cereals, fruit (especially oranges) nuts, vegetables (especially peas, beans and carrots).
- A high-fibre diet has other beneficial effects: it lowers blood cholesterol, helps weight reduction, and may deter haemorrhoids and varicose veins.
- Not all forms of constipation are due to lack of fibre in the diet. You should consult your doctor about any change in your normal bowel habits: this is, on rare occasions, a sign of serious disease, which may well be treatable if detected early.

PATIENT'S EXPERIENCE
"I had always tended towards constipation, but after the birth of my third child it got really bad. I developed piles, and had to have enemas from the district nurse for several days. She persuaded me to persist with a really high-fibre diet, much more bran and vegetables than I had been eating before. After three or four weeks my motions began to be quite soft: I went regularly – twice a day. She told me one doctor's definition of an ideal stool: 'twice round the pan and pointed at both ends'."

IRRITABLE BOWEL SYNDROME

Anticholinergics, antispasmodics, bulk-forming agents, tranquillizers, antidiarrhoeal drugs

NAMES YOU WILL HEAR
Anticholinergics
Chemical name: dicyclomine hydrochloride; **trade names:** Merbentyl, Procyclomin, Wyovin, Clomin. **Chemical name:** propantheline; **trade names:** Pro-Banthine, Propanthel. **Chemical name:** hyoscine butylbromide; **trade name:** Buscopan.

Antispasmodics
Chemical name: peppermint oil; **trade name:** Colpermin. **Chemical name:** mebeverine hydrochloride; **trade names:** Colofac, Duspatalin. **Chemical name:** alverine citrate; **trade names:** Spasmonal, Profenil Faible.

Bulking agents
Common name: bran; **trade names:** Fybranta, Proctofibe, Trifyba. **Common name;** ispaghula husk; **trade names:** Agiolax, Fybogel, Isogel, Regulan. **Common name:** sterculia; **trade names:** Normacol, Inolaxine, Karagum, Prefil.

Tranquillizers
Chemical name: trifluoperazine and isopropamide; **trade name:** Stelabid. **Chemical name:** fluphenazine and nortiyptyline; **trade name:** Motipress.

Antidiarrhoeal drugs
Chemical name: codeine phosphate; **trade names:** Codlin, Diarrest, Kaodene, Paveral, Todlin. **Chemical name:** loperamide; **trade name:** Imodium. **Chemical name:** diphenoxylate hydrochloride; **trade name:** Lomotil.

WHAT IS IRRITABLE BOWEL SYNDROME (IBS)?

The common symptoms include: alternating constipation and diarrhoea, sometimes with mucus; pain – dull or gripping – usually in the lower abdomen, but sometimes spreading all over the abdomen, and followed by diarrhoea; wind, nausea, flatulence and feeling bloated; suddenly needing to empty the bowel. All these may be intermittent or continuous.

Symptoms *not* due to IBS are: loss of weight; *sudden* change in bowel habit; passing blood in faeces. If you have these you *must* be investigated – your doctor may order hospital tests.

CAUSES Uncertain. The symptoms are thought to be due to abnormal bowel contractions, uncoordinated bowel movements and distension of the bowel. These may be due to lack of fibre in the diet, food intolerance or allergy, or stress. IBS can be triggered off by an attack of gastroenteritis, or bowel infection. In women, symptoms may be worse before periods.

PRESCRIPTION DRUGS

Anticholinergics theoretically lessen bowel activity. Effect may be delayed – see antispasmodics.
How they work: *see* **peptic ulcer,** *page 26.*
Antispasmodics can relax the bowel. Both these and anticholinergics may take a couple of weeks to show an effect: in many people they are unhelpful anyway.
How they work: by acting directly on the bowel muscle, causing it to relax.
Bulk-forming agents add bulk to the faeces which makes bowel action more regular and co-ordinated. Bran may be taken as natural bran or as bran tablets. Other fibre, for example isphaghula husk, comes in granules which should be dissolved in plenty of water and swallowed after meals.
Tranquillizers (and antidepressants) may be prescribed on the basis that IBS is associated with and worsened by stress. However they are not very helpful and tranquillizers can be addictive – *see* **anxiety,** *page 84.* It is better to deal with the causes of stress than to take tranquillizers.
How they work: *see* **anxiety,** *page 84.*
Antidiarrhoeal drugs are mainly useful if IBS is accompanied by extremely frequent bowel action.
How they work: *see* **diarrhoea,** *page 28.*

OVER-THE-COUNTER TREATMENTS

Bulk-forming agents and anti-diarrhoeal drugs are

widely available from chemists. *See **constipation** page 30* and ***diarrhoea**, page 28*, for details.

QUESTIONS TO ASK THE DOCTOR
■ Do I really need a prescription, or is it best to try natural remedies and self-help first?
■ Will the tablets work, and how soon?
■ How long should I take the tablets/keep up the special diet/high roughage intake?
■ Will the tablets have any side effects?
■ Am I likely to have IBS for life?

SIDE EFFECTS
Anticholinergics can cause a dry mouth, and, rarely, blurring of vision or inability to pass urine.
Antispasmodics have few side effects, although peppermint oil may cause heartburn.
Bulk-forming agents should be introduced slowly; if introduced too fast, they worsen flatulence. Start with one tablespoon a day of bran or one sachet or tablespoon of ispaghula husk and increase over a few days until faeces are soft and not too frequent.
Tranquillizers: *see **anxiety**, page 84.*
Antidiarrhoeal drugs: *see **diarrhoea**, page 28.*

SELF-MANAGEMENT
■ **Diet:** Eat plenty of vegetables and roughage. Bran can be bought from chemists or health food shops, and added to cereal, stews and soups. Eat wholemeal bread and use brown rice.
■ **Certain foods may trigger IBS.** Common culprits include: milk products, wheat, coffee, tea, nuts, peas, beans and even, occasionally, meat. Certain food flavourings and dyes may cause problems too, particularly yellow or red. If you want to find out whether a food affects you, you must exclude it completely from your diet for at least three weeks: if symptoms do not improve in this period, think again. Consult your doctor if in doubt.
■ **Stress:** If you suffer from IBS it is important to find time to relax regularly. Consider taking up yoga, swimming or aerobics and find a regular time *each day for relaxing your body completely*. Identify causes of stress in your life and change them if possible.

SELF-HELP IN AN ATTACK
■ Rest, and avoid stressful situations.
■ A hot water bottle often helps.
■ Continue to eat regular small amounts, maintaining the roughage in your diet.

PATIENT'S EXPERIENCE
"I had four years of nausea and feeling bloated. My GP said it was all psychological; but eventually I had severe pains and was going to the lavatory every couple of hours. A specialist diagnosed irritable bowel and advised me to take more roughage and try reducing dairy products. I've given up milk, tea and coffee; I eat quantities of vegetables, take regular bran and go swimming three times a week, and hardly have any problems now ... maybe just a couple of bad days every six months if I eat something I shouldn't."

HAEMORRHOIDS (PILES)

Local anaesthetics, astringents

NAMES YOU WILL HEAR
(All are available both as suppositories and ointment)

Local anaesthetics
(Steroid also present in those with a letter in brackets:
(B) = betamethasone
(H) = hydrocortisone
(F) = fluocortolone
(P) = prednisolone
Other ingredients are present in all these preparations)
Chemical name: lignocaine; **trade names:** Xyloproct(H), Betnovate Rectal(B). **Chemical name:** cinchocaine; **trade names:** Proctosedyl(H), Scheriproct(P), Ultraproct(F), Uniroid(H). **Chemical name:** pramoxine; **trade names:** Anugesic-HC(H), Proctofoam (H).

Astringents
Chemical name: bismuth subgallate; **trade names:** Anusol, Anusol-HC(H), Anugesic-HC(H).

See also **constipation**, page 30.

WHAT ARE HAEMORRHOIDS?

There are two distinct sorts of haemorrhoids: internal and external. Either can cause pain in the back passage, bleeding, or swellings at the anus called piles.

External haemorrhoids are extremely painful swellings at the margin of the anus, which appear suddenly, sometimes after straining. They may bleed, but not profusely. They look purplish, measure about $\frac{1}{4}$-$\frac{1}{2}$ in (0.5-1 cm) in diameter, and subside in 3-4 days.

Internal haemorrhoids originate deep inside the anal canal, where the normal mechanism for holding the bowel closed consists of three cushions – pads formed from the bowel lining and containing large veins. A haemorrhoid forms when one or more of these cushions bulges down towards the anal canal. They may then appear as red swellings at the anus. Because of the large veins inside them, internal haemorrhoids bleed readily, indeed they are the most common cause of bleeding from the back passage.

CAUSES With external haemorrhoids, a blood clot forms in one of the veins lying just under the skin of the anus, leading to congestion, swelling and pain.

Internal haemorrhoids are probably caused by constipation and straining. In pregnant women they arise from pressure on veins in the lower abdomen.

PRESCRIPTION DRUGS

Drugs have only a small part to play. External haemorrhoids are often treated by cooling with ice packs. In acute cases, a doctor, using a local anaesthetic, can cut open the 'thrombosed' vein and release the blood clot. The skin heals up quickly, and no other treatment is needed. One of the **local anaesthetic ointments** listed may be used for a few days without harm (see SIDE EFFECTS) if soreness persists, or if incision is thought unnecessary.

How they work: By blocking the nerves to the area. Internal haemorrhoids must be examined by a doctor in order to determine whether further tests are necessary to exclude other more dangerous causes of bleeding from the back passage. Most internal haemorrhoids will subside in a few days, and the local anaesthetic preparations listed may be used to relieve pain during this time. A cooling lotion may be prescribed, and regular salt baths recommended. More important are diet and/or laxatives to promote the easy passage of soft stools. See **constipation**, page 30.

Persistently bleeding haemorrhoids, or those internal

34

haemorrhoids which protrude outside the anus, will be referred to a specialist. Several treatments are used: injection of the base of the haemorrhoids, causing them to shrink; stretching the anal canal under anaesthetic; removal by tying them off; surgery.

Astringents protect raw surfaces and may aid healing.

How they work: by sealing exposed tissue. The steroid content of many of these preparations (see drugs list in margin) reduces inflammation and itching, but increases the risk of infection in the skin.

How they work: by suppressing the body's reaction to infection and allergy. Actually, their use in haemorrhoids has no rational basis.

QUESTIONS TO ASK THE DOCTOR
- Can I prevent them happening again?
- Is there any risk that it could be cancer?

OVER-THE-COUNTER TREATMENT
Piles are a common complaint, and many creams, ointments and suppositories are available without prescription. The same risk of sensitization applies to these, and they should be used with caution, not for more than two weeks at a time.

SIDE EFFECTS
There is a risk with all the preparations that the skin will develop sensitivity (allergy) to one or more of the components of the ointment or suppository. Sensitivity is manifested in further irritation and soreness.

SELF-MANAGEMENT
If you have bleeding from the back passage, whether or not it is painful, you should consult a doctor. However, local soreness, itching, or small swellings which subside, can be treated by simple home remedies.

- Avoid putting creams or ointments on to the skin around the anus: the risk of developing sensitization, and making it worse, is too great. The simplest solution is to sit in a bath or basin of warm salty water, several times a day if possible. Frequent washing of the anal skin in this way helps prevent the cycle of irritation, soiling, rubbing, leading to more irritation, and so on. After washing, the skin must be dried thoroughly, by dabbing, not rubbing, with a towel. A pad of cotton wool helps to keep the skin of the buttocks apart and promotes healing.

- To prevent recurrence of these problems, increase the fibre in your diet – see **constipation**, page 30.

see **constipation**, page 30.

PATIENT'S EXPERIENCE
"When I suddenly developed pain while going to the lavatory and noticed some blood in the pan, I was scared I had cancer. My mother said it was piles, and recommended a tube of cream from her chemist. Because of my fear, and the pain, I saw my doctor, who examined me and said it was a fissure: a crack in the skin at the anus. He prescribed lignocaine ointment, and told me to eat bran and also to take a laxative. (I had been rather constipated.) After two days the pain and bleeding stopped. I used to think the only place you found fissures was in your teeth."

PAIN RELIEF
The pain of external haemorrhoids or prolapsed internal haemorrhoids can be relieved by applying ice packs – enclose crushed ice in a plastic bag.

WHAT IS MALABSORPTION?

– A term covering a group of conditions in which there is failure to absorb one or more nutrients from the diet. It can take the form of an isolated defect, such as failure to absorb lactose; this results in diarrhoea after drinking milk, but few other symptoms. Or, at the other extreme, there may be total gut failure and inability to absorb all nutrients. This occurs typically after surgical removal of the small bowel and results in gross malnutrition and emaciation.

CAUSES These may be divided into two main groups.

First, failure to digest the food. This may occur if pancreatic juices are reduced by chronic inflammation (pancreatitis) or by cancer, or if the bile flow is impaired through liver disease or blockage of the bile ducts. It may also happen if food rushes through the intestine without time to mix with digestive juices, as happens after gastric operations.

Second, failure to absorb digested food. This happens in disease of or removal of, the small intestine itself. Important examples include Coeliac disease, an allergy to a constituent of wheat, and Crohn's disease (regional enteritis) in which there is chronic inflammation of the small intestine. Some infections may be responsible too, especially giardiasis.

The consequences of malabsorption are:

Weight loss: the simple result of loss of calories. Fat is particularly rich in calories (twice that of protein and carbohydrate per gram) and so fat malabsorption, prominent in pancreatitis, results in early weight loss.

Diarrhoea: undigested food reaching the colon or large bowel is broken down by bacteria, resulting in a laxative effect. In the case of fat, malabsorption causes pale, fatty liquid and offensive faeces.

Anaemia – see page 224. When the upper small intestine is diseased, there is failure to absorb folic acid and iron. Vitamin B12 is absorbed specifically from the last foot of the small intestine with the help of a chemical produced in the stomach. Disease or surgical removal of either of these may cause anaemia related to B12-deficiency.

Skin rashes: These often follow failure to absorb certain vitamins and minerals.

Thin bones – resulting from failure to absorb calcium and vitamin D.

PRESCRIPTION DRUGS

Pancreatic enzymes, extracted from animal pancreas, are

the mainstay treatments, along with dietary measures, of treating chronic pancreatitis.

How they work: by replacing the body's own pancreatic digestive enzymes in the small intestine. Unfortunately they are inactivated by stomach acid, and so have to be well mixed with food (often making food unpalatable) or given in capsules that dissolve in the duodenum. Alternatively, drugs such as cimetidine or ranitidine may be given to reduce stomach acid *(see **peptic ulcer**, page 26)*. They are not totally effective, and must be combined with a low-fat diet to prevent fatty diarrhoea.

Vitamins and **minerals** are prescribed to replace potential deficiencies. Needs will vary from patient to patient. More commonly needed are vitamins B, C, D and folic acid; iron, calcium and zinc.

Antibiotics: metronidazole is usually effective in giardiasis. It is important not to take alcohol at the same time. For further information on antibiotics, *see pages 78-9 and 134-7*.

OVER-THE-COUNTER TREATMENTS

Although vitamins and minerals are widely available, self-treatment should not be attempted.

DIET

Those with Coeliac disease, must, of course, avoid wheat entirely. The diet, in fact, needs to be obsessively strict: eating out can be a real problem. For instance, gravy thickened with flour is enough to damage the small intestine. Other causes of malabsorption, such as chronic pancreatitis and bowel resection, are more generalized in their effect and the diet may thus be just as awkward to maintain. Fat, because it is often poorly absorbed, usually has to be restricted. Sometimes calories can be supplemented by MCT (medium chain triglycerides), a liquid form of fat easily absorbed.

SELF-MANAGEMENT

In general:

■ It is worth following any prescribed diet carefully. Look at the labels of foodstuffs and become familiar with the constitutents of food. Eating at home is easiest. Try to maintain a varied diet.

■ You are susceptible to gastroenteritis, and foreign travel is therefore risky.

■ Join any appropriate club or society: discuss your day-to-day problems with others who share the same experience. Understand your condition and keep informed about new developments in treatment.

NAMES YOU WILL HEAR

Steroids
Chemical name: betamethasone valerate; **trade names:** Betnelan, Betnesol. **Chemical name:** prednisolone; **trade names:** Codelsol, Delta Phorical, Deltacortril, Deltalone, Deltastab, Precortisyl, Prednesol, Sintisone, Nisolone, Delta-Cortef, Deltasolone, Prelone, Lenisolone, Meticortilone, Predeltilone.

Sulphasalazine
Chemical name: sulphasalazine; **trade name:** Salazopyrin.

Antidiarrhoeal drugs
Chemical name: codeine phosphate; **trade names:** Codeine Linctus, Codeine Syrup, Galcodine, Uniflu, Codlin, Diarrest, Kaodene, Paveral. **Chemical name:** diphenoxylate hydrochloride; **trade name:** Lomotil. **Chemical name:** loperamide; **trade name:** Imodium. **Chemical name:** kaolin and morphine; **trade name:** usually prescribed by chemical name.
*See also **diarrhoea**, page 28.*

WHAT IS ULCERATIVE COLITIS?

– An inflammatory condition affecting the colon (large bowel) which is usually chronic. Common symptoms are diarrhoea, blood and mucus in the faeces and abdominal pain. Symptoms vary from patient to patient according to the amount of colon affected: if the inflammation is confined to the rectum, the stools may be solid but mixed with fresh blood and jelly-like mucus and there will be great urgency to open the bowel; more extensive colitis produces copious liquid stools and may cause chronic ill-health. Occasionally the illness starts acutely and may need emergency surgery to remove the colon before it bursts.

CAUSE Unknown. Dietary factors and infective triggers have been suggested. Crohn's disease is a closely allied condition which may produce an identical colitis, managed the same way, but can affect other parts of the gut as well.

Bleeding from the bowel and diarrhoea are serious symptoms that can be caused by other conditions such as dysentery and cancer of the colon, and so investigation before treatment is mandatory.

PRESCRIPTION DRUGS

Steroids are used in tablet or injection form during severe and extensive attacks. They work by damping down the body's inflammation response and are also particularly useful when applied locally to the lining of the colon.
How they work: by damping down inflammation.
Sulphasalazine: This is the mainstay of treatment of ulcerative colitis in remission and relapse, taken as tablets. In the colon it is split into two parts, the active one being called 5-ASA. There are recent developments where the 5-ASA itself can be given by mouth in a form which is released in the colon.
How they work: by settling inflammation.
Antidiarrhoeal drugs: Agents such as codeine phosphate, loperamide and kaolin + morphine mixture may slow down the gut and hence reduce diarrhoea but have no effect on the underlying inflammation.
How they work: *see **diarrhoea**, page 28.*

OVER-THE-COUNTER TREATMENTS

Some of these antidiarrhoeal drugs may be available without prescription, but there are risks attached to using 'chemical stoppers' for this condition: don't take them without medical advice.

QUESTIONS TO ASK THE DOCTOR
■ How soon should I see an improvement?
■ Will I need long-term treatment?
■ Are there alternatives if this treatment fails?
■ What are the warning signs that I need medical help?
■ What should I do about diet?

SIDE EFFECTS
Steroids: These are very effective in controlling a severe attack but have no place in preventing a relapse while the patient is well and in remission. When taken by mouth or injection, particularly in high dosage, they may cause weight gain, a 'moon' face, easy bruising and acne, but your doctor will be aware of these problems and do everything possible to minimize them. *See also* **anaemia,** *page 224.* Steroids must not be stopped abruptly or their dose varied at will by the patient. Side effects are minimal when steroids are given topically as enemas or suppositories, although small amounts will be absorbed into the bloodstream.

Sulphasalazine: This tablet, and its newer forms, is effective not only in treating an acute attack but also as prevention. It may therefore be prescribed for months or even years, with appropriate blood count checks. It may induce a certain amount of indigestion, and this can be reduced by building up to the prescribed dose over a few days. Some people may be allergic to the sulpha-component and get a skin rash, in which case the new 5-ASA preparations may be the answer. It is used in with caution in pregnancy. **Antidiarrhoeal drugs:** *see* **diarrhoea,** *page 28.*

SELF-MANAGEMENT
■ A few patients with ulcerative colitis seem to be sensitive to milk, so trying a milk-free diet is worthwhile.
■ When only the lower colon (rectum and sigmoid) are affected, the stool may be paradoxically hard and difficult to pass. Such constipation makes the colitis worse and may prevent the sulphasalazine getting to where it is needed. A high fibre diet is the best way to avoid this problem.
■ It is tempting to stop sulphasalazine once the attack of colitis settles, but it is crucial to continue a maintenance dose against relapse unless otherwise advised
■ Time the use of a steroid enema so that it is kept in for as long as possible. This is usually last thing at night. If used twice a day, lie down for an hour after inserting it in the morning. Many patients find the foam enemas easier to put in and keep in than the fluid ones.

NAMES YOU WILL HEAR
Viral hepatitis vaccine; gamma globulin injection. No specific drug treatments except these preventive injections. *See also alcholism, page 94 and cirrhosis, page 42.*

WHAT IS JAUNDICE?
– Yellow discoloration of the skin and of the whites of the eyes. It occurs when the amount of bilirubin pigment in the blood is raised. It often causes no symptoms, and may first be noticed by a friend or relative. Sometimes, when jaundice is severe, there is itching, the urine may be dark and the faeces paler than usual.

CAUSES Normally, bilirubin pigment, which is produced by the regular turn-over of red blood cells, is secreted by the liver as a waste product in bile. When the flow of bile is blocked or slowed due to a liver problem, jaundice results. Bile flow may be blocked within the liver or outside it. In adults, common problems *within* the liver are: viral hepatitis, alcoholic hepatitis and primary biliary cirrhosis. Certain drugs may also be responsible. Causes of jaundice *outside* the liver are: gallstones blocking the main bile duct; inflammation of the pancreas, and cancer of the pancreas or bile ducts. Sometimes an infection within the bile ducts may cause jaundice; the onset is usually sudden with fever, abdominal pain, sweating and vomiting. Seek medical help urgently.

Gilbert's Syndrome, a mild, hereditary form of jaundice, affects about 5 per cent of the population. The jaundice becomes more prominent during illness or when dieting or fasting. It does not require treatment.

PRESCRIPTION DRUGS
There are no specific prescription drugs.

However, a **vaccine** is available against one of the four different hepatitis viruses (B). A doctor may advise it for close contacts.

Other regular social and business contacts may in addition be well advised to have an injection of **gamma globulin** to boost their immunity against hepatitis. *See also alcoholism, page 94.*

Because jaundice is caused by so many different diseases, it is important that an accurate diagnosis is made as soon as possible.

QUESTIONS TO ASK THE DOCTOR
■ What is the cause of my jaundice?
■ Do I need special tests?
■ If viral hepatitis is suspected, and there is a delay in results of the tests, do I need to take any precautions?

OVER-THE-COUNTER TREATMENTS
None.

SELF-MANAGEMENT

Without the help of special blood tests, and sometimes a needle biopsy of the liver, it is virtually impossible to decide whether the jaundice is caused by one of many viruses, alcohol, a bacterial infection in the bile ducts, gall stones, or a reaction to medication being taken as treatment for another condition.

There are at least four different viruses which cause hepatitis (labelled, A, B, D and non-A non-B). Apart from jaundice, the early symptoms resemble a 'flu-like illness: fatigue, mild fever, muscle and joint aches and pains, loss of appetite, nausea, vomiting and vague abdominal pain. These symptoms often lessen when the jaundice appears. Also, viral hepatitis may occur without jaundice ever developing.

If you suspect you have viral hepatitis, consult your doctor. If the diagnosis is confirmed (or while you await the results of tests):

■ Avoid excessive exercise, though rest in bed is not necessary unless you feel weak.

■ Avoid physical contact with other people (including kissing). This includes those living with you, and visitors. Sexual activity does not affect recovery from hepatitis, but you may pass on the infection.

■ Avoid alcohol during acute phases.

■ Since hepatitis viruses are passed on by blood, body fluids and secretions, do not share items such as razor blades, scissors and toothbrushes. Cover any cuts.

■ A well-balanced diet is usually sufficient during the illness: vitamin supplements are not normally necessary. If there is nausea, it is best to have a large breakfast: nausea is generally least troublesome in the morning.

■ Avoid preparing meals for others, especially if you have hepatitis A. However, by the time the hepatitis is diagnosed, you will have already passed the most infectious phase and infection of close contacts may have already occurred.

■ Symptoms should clear up within a couple of months, but some require six months to recover fully.

■ In a very few, hepatitis may become chronic, causing liver damage and cirrhosis.

Only viral hepatitis requires these precautions.

Drug-induced liver injury is rare, but has been found with nearly every known drug. Most medicines which damage the liver do so in an unpredictable manner. An allergic type of reaction is found in many people. The diagnosis is often circumstantial: there are no specific tests. Once the offending drug is stopped, recovery rapidly occurs over a few weeks.

PATIENT'S EXPERIENCE

"I had had a cold for about two weeks, and couldn't shake it off. It was my neighbour who noticed that my eyes had turned yellow; the next day I could see that my skin had gone a similar colour.

My arthritis, which began some years ago, had also seemed more active. So for a week I took a few extra arthritis tablets. They were the new ones my doctor had recently given me.

After the jaundice appeared, I saw my doctor who arranged some blood tests; he also recommended some precautions at home, and suggested I stayed at home until the results came through. Three days later, the results for viral hepatitis were negative, but my jaundice was much worse. My doctor suggested stopping the arthritis tablets. Within a week, the jaundice had cleared and so had the 'flu-like symptoms. We assumed the jaundice was an allergic reaction to the tablets."

CIRRHOSIS

WHAT IS CIRRHOSIS?

– A chronic liver disease in which damage occurs to normal liver cells, which are then replaced by scar tissue. This process reduces the number of normal liver cells so that liver function becomes less efficient and flow of blood through the liver is partly blocked.

The liver is the single largest organ in the body. It is, with justice, called the body's chemical factory, and it has thousands of functions, the important ones being: maintenance of the blood clotting mechanism, production of many blood proteins, blood enzymes, the production of bile, metabolism of fats, maintenance of a normal blood sugar level, the storage of energy, the regulation of hormones, and eliminating drugs and poisons (including alcohol) by converting them into inactive compounds.

Cirrhosis often develops insidiously, but once liver function is impaired, the following may appear: loss of appetite; weight loss; nausea and vomiting; enlargement of the liver; jaundice; itching; abdominal swelling due to fluid accumulation (ascites); vomiting of blood (from an ulcer in the stomach or ruptured veins in the gullet); increased sensitivity to drugs; and mental changes progressing to confusion and coma.

CAUSES Excessive alcohol intake is the commonest cause of cirrhosis. Some patients with viral hepatitis may also develop cirrhosis. See **jaundice**, *page 40*. Other rare causes are: inborn abnormalities where excessive iron or copper is deposited in the liver; severe reactions to drugs; some forms of heart disease; disease of the bile ducts (biliary cirrhosis). Alcohol can be readily identified as the cause of cirrhosis, especially if a tiny piece of liver tissue is examined under the microscope. The development of cirrhosis is related to the amount of alcohol consumed, its regularity, and perhaps the individual's state of nutrition. Females are more prone to liver injury from alcohol.

PRESCRIPTION DRUGS

There is no cure and the scarring process cannot be reversed. Treatment is aimed at reducing the extent of liver damage and controlling complications such as accumulation of fluid.
Diuretics such as spironolactone and frusemide taken as tablets once or twice a day may help reduce fluid accumulation.
How they work: by increasing loss of fluid through the kidneys.

Steroids: Prednisolone is the most-used for damping down inflammation in the liver caused by some forms of chronic hepatitis. For the majority of cases of cirrhosis, however, steroids are unhelpful, and may be harmful, because of fluid retention.

How they work: by blocking inflammatory reaction.

Azathioprine: this is a more powerful suppressant of inflammation than steroids. It is used only under expert guidance in patients with primary biliary cirrhosis.

How it works: see *organ transplants, page 216.*

QUESTIONS TO ASK THE DOCTOR

■ What is the cause of my cirrhosis?
■ Do I need special tests?
■ Is specific treatment needed?
■ Will cirrhosis affect my job, diet or activities?
■ Are any special precautions necessary?

OVER-THE-COUNTER TREATMENTS

None.

SIDE EFFECTS

See *heart failure, page 54, anaemia page 224* and *organ transplants, page 216.*

SELF-MANAGEMENT

The cause of cirrhosis can only be found by blood tests, and sometimes a ''needle biopsy'' of the liver. If you suspect you may have cirrhosis, consult your doctor. However, alcohol is by far the commonest cause.

■ Stop drinking alcohol completely.

■ Avoid excessively high protein in your diet. However, a well balanced diet is essential. You may also have to limit the total quantity of fluid you drink. This may in turn lessen the need for diuretics.

■ If viral heptatis is suspected, or found to be the cause of cirrhosis, and you are a carrier of the virus, you may have to follow the same precautions as for viral hepatitis *(see jaundice, page 40).*

■ Cirrhosis reduces the body's response to infection, so if a mild infection persists, you should seek the advice of your doctor.

■ Avoid taking any tablets or other medicine which are not essential. They may overload an already overworked liver, and the action of most medicines is greatly prolonged in chronic liver disease such as cirrhosis.

■ Aspirin and similar analgesics are best avoided. They can worsen bleeding from the oesophagus, or from stomach ulcers.

Cardio-vascular disease

At the centre of the cardio-vascular system is the heart which acts as a pump to drive blood around the body. The left ventricle receives oxygenated blood from the lungs via the left atrium and then pumps the blood, under pressure, to the organs of the body through the arteries. From the main arteries the blood passes into a branching network of smaller and smaller blood vessels ending in capillaries which allow the nutrients and oxygen in the blood to reach every cell in the body. The right ventricle receives non-oxygenated blood returning to the heart from the peripheral circulation, via the veins and right atrium, and pumps it at relatively low pressure to the lungs. The heart receives its own circulation of blood via the coronary arteries.

ANGINA	**46-47**
HYPERTENTIONS	**48-51**
MYOCARDIAL INFARCTION	**52-53**
HEART FAILURE	**54-55**
Disorders of **HEART RHYTHM**	**56-59**
STROKE	**60-61**
Disorders of the **CIRCULATION**	**62-63**
BLOOD CLOTS	**64-65**

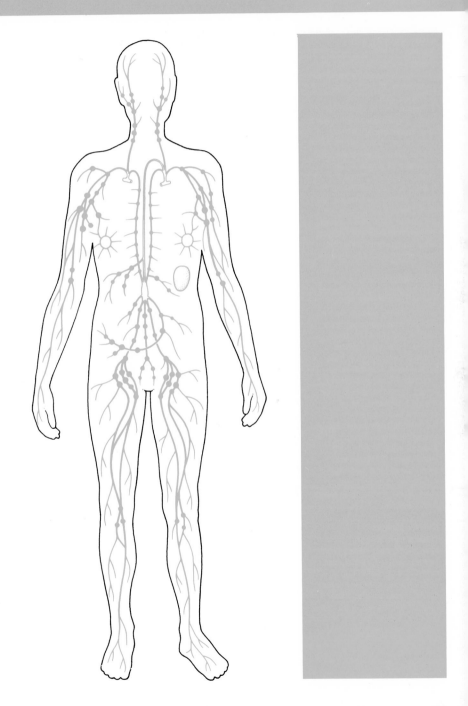

NAMES YOU WILL HEAR
Nitrates

Chemical name: glyceryl trinitrate (GTN) as tablets, spray or ointment; **trade names:** Coro-nitro spray, Nitrolingual spray, Natirose, Nitrocontin Continus, Suscard Buccal, Sustac, Percutol ointment, Transiderm nitro, deponit (plaster), Nitrolate, Nitrol, Nitrong, Nitrostabilin, Nitrostat, Angised, **Chemical name:** isosorbide dinitrate; **trade names:** Caravasin, Cedocard, Vascardin, Sorbichew, Isoket, Sorbid SA, Soni-Slo, Isordil, Isotrate, Novosorbide, Coronex, Apo ISDN. **Chemical name:** isosorbide mononitrate; **trade names:** Elantan, Monorit, Mono-Cedocarol. **Chemical name:** pentaerythritol tetranitrate; **trade names:** Cardiacap, Mycardol.

Beta-blockers

Chemical name: propranolol; **trade names:** Angilol, Apsolol, Bedranol, Berkolol, Inderal, Sloprolol, Cardinol. **Chemical name:** acebutolol; **trade name:** Sectral. **Chemical name:** atenolol; **trade name:** Tenormin. **Chemical name:** betaxolol; **trade name:** Kerlone. **Chemical name:** metoprolol tartrate; **trade names:** Betaloc, Lopresor. **Chemical name:** nadolol; **trade name:** Corgard. **Chemical name:** oxprenolol hydrochloride; **trade names:** Apsolox, Laracor, Slow-Pren, Trasicor. **Chemical name:** pindolol; **trade name:** Visken. **Chemical name:** sotalol hydrochloride; **trade names:** Beta-Cardone, Sotacor. **Chemical name:** timolol maleate; **trade names:** Betim, Blocadren.

Calcium blockers

Chemical name: diltiazem hydrochloride; **trade names:** Tildiem, Cardizen, Tilazem. **Chemical name:** nifedipine; **trade name:** Adalat. **Chemical name:** nicardipine; **trade name:** Cardene. **Chemical name:** verapamil hydrochloride; **trade names:** Berkatens, Securon, Cordilox, Isoptin. **Chemical name:** lidoflazine; **trade name:** Clinium. **Chemical name:** prenylamine; **trade names:** Synadrin, Segontin.

WHAT IS ANGINA?

Constricting pressure-like pain felt behind the breast bone sometimes spreading to the arms or throat, usually brought on by exertion or emotional upset and relieved after a few minutes' rest.

CAUSES Usually a narrowing of the coronary arteries which restricts blood flow to the heart muscle. At rest the blood supply to the heart is adequate despite the coronary artery narrowing, but when the heart has to beat faster or more forcefully during exercise or emotional stress the heart muscle becomes starved of the extra blood it needs and angina results. Resting reduces the heart's rate of beating and hence its need for extra blood and consequently the pain disappears.

Angina is also a warning pain: if an already narrowed artery becomes completely blocked, typically by a blood clot, a heart attack *(page 52)* – results.

Arterial disease is ultimately caused by a number of factors, all now well publicized: *see page 52.*

PRESCRIPTION DRUGS

Three groups of drugs are used. They act in different ways, and may be used alone or in combination.

Nitrates: used to treat an attack as it occurs (a small tablet placed under the tongue or lip – 'sub lingual' or 'sub-buccal' – or a spray under the tongue). Long-acting nitrates are available as tablets or as an impregnated plaster applied to the skin, or a paste rubbed into the skin, and are used to reduce the frequency and severity of attacks.

How they work: Nitrates probably widen the coronary arteries and reduce the amount of blood flowing into the heart, allowing the heart to pump more easily.

Beta-blockers: commonly used to reduce the frequency and severity of attacks. Taken as tablets, they allow patients to take exercise before the pain comes on.

How they work: by slowing the heart rate and reducing the blood pressure thereby allowing the heart to pump more efficiently.

Calcium blockers: used in same way as beta-blockers.

How they work: by reducing the force at which the heart pumps, by lowering blood pressure and by widening the coronary arteries.

OVER-THE-COUNTER TREATMENTS

Some nitrates may be purchased direct from a chemist in an emergency, but only for angina patients under medical care.

QUESTIONS TO ASK THE DOCTOR

■ How often can I take the tablets under the tongue/ use the spray?
■ How quickly will they work?
■ What should I do if they don't work?
■ Can I take beta-blockers and calcium blockers just when I need them?
■ Can I stop taking beta blockers and calcium blockers if they upset me?
■ Does angina inevitably lead to a heart attack?

SIDE EFFECTS

Nitrates often cause headaches which become less severe as you get used to the medication. Sometimes in older patients, they may cause light-headedness; sit or lie down if this develops.

Beta-blockers may cause cold hands and feet, aching muscles, particularly in the legs, feelings of mental and physical slowing and vivid dreams. Occasionally they cause asthma – seek immediate medical advice.

Calcium blockers may cause headache, flushing of the face, minor ankle swelling and bowel upset (constipation or diarrhoea). All these side effects are infrequent and usually minor compared with the consequences of untreated angina. But of course, prevention is better than cure – see **SELF-MANAGEMENT.**

SELF-MANAGEMENT

Sublingual tablets or spray to relieve an attack can be taken as often as necessary. They should be taken immediately pain starts, or when you are in a situation in which the pain is likely to occur – prevention is better than cure. These drugs are not painkillers; they help put right the cause of the angina. Relief should be obtained within 15 minutes. If the attack recurs, or your need for tablets or spray increases over a few days, seek medical advice.

The sublingual tablets lose their effect on storage and should be renewed every three months.

Smoking is forbidden as it may bring on an attack and is a major cause of coronary artery narrowing (atheroma). Dieting to reduce weight or blood fats may be useful: discuss with your doctor.

SELF-HELP IN AN ATTACK

At the first warning of an attack, sit down and try to relax. Take a sublingual tablet or spray. Do *not* try to manage without your medication. When the attack has subsided you can spit the tablet out.

WHAT TO AVOID

Try to avoid situations known to bring on angina, for example arguments, walking into a cold wind or walking after a heavy meal. If you cannot avoid a provocative situation, take a sublingual tablet (or spray) immediately beforehand. Try to lead an ordered, regular life. Plan your day to avoid rushing. Sometimes sexual intercourse (emotion and exercise) may bring on an attack; a sublingual tablet or spray before sex may prevent this.

WHAT IS HYPERTENSION?

The technical term for high blood pressure in the arteries, a relatively common condition affecting about one in ten of the population, particularly in middle age. (Each time the heart beats it produces a pressure wave consisting of a maximum – systolic – and minimum – diastolic – pressure.)

There is no clear division between normal and raised blood pressure although doctors usually define one for the sake of convenience. There are borderline values which some doctors would define as hypertensive and others would not. Systolic blood pressure normally rises with age and therefore most doctors use the diastolic pressure to define hypertension. A diastolic pressure greater than 100 millimetres of mercury is frequently quoted as abnormal. Blood pressure is not a fixed property but varies from time to time depending on activity and time of day. Anxiety and stress (caused, for example, by consulting a doctor) make it rise and allowance must be made for this. Only a persistently elevated blood pressure is abnormal.

Most patients with high blood pressure have NO SYMPTOMS so the condition can go undetected. To identify hypertenstion you must have your blood pressure measured.

CAUSES Ninety per cent of patients have 'essential hypertension', meaning no obvious cause. Rarely it may be due to kidney disease, narrowing of important blood vessels or abnormal hormone production. Oral contraceptives can occasionally cause hypertension, hence the importance of monitoring blood pressure in women who use them. Hypertension may also develop in pregnancy (pre-eclampsia). Heredity is an important factor; if your parents' blood pressures were high, the chances of you being hypertensive are greater.

Measuring blood pressure: The instrument normally employed is called a sphygmomanometer. A cuff with an inflatable rubber lining is wrapped around the upper arm and inflated so that no blood can get through. The pressure is then slowly decreased while the doctor/nurse listens over the artery at the elbow. When blood starts to flow it creates a thumping noise (systolic pressure). As the pressure continues to fall the sound becomes muffled and then disappears (diastolic pressure). Equipment is available for patients to measure their own pressure, but it is usually preferable for a trained person to do it.

Does high blood pressure matter? People with untreated hypertension have a greater than normal chance of developing strokes, heart and kidney disease with a consequent reduction in life expectancy. Drugs to lower blood pressure will help to reduce these risks considerably.

PRESCRIPTION DRUGS
Your doctor will aim to lower your blood pressure gradually over a period of weeks. He will start with a low dose of tablets and slowly increase it. If this is not sufficient, another type of drug may be substituted or added.

How they work: Beta-blockers affect nerves which control the circulation; **diuretics** cause the kidneys to lose salt and water and produce some reduction to tension in the arteries; **vasodilators** reduce tension in the arteries. **Converting enzyme inhibitors** reduce production of the hormone which raises blood pressure; others act on the brain; and sometimes drugs working in different ways are combined (see **Combinations** under **NAMES YOU WILL HEAR**).

OVER-THE-COUNTER TREATMENTS
None. Various non-drug treatments (meditation, biofeedback, relaxation exercises) may be helpful in lowering blood pressure, but they involve regular therapy and a large individual commitment. They are only useful for mild hypertension and their long-term overall benefit is unproven.

QUESTIONS TO ASK THE DOCTOR
■ What tests (if any) do I need?
■ Should other members of my family have their blood pressure checked?
■ Will raised blood pressure interfere with my job?
■ Will I be refused life insurance?
■ Will my pregnancy be affected?
■ What happens if I forget to take my medication?
■ For how long do I have to take tablets?

SIDE EFFECTS
Treatment for hypertension is usually long-term (often 'for life'), so the drugs should be simple to take and as free as possible from side effects. Although no drug is completely free of side effects, modern ones go close to this ideal.

It is important that you discuss any symptoms you may experience after starting treatment with your doc-

Combinations
Chemical name: amiloride + hydrochlorthiazide; **trade name:** Moduretic. **Chemical name:** triameterene + hydrochlorthiazide; **trade name:** Dyazide. **Chemical name:** amiloride + frusemide; **trade name:** Frumil. **Chemical name:** rusemide + spironolactone; **trade name:** Lasilactone.

tor. These are not always related to the treatment. Dizziness or light-headedness may occur if blood pressure is lowered suddenly or excessively; **beta-blockers** may cause cold hands and feet, tiredness and may not be suitable for patients with asthma or bronchitis; **diuretics** may occasionally cause gout and sometimes sexual difficulties. *See also **heart failure**, page 54*. The great majority of people experience no side effects while on these drugs. Many of the drugs can now be given once or twice daily, avoiding a midday dose. Most drugs are best taken prior to breakfast and/or the evening meal, making it easier to remember. *For side effects of vasodilators see page 55.*

SELF-MANAGEMENT
In order to help control your blood pressure, you should be aware that:

■ There is a relationship between dietary salt intake and hypertension. Although salt restriction may not prevent high blood pressure, it is advisable for patients with hypertension to reduce their salt intake by avoiding foods with a high salt content and not using salt at the table. Salt substitutes for cooking are available, although there is generally no harm in using ordinary salt in cooking.

■ High blood pressure is commoner in people who are overweight. Such patients should loose weight by careful and sensible dieting.

■ Heavy alcohol intake raises blood pressure: hypertensive patients should not exceed two pints of beer (or the equivalent) per day.

■ As people with hypertension have a higher risk of coronary heart disease and arterial disease of the legs, they should STOP SMOKING. Similarly, a reduction in fat consumption (particularly animal fat) will help.

■ Don't forget to take your tablets, although missing an occasional one will not cause serious problems. Poor compliance will result in poor blood pressure control. If you do forget your tablets, do *not* take twice the dose next time but continue as usual.

■ Regular measurement of blood pressure by a nurse or doctor should be perfomed every three to four months. Only if your blood pressure is poorly controlled should more frequent checking become necessary. Be aware of your condition, but do not let it rule your life.

■ There is a small amount of evidence that regular exercise will also help to lower blood pressure. Dynamic exercise (for example, walking, running, swimming, cycling) is therefore to be recommended; isometric ex-

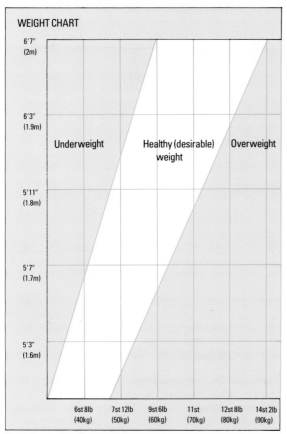

WEIGHT CHART

	6st 8lb (40kg)	7st 12lb (50kg)	9st 6lb (60kg)	11st (70kg)	12st 8lb (80kg)	14st 2lb (90kg)

6'7" (2m)

6'3" (1.9m)

Underweight   Healthy (desirable) weight   Overweight

5'11" (1.8m)

5'7" (1.7m)

5'3" (1.6m)

Chart shows generally accepted ranges

ercise (for example, weightlifting) is usually not a good idea for hypertensive patients. In the long run, most patients with hypertension should be able to lead a perfectly normal life with few restrictions.

SELF-HELP

Hypertension is a long-term problem and you must therefore get repeat prescriptions from your doctor. Be careful not to run out of tablets even when your blood pressure is controlled.

It is wise to be cautious when starting additional drugs for other conditions, as they may occasionally interfere with the blood pressure tablets. This is particularly true of certain drugs used for treating arthritis. If in doubt, consult your doctor or chemist.

NAMES YOU WILL HEAR

Analgesics
Chemical name: morphine; **common name**: heroin; **trade names**: Cyclimorph, MST-continus, Nepenthe. Chemical name: pethidine; **trade names**: Pethilorfan, Pamergan, Pethoid, Demerol, Demer-Idine. Chemical name: pentazocine; **trade names**: Fotral, Talwin, Sosegon. *See also pain, page 106.*

Diuretics
Chemical name: frusemide; **trade names**: Lasix, Frumil, Dryptal, Aluzine, Lasix, Aquamide, Uremide, Urex, Lasic, Furoside, Neorenal, Novosemide, Uritol, Aquasin. Chemical name: bumetanide; **trade names**: Burinex, Burinex. Chemical name: ethacrynic acid; **trade names**: Edecrin, Edecril, Edecrin, Edecrin. *See also hypertension, page 48.*

Antiarrhythmic drugs
Chemical name: lignocaine; **trade names**: Xylocaine, Xylocard, Xylocaine, Leostesin, Nurocain, Sarnacaine, Xylocaine, Democaine, Leostesin, Peterkaien, Remicane, Remicard. Chemical name: disopyramide; **trade names**: Rythmodan, Dirythmin, Norpace, Rythmodan, Norpace. Chemical name: verapamil; **trade names**: Cordilox, Securon.

*46 (for beta-blockers), **heart failure**, page 54. **lipid disorders**, page 162 **disorders of heart rhythm**, page 56 and **hypertension**, page 48.*

WHAT IS MYOCARDIAL INFARCTION?

The technical term for heart attack. (An attack of ***angina**, page 46* , is by contrast a warning pain from your heart that it may be prone to a heart attack.) Myocardial infarction occurs when the blood supply to the heart (via the coronary arteries) is totally obstructed (as opposed to simply restricted, as in angina): an area of heart muscle actually dies. This obstruction is known as thrombosis – hence coronary thrombosis – a term used interchangeably with myocardial infarction.

A heart attack usually presents like a severe attack of angina. Pain in the centre of the chest is often vice-like and may spread to the arms or neck. Often the patient feels sick, dizzy and short of breath. Sometimes there may be no pain at all and shortness of breath or palpitations may be the only features.

CAUSES Most commonly, a blood clot blocks an already narrowed artery. Narrowing of the arteries is due to atheroma, also known as atherosclerosis, in which fat-like materials are deposited in the linings of blood vessels, decreasing their width.

Smoking is undeniably important. Women are relatively protected from heart attack before reaching the menopause. It is very unusual for a woman under 50 to have a heart attack unless she smokes. So both men and women should do everything they can to stop smoking.

Overweight: The more overweight you are the more likely you are to have a heart attack *(see pages 50-51)*.

High blood pressure: Men and women who have high blood pressure are more likely to have a heart attack although the risk is less in women. Attention is now given to measuring blood pressure in young people and to taking action early. *See **hypertension**, page 48.*

Cholesterol: People with high cholesterol levels are more likely to have heart attacks, as are diabetics.

Family history.

PRESCRIPTION DRUGS

The first thing a doctor will do for the heart attack patient is to give a powerful **analgesic** by injection. This will ususally be morphine or heroin and will work within ten to 20 minutes. The patient may also be given a **diuretic** to make them pass more urine – *see page 54.* Sometimes drugs are also given to steady the rate of the heart beat (**antiarrhythmic** drugs). These may be given by injection or by mouth. In order to prevent a further heart attack, particularaly in people under the age of 60, beta-blocking drugs are sometimes used. In the long term, after blood tests, the patient may be given a diet and a course of drugs to reduce fats in the body; alternatively, a drug to lower the blood pressure may be prescribed – see **lipid disorders** and **hypertension**, pages 162 and 48.

How they work: analgesics, see page 106; **diuretics,** see page 54; **antiarrhythmic drugs,** see page 56.

OVER-THE-COUNTER TREATMENT
None, but some patients may be given a small daily dose of aspirin to try and prevent future heart attacks. Although aspirin is easily available, it only works in some individuals and often causes side effects such as **indigestion** (page 22). So ask your doctor before you use it regularly

QUESTIONS TO ASK THE DOCTOR
■ What can do to stop this happening again?
■ When can I start having sexual intercourse again?
■ What is the long-term damage to my heart?
■ How likely is another heart attack?
■ Can I resume a normal life when I have recovered?

Heart attacks, of course, are serious, but must not be regarded as 'terminal'. On the contrary, the patient's best chance of long-term survival is using the experience as motiivation to return to a full life through correct diet and exercise.

SIDE EFFECTS
See **analgesics,** page 106; **diuretics,** page 54; **antiarrhythmic drugs,** page 56,

SELF-MANAGEMENT
■ Watch your weight – try to get as close to your ideal weight as possible (see table, page 51).
■ Exercise in moderation is fine. Usually you should be able to return to full activities within six weeks of leaving hospital. It is a good idea to try to take exercise, such as walking, every day.
■ Stop smoking. If you are a regular smoker this is the best thing you can do.
■ You may be given a diet to lower the fats in your blood. Even if this is not specifically recommended, it is sensible to try to reduce the amount of fat in your diet. Most Westerners eat far too much fat from animal sources. Reduce the amount of fatty meat and bacon you eat, substitute a low fat spread for butter and use vegetable oil rather than lard or dripping.

PATIENT'S EXPERIENCE
"When I got the attack of pain in my chest I thought I was going to die. The relief that the injection gave was almost magical. I was rushed to hospital and stayed in the coronary care unit for two days with various tubes and wires connected to me. After that I was sent to the general ward and was soon up and about. I went home ten days after going into hospital. I was a bit tired for a few days after going home but within six weeks I was doing everything I did before and within two months I was back at work. I even think my angina is better than it was but that may be because the shock of the heart attack gave me the will power to stop smoking."

SELF-HELP IN AN ATTACK
At the first warning of chest pain, sit down and try to relax. If you have a supply of nitrate preparation for **angina** (see page 46), put a tablet under your tongue or use your spray. It is quite alright to use a second or third dose after ten minutes if the first is not effective. If you suffer from angina and the pain is not relieved within 30 minutes, call your doctor, or if he is not available, call an ambulance and go to hospital. If you have never experienced angina before, call a doctor or ambulance earlier.

HEART FAILURE

Diuretics, vasodilators, ace inhibitors, digoxin

WHAT IS HEART FAILURE?

Not to be confused with heart attack, *page 52,* it occurs when the heart cannot pump adequate amounts of
blood to the rest of the body, or can only do so by
enlarging or by generating abnormally high pressures
within the heart cavities during its filling phase. Symptoms are shortness of breath during exercise and, in
severe cases, at rest and when lying flat. Sometimes
ankle-swelling and tiredness are symptoms, too.

CAUSES The commonest causes are coronary heart
disease and its outcome, heart attack. Untreated high
blood pressure, damaged heart valves and occasionally
disease of the heart muscle are also sometimes to
blame.

PRESCRIPTION DRUGS

Diuretics: Two types are commonly used: thiazides long-
acting, taken once per day; and loop diuretics, shorter-
acting, more potent than thiazides.
How they work: by acting on the kidneys, causing loss of
salt and water from the body. By reducing the fluid in
the circulation, the pressure in the heart and lungs is
also reduced. Diuretics cause loss of potassium from
the body, so potassium tablets are usually prescribed
as well in order to make good the shortage.
Vasodilators: often added if diuretics are inadequate.
How they work: by dilating the arteries and veins, so
reducing the pressure on the filling and pumping sides
of the heart (see diagram). Their effect tends to lessen
after a few weeks.
Ace inhibitors: a relatively new and promising treatment
acting in some ways like diuretics and vasodilators
combined.
How they work: Like vasodilators they dilate arteries and
veins, but they also have a beneficial effect on hormones (the body's chemical messengers) which
reduces the amount of fluid in the circulation.
Digoxin: not now used as first-line treatment for heart
failure in the UK, Australasia or the USA. This is a
centuries-old drug derived from the foxglove plant.
How it works: This is the only orally-taken drug which
makes the heart beat more forcefully. Its key role is in
controlling the chaotic heart rhythm that occurs in atrial
fibrillation *(see page 57).* If this is the cause of heart
failure, digoxin is the drug of first choice.

OVER-THE-COUNTER TREATMENTS
None.

QUESTIONS TO ASK THE DOCTOR

■ How much will 'water tablets' (diuretics) interfere with my daily activities?
■ Will I need to drink more fluid to replace what is lost by taking diuretics?
■ How long will I have to take the tablets?
■ When and how often do I need to take the potassium tablets?

SIDE EFFECTS

Diuretics cause an increase in frequency and volume or urine passed – inconvenient at work, on long journeys or when out of the house. Loop diuretics act within about 30 minutes of ingestion, the effect diminishing four to six hours later. Take the pills at times which suit your daily routine. Thiazides act more gradually throughout the day; the effects are most noticeable during the first few days of therapy.

Diuretics do make people thirsty. Counteract this by drinking freely, but avoid salty foods, and adding salt to your food, as this reduces the effectiveness of the treatment. Loss of potassium due to diuretics may jeopardise the proper working of muscles, including the heart; however it is easily replaced by taking potassium tablets. Gout and sexual problems are rare side effects.

Vasodilators may cause flushing of the face, headaches and sometimes palpitations.

Ace inhibitors may cause skin rashes and upset of kidney function. These drugs are a promising advance in the treatment of heart failure, but as with all other treatments, medication is usually required long term.

SELF-MANAGEMENT

Only exercise within your limitations, and take adequate rest. Smoking is forbidden. Alcohol can aggravate symptoms in some people by reducing the heart's efficiency. A low-salt diet is helpful in some people and may allow a reduction in medication. Discuss this with your doctor – don't attempt it without proper supervision.

SELF-HELP IN AN ATTACK

Attacks of breathlessness sometimes occur at night in bed. **1** Sit up. **2** Put a nitrate tablet under the tongue *(see **angina**, page 46)*. **3** Consider taking an extra diuretic tablet, bearing in mind that this will keep you awake passing water. **4** If the attack settles quickly, consult your doctor next day. If the breathing difficulty persists, send for the doctor immediately.

NAMES YOU WILL HEAR
Class I
Chemical name: quinidine; **trade names:** Kiditard, Kinidin Durules, Quinidoxin, Biquin, Kinidine. **Chemical names:** lignocaine hydrochloride, lidocaine hydrochloride; **trade names:** Xylotox, Lidothesin, Lignostab, Xylocaine. **Chemical name:** procainamide; **trade names:** Pronestyl, Procainamide Durules. **Chemical name:** disopyramide; **trade names:** Norpace, Rythmodan, Dirythmin. **Chemical name:** mexiletine; **trade name:** Mexitil. **Chemical name:** tocainide; **trade name:** Tonocard.

Class II – Beta-blockers
Chemical name: propranolol; **trade names:** Angitol, Apsolol, Bedranol, Berkolol, Inderal, Sloprolol, Cardinol. **Chemical name:** acebutolol; **trade name:** Sectral. **Chemical name:** alprenolol; **trade name:** Betacard. **Chemical name:** atenolol; **trade name:** Tenormin. **Chemical name:** metoprolol tartrate; **trade names:** Betaloc, Lopresor. **Chemical name:** nadolol; **trade name:** Corgard. **Chemical name:** pindolol; **trade name:** Visken. **Chemical name:** sotolol hydrochloride; **trade names:** Betacardone, Sotocor. **Chemical name:** timolol maleate; **trade names:** Betim, Blocardren.

Class III
Chemical name: amiodarone; **trade name:** Cordarone X.

Class IV – Calcium blockers
Chemical name: verapamil hydrochloride; **trade names:** Berkatens, Securon, Cordilox, Berkatens, Securon, Isoptin.

Cardiac glycosides
Chemical name: digoxin; **trade names:** Lanoxin, Cardiox, Natigox, Prodigox, Purgoxin. **Chemical name:** digitoxin; **trade names:** Digitaline Nativelle, Digitox.

WHAT IS NORMAL HEART RHYTHM?

The adult heart normally beats at a rate of 70-80 beats per minute (bpm). In young children the rate may exceed 90 bpm and in athletes it may fall to below 60 bpm. The regular rhythmic beating of the healthy heart (called sinus rhythm) is automatically controlled from centres within the nervous system which transmit electrical impulses to the heart. In response to exercise or anxiety, the rate increases; during sleep or rest, it decreases. The electrical impulses are transmitted through the chambers of the heart (the atria and the ventricles – *see diagram, page 59*) and through the heart muscle to give a co-ordinated pumping action.

WHAT IS ABNORMAL HEART RHYTHM?

There is a wide range of disturbances of heart rhythm from the harmless to the potentially lethal. Paradoxically, the harmless rhythm disturbances – the odd ''missed'' or ''jumped'' beat, also called palpitations – are often the ones which cause the patient most alarm; whereas more serious rhythm disorders, which require medical treatment, may be completely unnoticed.

Disorders of rhythm (dysrhythmias) may be subdivided into two main categories depending on whether the heart is beating too slowly (less than 60 bpm) or too quickly (more than 100 bpm). The first, **bradycardias,** do not respond well to drug treatment; if treatment is required, they respond best to a pacemaker which can prevent the heart rate falling too low. The second, **tachycardias,** are more common, and can be due to a number of different types of dysrhythmia.

Diagnosis of a specific type of dysrhythmia depends on examining an elctrocardiograph (ECG). Occasionally it is possible to make a precise diagnosis by taking the pulse, and if the dysrhythmia is intermittent, the patient can give useful information if he/she counts the pulse rate at the wrist and judges whether the rhythm is at a constant, albeit rapid, speed with each beat of approximately equal force.

CAUSES A minor disturbance, such as a ''missed'' or ectopic beat, usually has no serious underlying cause and can be considered a simple variation of normality. Even frequent ectopic beats or short-lived palpitations are often normal; however, they are sometimes caused by an excessive intake of stimulants such as caffeine, alcohol or nicotine. Clearly, if the heart is diseased or damaged, the whole range of cardiac dysrhythmias can occur, but even the more serious types of dysrhythmia do not always reflect irreversible heart disease or damage.

The diagnosis of a dysrhythmia does not necessarily indicate the need for treatment. The doctor's decision about treatment depends upon the nature of the dysrhythmia, the potential complications and the level of accompanying symptoms.

PRESCRIPTION DRUGS

The following are some of the more common types of dysrhythmia, usually forms of tachycardia, with examples of typical treatments. The terminology used related to the part of the heart from which the dysrhythmia originates: either from the ventricles (ventricular) or from the atria (atrial or supraventricular). The terminology also describes the nature of the abnormality: if there is a ''missed'' or ''jumped'' beat it is called an ectopic beat; if there is rapid but co-ordinated beating, then the straightforward term *tachycardia* applies; if there is rapid but un-cordinated activity of the atria or ventricles, *flutter* or *fibrillation* apply.

Atrial (supraventricular) tachycardia: This dysrhythmia is not usually serious (in most cases the heart is structurally normal), but the heart rate may be sufficiently fast (ranging from 120 to 240 bpm) to cause uncomfortable palpitations and symptoms such as breathlessness, chest tightness and light-headedness. The patient may also need to empty the bladder frequently. Paroxysms are often recurrent, but with a variable duration (minutes to hours) and a variable frequency (from several episodes per day to only one or two per year). Occasional paroxysms may respond to the Valsalva Manoeuvre (see **SELF-MANAGEMENT**), but if long-term treatment is required, the calcium antagonist drug, verapamil, or one of the beta-blockers is usually effective. Alternative medications include disopyramide and amiodarone.

Atrial fibrillation or atrial flutter: These have similar symptoms to atrial tachycardia but they are typically seen in patients who have an abnormality of one of the heart valves. With both dysrhythmias, but especially atrial fibrillation, the overall heart rate is not only fast (about 160 bpm) but irregular. Conversion to normal sinus rhythm is only occasionally possible and the usual aim of treatment is to keep the heart rate under control at about 80 bpm with one of the cardiac glycosides.

Ventricular ectopic beats: Ectopic beats, both ventricular and supraventricular, occur occasionally in most normal individuals (''My heart missed a beat''). Treatment

PATIENT'S EXPERIENCE

"My elderly mother had been tired for some time, breathless, too, even when she walked short distances, and her feet began to swell. She complained that she felt her heart beating very fast at times. I am a trained nurse, so I checked her pulse. It was slow. I was taken aback by her doctor's verdict: he told her not to worry — she was just getting old.

My fears were confirmed when she blacked out while shopping. She was fine almost immediately afterwards, but I took her back to the doctor and said I thought she should see a specialist about her heart.

The cardiologist said that she needed a pacemaker and admitted her straight into hospital. She was anxious about having a pacemaker fitted, but the specialist assured her it was a simple operation which, even at her age, shouldn't cause complications. The pacemaker box was put under her skin below the collar bone. The wires led into a vein, then to the heart. She had to have antibiotics for a few days to prevent infection of the operation site.

The improvement was dramatic. She passed an enormous amout of urine, her feet went back to normal, and the dreadful tiredness eased. She has to have the pacemaker checked regularly, but it will probably last a few years."

is not necessary. But ventricular ectopic beats also occur in association with a heart attack *(see **myocardial infaction**, page 52)* in which case a short course of treatment may be given. Ectopic beats sometimes also occur in long-standing heart disease; long-term drug treatment will be given to suppress them. The drugs in class I are often used for this purpose, with amiodarone as an alternative.

Ventricular tachycardia: The effects of this dysrhythmia range from minor upset to shock and cardiac arrest. The rate falls in the range 120-250 bpm. Ventricular tachycardia usually reflects an underlying cardiac problem and if the episodes are frequent or associated with severe symptoms, then treatment with a class I or class III drug is usually given.

How the drugs work: There is considerable overlap in function: see below. In general though, they dampen down electrical impulses to the heart, or their transmission from the atria to the ventricles, or their transmission through the heart muscle. See above for reasons underlying the choice of drug. See under NAMES YOU WILL HEAR for drug names.

Class I drugs stabilize the electrical activity within cardiac muscle cells.

Class II – beta-blockers – block the effects of excess nervous activity to the heart. They' are often used to slow the heart, or to prevent the development of rapid heart rhythms arising from the atria. Generally, these drugs are used for the less serious types of dysrhythmia.

Class III – amiodarone – has a similar action to Class I drugs. It tends to be reserved for particular types of dysrhythmia arising from either the atria or the ventricles. It is often used when there has been a poor response to some of the other drugs.

Class IV – calcium antagonists – suppress the excitability of the heart muscle and the transmissions of electrical impulses.

Cardiac glycosides work mainly by interfering with the transmission of electrical impulses from the atria to the ventricles.

OVER-THE-COUNTER TREATMENTS
None.

QUESTIONS TO ASK THE DOCTOR
- Is there a serious underlying heart problem?
- What can I do to prevent an attack coming on?
- Will I need to take tablets for ever?

- What are the risks if I run out of tablets?
- Do the tablets have serious side effects?

SIDE EFFECTS

With all these drugs, side effects may be common, even expected, but are not always serious: thus treatment can be continued if the effects are not too troublesome. Alternatively side effects may indicate overdose or a potentially serious adverse effect which should be reported to a doctor so that the dosage can be reduced or the treatment withdrawn.

Common side effects: Minor stomach upsets occur with **quinidine** and **mexiletine;** dry mouth, urinary retention and blurred vision with quinidine and **disopyramide;** tiredness, cold hands and feet, and sometimes breathing difficulties, with **beta-blockers;** skin rashes and skin pigmentation with **amiodarone;** constipation with **verapamil.**

Effects of overdosage (requiring a dosage reduction): **Class I** drugs can cause disturbances of the central nervous system including mental confusion, twitching, tremor, slurred speech and dizziness. **Digoxin** often causes nausea and vomiting. Adverse effects with **procainamide** which may require the drug to be stopped: skin rash, joint stiffness and malaise.

SELF-MANAGEMENT

This is only occasionally possible and worthwhile, and for only one type of dysrhythmia: paroxysmal atrical tachycardia – see PRESCRIPTION DRUGS. If the paroxysms are only occasional, a breathing technique called the Valsalva Manoeuvre may enable the patient to ''switch off'' the paroxysm and restore a normal sinus rhythm. Take in a deep breath and then slowly, but forcibly, blow the breath out through tightly pursed lips: rather like blowing up a balloon. Your doctor will rehearse the technique with you.

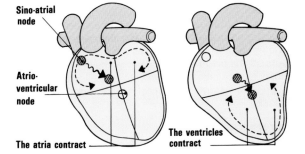

Sino-atrial node

Atrio-ventricular node

The atria contract

The ventricles contract

The heart is a muscular pump *which works by contraction and expansion of its muscle fibres. A natural pacemaker, the sino-atrial node, initiates each pumping action by transmitting impulses. These make the atria contract; they also pass through the atrial walls to the atrio-ventricular node, which relays the impulses to the ventricles, causing them to contract in turn.*

STROKE

Aspirin

WHAT IS A STROKE?

– The term used to cover a group of disorders which affect the blood supply to the brain with loss of function elsewhere in the body. Stroke can also be described as a cerebrovascular accident.

When the blood supply to any part of the brain is cut off, the brain cells stop working and the area of the body controlled by those brain cells is also unable to function. The right side of the brain controls the left side of the body and vice versa. The most common problem is weakness or paralysis of one side of the body. Speech may also be affected. In less severe cases, only one arm or one leg may be affected, or perhaps there may be an effect on sensation, vision or balance.

If the blood supply to the brain is restored within a short time, then function also recovers. This type of stroke lasts less than 24 hours and is called a transient ischaemic attack. If the blood supply is not restored, then the affected part of the brain dies and recovery depends on the ability of other parts of the brain to take over the role of the damaged part. If damage is mild, good recovery occurs over several months. In severe cases, however, there is permanent disability. Some patients may suffer from epilepsy following a stroke.

CAUSES Blood supply may be affected by:
Thrombosis: arteries narrow because of atherosclerosis *(see page 52)* and eventually shut off the blood supply completely. Onset of symptoms may be sudden, but is usually graded over several hours or days. Recovery of physical function in major strokes of this type is often poor because other arteries are also diseased, thus making it difficult for other parts of the brain to compensate to any useful extent.
Haemorrhage: One of the small arteries bursts and leaks blood into the brain tissue. Damage is caused by the resulting blood clot as well as by a reduction in the blood supply. Onset of symptoms is usually sudden.
Embolus: A small blood clot or clump of cells which breaks off from one part of the circulation (often the heart) and travels via the bloodstream to stick in another part where the arteries are smaller. This in turn cuts off the blood supply to part of the brain. If the embolus is very small, it breaks up and allows the blood supply to return to normal (a transient ischaemic attack).

PRESCRIPTION DRUGS

There are no drugs which will cure a stroke once it

develops. Thrombotic and haemorrhagic strokes are more common in patients with high blood pressure and in such cases treatment to lower blood pressure may help to prevent a stroke – see **hypertension**, page 48.

Aspirin or similar drugs in small daily doses (300-600 mg/day) may reduce the frequency of transient ischaemic attacks. However, clinical trials have not been entirely convincing and little benefit has been seen with this treatment in women.

How it works: By making platelets (small blood cells) less likely to stick together and therefore less likely to form clumps within the circulation.

OVER-THE-COUNTER TREATMENTS

Aspirin as a treatment for stroke patients should be taken only under medical advice;

QUESTIONS TO ASK THE DOCTOR

Major stroke:
- When am I likely to see some improvement?
- How long can I expect to continue to improve?
- How can I prevent another stroke?

Transient ischaemic attack:
- How long should I take aspirin?
- How will I know when it is working?
- What happens if I am allergic to aspirin?

SIDE EFFECTS

If **aspirin** is necessary, treatment is for life. The problem is that in substantial, long-term dosage, the drug loses some of its effect, and side effects are more likely. The main side effect is a mild stomach upset such as heartburn. More severe effects such as an ulcer or bleeding from the stomach are rare with small doses. *See also* **pain**, *page 106*.

For the one per cent allergic to aspirin, other drugs such as warfarin may be used. *See page 64.*

SELF-MANAGEMENT

Prevention is the key.
- Do not smoke.
- Have your blood pressure checked once a year.
- Reduce your intake of saturated fat and salt.
- Take regular exercise.

SELF-HELP IN AN ATTACK

1 Get medical help as soon as possible. **2** Lie down and keep calm. **3** Accept that you may have to go into hospital for help with your recovery.

AFTER A STROKE
Having had a stroke, you will be treated as necessary with physiotherapy, speech therapy and occupational therapy while still in hospital. After you get home it is important to continue exercises you learned from the physiotherapist to maintain maximum functional improvement. Although most improvement occurs in the first six months, function can continue to improve over several years.

Several important disorders of circulation are featured elsewhere in this book: for example angina *(page 46)* and stroke *(page 60)*. Here are covered circulatory problems affecting the legs and, to a lesser extent, the arms. Three relatively common types are covered.

PERIPHERAL VASCULAR DISEASE

Narrowing of the arteries with reduction of the blood supply to the tissues in the legs. It is most noticeable when exercising. On walking, a cramp-like pain (intermittent dilation) occurs (most often in the calf muscles) after going a certain distance. It ceases a few minutes after stopping. The distance that can be walked before the onset of pain is less when going uphill or walking into the wind. The skin becomes dry, scaly and cold and there is loss of surface hair on the legs. Gangrene may develop in severe cases.

CAUSE Atherosclerosis *(see page 52)*.

PRESCRIPTION DRUGS

There are no really effective drugs for this problem, but you may get a little help from one of the vasodilators. Self-help is therefore essential. Some severe cases require surgery (replacement of a narrowed artery).

QUESTIONS TO ASK THE DOCTOR
■ Will the medicine help me much?

SELF-MANAGEMENT

Prevention is the key. See **angina**, page 46.

SELF-HELP IN AN ATTACK

If leg pain comes on while exercising, stop until it passes away. If black spots appear on your toes or legs, consult your doctor immediately.

VARICOSE VEINS

Veins carry blood back to the heart. In the legs this process is helped by the pumping action of the muscles and the valves within the veins which (when healthy) prevent blood flowing backwards. Veins are said to be varicose when they become distended and tortuous and the valves are not working properly. The main problem is often cosmetic, but ankle swelling and aching in the legs may occur. Occasionally, there is ulceration.

CAUSES A defect in the valves, or obstruction to venous blood flow caused, for instance, by obesity.

PRESCRIPTION DRUGS

Varicose veins are not helped by drug treatment. Some patients require surgery.

QUESTIONS TO ASK THE DOCTOR

■ Will any treatment be necessary?
■ What can I do to minimize the problem?

SELF-MANAGEMENT

If you are overweight, diet. Avoid long periods of standing and raise your feet on a support when sitting. Wear support stockings if advised by your doctor. Avoid tight garments round the abdomen. Take regular exercise. If an ulcer develops, contact your doctor.

RAYNAUD'S PHENOMENON

A disorder of blood vessels in the hands (or occasionally the feet) which results in constriction of small arteries in response to cold or emotion. In most patients this is simply an exaggeration of the normal response to cold. Sometimes it may occur due to the arms being exposed to excessive vibrations.

CAUSES Usually unknown. Occasionally a diseased blood vessel, or some other disease elsewhere in the body is implicated. Drugs, including beta-blockers, can cause Raynaud's phenomenon.

PRESCRIPTION DRUGS

Vasodilators may help some people. They are often prescribed on a trial-and-error basis: if the first does not work, another is tried. Several types are available, but there is no single ideal drug at present. Drugs are only necessary in severe cases.

How they work: by making the small arteries and arterioles increase in diameter and less likely to constrict.

QUESTIONS TO ASK THE DOCTOR

■ Do I need drug treatment?
■ Is there likely to be an underlying cause?
■ What is the long-term outlook?

SIDE EFFECTS

See page 55.

SELF-MANAGEMENT

Wear warm clothing, especially gloves and footwear. Avoid working in the cold with vibrating machinery.

Anticoagulants

WHAT IS A BLOOD CLOT?

Usually a normal process essential to stop excessive bleeding from an injury. However, blood clotting can occur where it is unwanted – typically within the deep veins of the legs (deep venous thrombosis). The clot (thrombus) impairs the flow of blood to the heart and fluid builds up in the leg below the site of blockage. The leg becomes swollen, painful and warm. Sometimes part of the clot breaks off and travels in the blood stream elsewhere in the body, usually to the lungs (pulmonary embolus). This may cause chest pain (which is often worse on taking a deep breath or when coughing). Breathlessness, a fast pulse, coughing up blood and fever may also occur.

CAUSES 1 Obstruction or slowing of blood flow in the legs: this can occur after lying several days in bed, especially with a pillow under the knees, or after a long flight or other journey. **2** Damage to the wall of a vein occurring as a result of an accident, an operation, or inflammation around the vein. **3** Taking oral contraceptives *(see page 179)*. **4** A rare genetic defect in the clotting mechanism.

PRESCRIPTION DRUGS

Heparin is used in most patients as soon as the diagnosis is made. It is usually given by injection and is thus mainly used in hospital.
How it works: by improving the effect of a natural anticoagulant in the blood, which in turn stops the action of natural blood clotting factors. This is a fast-acting remedy.
Warfarin is usually also started when the diagnosis is made or a few days thereafter: it takes a few days to work properly. It is taken as tablets, coloured for different strengths, and may constitute life-long treatment if the problem is recurrent.
How it works: by reducing the amount of vitamin K in the liver – this vitamin being necessary for the activation of clotting factors.
Phenindione is given in rare cases of a patient being allergic to warfarin. **Nicoumalone** is an increasingly little-used alternative to warfarin.

OVER-THE-COUNTER TREATMENTS

None.

QUESTIONS TO ASK THE DOCTOR

■ How long will the treatment take?

- How will treatment be controlled?
- What exercise should I take?
- Do I need to be careful with diet?
- Can I take other medication? Are my contraceptive pills implicated in my problem?
- What are the main side effects?

SIDE EFFECTS

Heparin's main side effect is spontaneous bleeding, typically from stomach, bowel or kidney, or into the skin (bruising). This is generally the result of an overdose. Careful dose control is essential to minimize the problem. Because the drug is administered under hospital supervision the risk is minimized, and in any case heparin's effect is quickly reversed.

Warfarin: As with heparin, the main side effect is spontaneous bleeding. Thus the dose must be carefully adjusted under hospital supervision for each individual. Blood samples are necessary, daily at the start of treatment but less often when the treatment has stabilized. Long-term warfarin users are at a small but significant risk and must be carefully counselled from the start in recognizing bruising and bleeding into the urine and into the bowel, and in reporting such facts immediately. Allergic reactions are rare.

SELF-MANAGEMENT

Take your warfarin tablets regularly at the same time each day to achieve a uniform effect. Avoid any major dietary changes, particularly foods rich in vitamin K (for example, cauliflower, spinach, brussel sprouts). Prevent recurrence of deep venous thrombosis by:
- Avoiding prolonged immobility: if you have to lie in bed, wriggle your toes and move your legs at least every 30 minutes while awake. If you are taking a long journey, get up and walk every hour.
- Regular gentle exercise such as walking or cycling.
- Avoid oral contraceptives, particularly the combined contraceptive pill.
- Wear support stockings if advised to do so.
- Avoid taking other drugs, particularly aspirin. You may use paracetamol for pain relief.

SELF-HELP IN AN ATTACK

If your leg swells up, consult your doctor as soon as possible and avoid exercise until your leg has been examined. If you need something for the pain, take a paracetamol tablet. If possible, go to bed, lying with your feet up: elevate the foot of the bed.

Respiratory and associated diseases

The lungs receive oxygen from air breathed in and this oxygen is transferred to the blood in the spongy tissue of the lungs. In exchange, carbon dioxide is transferred to the lung tissues, and then breathed out. Difficulties in breathing happen when the lung tissue is congested, inflamed, or otherwise damaged or if the air passages are narrowed, as in asthma.

COUGH   68-69
BRONCHITIS AND EMPHYSEMA   70-73
ASTHMA   74-77
PNEUMONIA AND PLEURISY   78-79
TUBERCULOSIS   80-81

See also: *Lung cancer, page 202.*

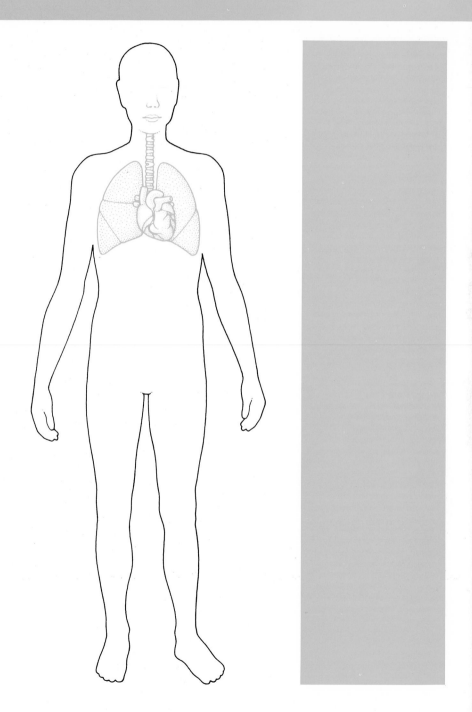

NAMES YOU WILL HEAR

Decongestants
Chemical names: pseudoephedrine hydrochloride: Actifed, Sudafed, Sudilex, Drixora Repetabs, Eltor.

Mucolytics
Chemical name: carbocisteine; **trade names:** Mucodyne, Mucosirop. Chemical name: bromhexine hydrochloride; **trade name:** Bisolvin.

Expectorants
There are many expectorants such as iodide, chlorides, bicarbones, squill and ipecacuanha. These are seldom used alone, but are often found in combination with bronchodilators or mycolytics.

Bronchodilators
Chemical name: theophylline hydrate; **trade names:** Neulin, Nuelin, Theocontin, Theo-Dur, Theograd, Iphylline, Elixophylline. **Chemical name:** orciprenaline sulphate; **trade name:** Alupent. **Chemical name:** salbutamol; **trade name:** Ventolin.

Antibiotics
Chemical name: amoxycillin sodium; **trade names:** Amoxil, Moxacin, Moxilean, Novamoxin, Penamox, Polymox. **Chemical name:** co-trimoxazole; **trade names:** Bactrim, Fectrim, Nodilon, Septrim. **Chemical name:** trimethoprim; **trade names:** Iprol, Monotrim, Syraprim, Trimopan.

Cough suppressants
Chemical name: codeine phosphate; **trade names:** Codeine Linctus, Codeine Syrup, Dimotane Co, Galcodine, Phensedyl, Tercoda, Terpoin, Unifly, Codlin, Diarrest, Kaodene, Paveral, Todlin. **Chemical name:** pholcodine tartrate; **trade names:** Dia-Tuss, Duro-Tuss, Pholtex, Copholco, Copholcoids, Davenol, Expulin, Galenphol, Pavacol D, Pholcomed, Rinurel.

WHAT IS A COUGH?

Muscular contraction of the diaphragm whose function is to expel mucus from the respiratory tract. A cough is usually useful and does not always require treatment. If a dry cough is due to thick secretions, these can be ''loosened'' so that they can be coughed up; a dry cough which is disturbing sleep can be ''suppressed''. Coughing at night may be an early sign of asthma *(see page 74)*.

CAUSES Mucus, produced by the respiratory tract as a response to infection or inflammation. It may be produced in the chest, or may arise in the nose and throat as in a common cold or hay fever. Smoking irritates the lungs and gives rise to cough, hoarseness, reduced lung function, bronchitis, heart disease and lung cancer.

PRESCRIPTION DRUGS

Decongestants will suppress mucus production in the nose in cases of infection or allergy.
Mucolytics are supposed to make mucus in the chest less thick and easier to cough up.
Expectorants stimulate coughing in order to clear mucus.
Bronchodilators will dilate constricted airways and also make mucus easier to cough up.
Antibiotics will kill bacteria if present.
Cough suppressants will act on the 'cough centre' in the brain and suppress the cough.

OVER-THE-COUNTER TREATMENTS

Simple linctus, decongestants, mucolytics, bronchodilators and cough suppressants can all be bought from chemists. Decongestants are often used when the upper airways are congested, and mucolytics and bronchodilators when mucus is being coughed up from the chest. There is, however, little evidence to support the use of decongestants and mucolytics.

Cough suppressants are rarely necessary and should only be used if there is no thick mucus in the chest, or if the patient is exhausted and needs rest. Bronchodilators are useful for wheeze and night cough in asthma sufferers *(see **asthma,** page 74)*.

It is better to choose medicines with only one active ingredient rather than those with multiple actions. *See **common cold,** page 134.*

QUESTIONS TO ASK THE DOCTOR

■ Which of these drugs do I really need?

- How long will they take to work?
- How long should I take the treatment?
- What will happen if I stop them too soon?
- Will it help to stop smoking?
- Have I got asthma?

SIDE EFFECTS

Antihistamines, which are usually found in **decongestants,** cause drowsiness in many people and should not be taken when driving or working in a potentially dangerous environment. For more information on the side effects of decongestants, *see middle ear infections, page 256* and *hay fever, page 260.* **Mucolytics** cause gastric irritation and should not be used by patients with a history of indigestion or peptic ulcer. **Bronchodilators** can cause tremor and palpitations, especially if the recommended dose is exceeded, or in sensitive individuals. *See asthma, page 74.* Antibiotics can cause nausea and lethargy; they may also give rise to an allergic reaction, usually a rash. Report it to a doctor immediately. *See also pneumonia and pleurisy, page 78.* **Cough suppressants** cause constipation.

SELF-MANAGEMENT

It is important to differentiate between **1** a cough caused by a post-nasal drip (from mucus production in the nose): this is best treated with a decongestant; **2** a cough caused by mucus production in the chest or asthma for which mucolytics or bronchodilators are the best treatment and **3** a dry, useless cough, for which a cough suppressant may be used. Inhalation of steam *(see sinusitis, page 262)* is often useful for patients with sticky mucus in the chest.
- Encourage children to blow their noses and cough up any mucus.
- Stop smoking – if smoker's cough is already a problem, you need to give up now.
- Dehydration can make secretions thicker, so it is important to drink plenty of fluids.
- Patients with recurrent attacks of wheezy bronchitis or asthma should seek advice on starting treatment with bronchodilators as soon as a cough starts.

Consult a doctor if:
- Mucus coughed up is green or yellow ■ Mucus contains blood ■ There is pain in the chest with coughing ■ A cough is accompanied by a high temperature ■ A cough is associated with shortness of breath or wheeze ■ A cough continues for more than ten days.

Antibiotics, bronchodilators, steroids, mucolytics, antitussives, inhalants

Continued on page 72

WHAT ARE BRONCHITIS AND EMPHYSEMA?

Acute bronchitis is characterized by cough, production of yellow or green phlegm and fever resulting from infection of the lower air passages (the bronchi). The infection usually spreads from the upper airways and in fit individuals is commonly a self-limiting viral infection which requires symptomatic treatment only. In patients with pre-existing lung disease, is more serious.

Chronic bronchitis and emphysema is an extremely common condition in industrialized countries, not unjustly known as the English disease: in the UK it is responsible for the loss of more than 13 million working days a year. Although separate pathological entities, chronic bronchitis and emphysema frequently develop together and can be impossible to distinguish; indeed they are here considered as one. The severity of the disease varies from a simple smoker's cough and morning phlegm to total breathless incapacitation.

Chronic bronchitis is characterized by long-term coughing and excess phlegm production due to damage to the airway.

Emphysema is enlargement of the air spaces in the lung tissue beyond the smallest airways (the bronchioles). A major feature of chronic bronchitis and emphysema is limitation of airflow which may produce wheezing, though the airflow obstruction is not usually as variable or as reversible as in asthma.

The term chronic obstructive airways disease, COAD (or chronic obstructive pulmonary disease, COPD) is used to describe the picture of chronic bronchitis and emphysema with airflow obstruction. Chronic bronchitis develops insidiously, starting usually in winter with a chronic cough and morning sputum, but eventually continuing year-long. The sufferer may be breathless on exertion, or when at rest. Wheezing may be prominent. In advanced cases there is a lack of oxygen reaching the tissues which become blue (cyanosed). Eventually respiratory failure can develop and the resulting strain on the heart can produce heart failure.

The progress of the disease is very variable. Some patients never have more than cough and phlegm; but there is usually a gradual deterioration in respiratory function with increasing breathlessness. In patients whose lungs are already damaged with chronic bronchitis and emphysema, acute infection should be treated seriously: resistance is lowered and lung function can rapidly deteriorate.

Although chronic bronchitis and emphysema is a progressive disease, it can be slowed or halted.

CAUSES The major factor is cigarette smoking, though other forms of atmospheric pollution are also implicated and in some people there may be an inherited predisposition to damage from inhaled pollutants.

Tobacco smoke causes swelling of the bronchial walls with enlargement of the mucous glands and damage to the fine hair cells which clear secretions from the lungs. Smoke also inhibits the action of certain enzymes which normally protect the lungs.

PRESCRIPTION DRUGS

Antibiotics: those listed are most commonly used for acute exacerbations of chronic bronchitis. Some patients with persistent or repeated infection require continuous antibiotics, particularly during winter.

How they work: by killing bacteria responsible for infection. Bacteria can become resistant to the action of some antibiotics and the choice of antibiotic from the large number available depends on resistance patterns.

Bronchodilators are widely used to alleviate chronic bronchitis and emphysema. However, they are only effective if there is reversible airways narrowing. There are three types: sympathomimetics, anticholinergics, and methylxanthines, taken as tablets or by inhalation.

How they work: the three groups act on different receptors to open up the airways and can be used in combination for additive effect. *See **asthma**, page 74.*

Sympathomimetics are chemically related to adrenaline and are best inhaled directly into the lungs since they act faster, with fewer side effects, by this route. They are usually prescribed as an aerosol inhaler but may also be available as a dry powder for inhalation (salbutamol rotacaps) for patients who have problems using an aerosol. The modern sympathomimetics listed are selective in their action on the lungs rather than the heart. Many are now available but all act similarly and none has a particular advantage. After inhalation the effect is usually seen within 30 minutes.

Anticholinergics: Ipratropium bromide is the only anticholinergic drug usually available for this condition, although others are being developed. It can only be taken by inhalation and takes longer to work than the sympathomimetics.

Methylxanthines are chemically related to caffeine and non-selective in action, with a stimulant effect on the heart as well as the lungs. The modern formulations are largely oral preparations.

Steroids are related to cortisone produced by the adrenal gland. They are sometimes given, by mouth or by injection, for acute flare-ups of chronic obstructive airways disease and in patients with advanced disease for whom all other therapies have proved ineffective. Since potential side effects are so great it is essential that they are only used when really necessary.

Inhaled steroids *(see also **asthma**, page 74)* are a valuable and safe long-term therapy for wheezy bronchitis, though they will only work if there is at least some degree of reversible airways narrowing. They are not effective during an acute attack since an inadequate amount of the drug reaches the bronchial wall: they must be used regularly to be effective. They are less effective in bronchitis than in asthma.

How they work: by reducing the inflammation in the bronchial wall which causes airway obstruction.

Expectorants ease removal of bronchial secretions.

How they work: theoretically by increasing the volume and reducing the stickiness of secretions; there is little hard evidence that they are of any value.

Mucolytics contain enzymes which reduce the stickiness of bronchial secretions.

How they work: by breaking down the structure of sticky phlegm. They may be of value in some lung diseases, but in chronic bronchitis their worth is very doubtful.

Antitussives will suppress coughing.

How they work: by acting on the brain to inhibit the cough reflex. Useful for a dry, non-productive cough.

QUESTIONS TO ASK THE DOCTOR
■ How often should I use the inhalers?
■ Can you check that I am using inhalers correctly?
■ Can I take extra puffs of a bronchodilator inhaler if my breathing is bad?
■ Should I have influenza vaccine?
■ Should I have a supply of antibiotics to start taking as soon as I develop an infection?

SIDE EFFECTS
Antibiotics can cause allergic reactions such as skin rashes. Report them to a doctor immediately. **Bronchodilators;** Sympathomimetics rarely have side effects. *See **asthma**, page 74.* Anticholinergics are usually free of serious side effects, though in high dose can cause retention of urine, glaucoma *(see page 270)* and a dry mouth. With **methylxanthines** there is little difference between the effective dose and the toxic dose. Nausea, abdominal discomfort and headaches are common side effects. A change in dose, timing of medication or drug formulation may help. The amount of drug in the blood

may need to be measured to ensure that the dose is both non-toxic and effective.

Steroids: inhaled doses are free of the major side effects of steroids *(see **asthma**, page 74)*, but they can lead to oral thrush which requires treatment with an antifungal agent. Washing the mouth out after use reduces the likelihood of thrush developing. Mild hoarseness may develop but it is reversible.

A short course of steroid tablets is unlikely to be harmful but prolonged therapy (more than a few weeks) does carry the risk of numerous side effects which have to be weighed against the benefits of treatment. Long-term steroids suppress the body's normal secretion of cortisol and it is essential that you do not change (or stop) the dose of steroids without your doctor's advice. *See **anaemia**, page 224.*

OVER-THE-COUNTER TREATMENTS

Numerous bronchodilator preparations are available, usually containing a mixture of ephedrine and theophylline. These are non-selective in their action and are likely to produce side effects including heart palpitations and generalized tremor. The formulation of these drugs is inferior to the prescription-only drugs which can be adjusted to the individual's body weight, age and specific needs – and cannot be recommended.

Many expensive antitussive compound formulations are available, and have no advantage over pholcodine and codeine linctus available on prescription.

Steam inhalation preparations are widely available. It is the steam which is of value, not the aromatic extras, though these can make inhaling more pleasant.

SELF-MANAGEMENT

■ *You must stop smoking.* Even in advanced disease, you may gain benefit. Various techniques such as nicotine chewing gum, hypnotherapy or acupuncture may help, but ultimately it comes down to willpower. Join (or form your own) no smoking group.

■ Avoid smokey atmospheres and sudden changes to extremes of air temperature.

■ Excess weight makes normal people breathless and contributes to breathlessness induced by lung disease. If overweight, diet. *See ideal weight table, page 51.*

■ While exercise will not necessarily improve lung function, regular exercise such as brisk walking can improve exercise tolerance and your feeling of well being.

■ Vaccination against influenza may be helpful in preventing acute attacks.

SELF-HELP IN AN ATTACK

■ As soon as you feel infection starting, with phlegm changing colour from white to yellow or green, see your doctor for a course of antibiotics. If these have already been provided, start taking them.

■ Stay indoors: do not try to work through the attack.

■ If phlegm is sticky and difficult to clear, steam inhalations may help. *See sinusitis, page 262.*

OXYGEN

Oxygen is usually given in hospital for severe acute attacks. In advanced disease, long-term oxygen at home for at least 15 hours a day has been shown to be of value in improving well-being and survival. This can be provided at home by oxygen concentrator, about the size of a small domestic refrigerator. However, only a minority of patients are suitable for this type of treatment and hospital assessment is essential.

Mast cell stabilizers, beta stimulants, methylxanthines, anticholinergics, steroids

Mast cell stabilizers
Chemical name: sodium cromoglycate; trade names: Intal, Lomusol, Nalcrom, Lomudal.

Beta stimulants
Chemical name: salbutamol; trade names: Ventolin. Chemical name: terbutaline; trade names: Bricanyl, Feevone. Chemical name: fenoterol; trade names: Berotec, Partusisten. Chemical name: oriciprenaline; trade names: Alupent. Chemical name: isoetharine; trade names: Numotac, Bronchilator, Bronkosol.

Methylxanthines
Chemical name: aminophylline; trade names: Phyllocontin, Theodrox, Anodrophylline, Cardophylline, Somophyllin, Aminophyl, Corophyllin, Euphyllin, Retard, Peterphyllin. Chemical name: theophylline; trade names: Neulin, Nuelin, Theocontin, Theo-Dur, Theograd, iphylline, Elixophyllin.

Anticholinergic
Chemical name: ipratropium bromide; trade names: Atrovent.

Steroids
Chemical name: beclomethasone propionate; trade names: Becotide, Vanceril, Viarox. Chemical name: betamethasone valerate; trade name: Bextasol. Chemical name: prednisolone; trade names: Codelcortone, Deltalone, Precortisyl, Adnisolone, Deltasolone, Lenisolone, Metricortelone.

WHAT IS ASTHMA?

Narrowing of the small air passages of the lungs (the bronchioles), so that it becomes difficult to move air in and out. The condition is reversible – meaning the bronchioles can recover from the spasm. The symptoms vary in severity from the mildly inconvenient to the potentially fatal. Wheeze and shortness of breath are the commonest symptoms, but severe persistent cough can also result from asthma, and in young children cough is often a symptom or a warning sign of an attack. Some asthmatics get infrequent attacks, while others may be affected nearly all the time. Although many cases of asthma start in childhood, the disease can start during adulthood.

CAUSES Asthma often runs in families along with associated conditions such as eczema and hay fever. The mechanism of asthma is not fully understood, but attacks can be triggered by any of the following:
■ Allergies: some asthmatics are allergic to such everyday items as house dust (strictly speaking, the house dust mite), pollen, fungal spores, dogs, cats or birds. Usually the allergy is to things *inhaled*, but occasionally asthma can be triggered by allergies to foods.
■ Emotion: stress can provoke attacks in some people who already suffer from asthma.
■ Viral respiratory infections: colds or flu are a common cause of asthmatic attacks, especially in early childhood (typically, before the age of four).
■ Sudden exposure to cold air.
■ Exercise can occasionally precipitate an attack.
■ Smoke (including cigarette smoke).
■ Some drugs, including beta-blockers *(see **hypertension**, page 48)* and aspirin.

PRESCRIPTION DRUGS

Mast cell stabilizers: Drugs such as sodium cromoglycate are useful for the *prevention* of attacks; they are of no use for the *treatment* of attacks. These drugs are usually only effective if inhaled, and there are several ways of taking them including aerosols, inhalation of fine powder from plastic cartridges, and nebulizers (see illustration).

How they work: by acting on the mast cells – the cells which release the chemicals which cause airway narrowing. Essentially, they prevent release of these chemicals.

Beta stimulants: used to *treat* attacks once in progress, and also to prevent them occurring. Beta stimulants can be given as tablets (or by injection) but are most commonly inhaled by means of an aerosol spray.

How they work: by stimulating the part of the nervous system which causes the muscles in the walls of the air passages to relax. Consequently, the air passage widens, allowing air to pass in and out more freely.

Methylxanthines can be useful for prevention and treatment. They are usually given as tablets or by injection.

How they work: by acting directly on the muscles in the walls of the air passages, causing them to relax.

Anticholinergics are usually used in addition to a beta stimulant or methylxanthine. This group of drugs is widely used to treat many conditions. The only one in common use in asthma is ipratropium bromide. It is available as an inhaler, and a solution of the drug can be used in a nebulizer.

How they work: by blocking the part of the nervous system which normally causes bronchial muscle to contract, thereby producing relaxation and widening of the bronchioles.

Steroids: powerful drugs, used in the treatment of many illnesses; in asthma, they can be used in small doses to prevent attacks, or in large doses to treat severe attacks. Usually steroids are taken in small doses by metered aerosol, or by inhalation of a powder. In bad attacks, a doctor may give a suitable dose in tablet form.

How they work: The action of steroids in asthma is complex, but basically they damp down inflammation in air passages and cause the muscle in the walls of the air passages to relax.

OVER-THE-COUNTER TREATMENTS
Don't try to treat yourself. Remember ASTHMA CAN KILL. All bad attacks should be reported to a doctor.

QUESTIONS TO ASK THE DOCTOR
■ Is this drug meant to *prevent* attacks, or help to *treat* an attack once it has started?
■ Is there a right and a wrong way to use the aerosol/spinhaler/nebulizer?
■ How long should I take the drug?
■ If the drug fails, is it safe for me to increase the dose?
■ Does it matter in which order I take my inhalers? (See **SELF MANAGEMENT**.)
■ Is it worth having an allergy test?

SIDE EFFECTS
Mast cell stabilizers, prescribed for *prevention* of attacks,

The trachea or windpipe *divides into two in the chest.*

The right and left *main bronchi.*

Right and left bronchi *divide into ever-smaller bronchi, and then into bronchioles.*

A *shows a (much magnified) normal bronchiole. The muscle is the thin band of surrounding cells. (Actual width may be as little as one mm.)*

In B the muscle has contracted, narrowing the air passage. In a really bad attack, the bronchiole may be blocked completely.

Inhalation devices

Pressurized inhaler: *effective, convenient to carry. You have to learn to synchronize breathing in with activating the puff; simple for all but the very young or otherwise incapable.*

Plastic chambers *like this can be used in conjunction with aerosol inhalers. The drug is puffed into the chamber, then breathed in at leisure – so avoiding the problem of synchronization. It enables children as young as three years to use an aerosol; the alternative is a nebulizer.*

Dry powder inhaler: *The drug comes in small plastic capsules which are impaled on a needle inside the device. When air is sniffed through the device, the drug is dispersed by a tiny propellor.*

are taken regularly even when free of asthma. Adverse effects are unusual, and are rarely serious; sore throat and cough are the most common.

Beta stimulants: much easier to use than previous generations of bronchodilators, modern beta stimulants such as Ventolin (salbutamol) have been developed to give insignificant side effects, though mild tremor and sore throat are not uncommon.

Methylxanthines are usually long-acting and prescribed once or twice daily. It is often sensible to take the last dose just before going to bed so that the drug is acting while you are asleep. Methylxanthines can be interfered with by other drugs including ulcer healing agents and some antibiotics. If you are on other medication it is important to tell your doctor. It is also very important NOT TO EXCEED THE PRESCRIBED DOSE of these drugs, as adverse side effects are not uncommon, and can be serious. Mild side effects include nausea, loss of appetite, headaches and anxiety; serious side effects include heart rhythm disturbance and fits.

Anticholinergic: patients with glaucoma (raised pressure in the eyeball) should not use this drug, nor should men with prostate trouble (usually older men who have difficulty passing water) – a doctor must advise in these cases. Anticholinergic inhaler side effects are not common but include glaucoma, constipation, difficulty passing urine, and heart palpitations.

Corticosteroids: long-term treatment with steroids worries people who have heard of the side effects of these drugs. But in asthma, the long-term treatment is usually with an inhaler, which delivers a comparatively small dose straight to the lungs. The only significant side effects reported are thrush, a fungal infection causing white spots in the mouth and throat. Steroid tablets and injections are another matter: they can cause serious side-effects, brittle bones, high blood pressure, sugar diabetes and depression. These take a long time to develop, and since steroid tablets and injections are a temporary measure, such side effects are not really an issue in asthma.

SELF-MANAGEMENT

■ If you have a child taking drugs by nebulizer (see diagram) heed the warnings given about over-using the apparatus. The very young can succumb to asthma quite quickly; doctors prefer patients to go to hospital before an attack builds up to a serious level.

■ Resolve to *contest* your asthma *all the time*; don't let it build up. Carry a salbutamol inhaler with you. Don't miss out on the steroid inhaler dose: long-term asthma can do you more damage than an inhaled steroid. Remember you can use a salbutamol inhaler to prevent attacks *as well as* treat them. Try to anticipate the onset of an attack – for example if about to take exercise, or visit a particularly dirty house; one puff gives relief for up to four hours.

■ If you use both a steroid inhaler and a salbutamol inhaler, take the salbutamol *first*: it will make the air passages widen, so allowing the subsequent steroid dose to penetrate better.

■ Discuss the possibility of allergy tests with your doctor. This is a complex area, but worthwhile for manypatients with long-term asthma. Once you know your allergies, you can take evasive action. In the case of allergy to house dust, this means, for example, keeping the bedroom and bed as dust-free as possible. Specialists have useful advice to offer in this area. Some specialists may suggest a course of desensitizing injections, but this is rarely useful.

■ If you are highly strung, and find that emotion brings on attacks, discuss the possibility of relaxation therapy with your doctor.

■ Avoid drugs which can bring on attacks, such as beta-blockers *(see **hypertension**, page 48 and **angina**, page 46)* and aspirin.

■ If you are a smoker, stop. You run the risk of permanent damage to your lungs, and your asthma attacks will be more frequent.

SELF-HELP IN AN ATTACK

■ Shake the salbutamol inhaler before use.
■ Breathe it in as deeply as possible, and try to hold your breath. If the attack persists, and particularly if you are getting tired or cannot speak, SEEK URGENT MEDICAL HELP. Many asthmatics now have nebulizers at home, and these deliver a larger dose than an inhaler. If it is not effective within the period specified by the doctor/hospital, seek medical help immediately.

Nebulizer: *These vary in design.The drug, in liquid form, is placed in the small container attached to the mask. When oxygen is passed through, a fine inhalable mist is produced. Portable nebulizer for use at home has air instead of oxygen.*

PNEUMONIA AND PLEURISY

Mucolytics, bronchodilators, cough suppressants, antibiotics, analgesics

WHAT ARE PNEUMONIA AND PLEURISY?

Pneumonia is an inflammation of the lungs. It causes fever, shortness of breath and cough. The coughing often results in the production of yellow or green sputum; occasionally blood can come up too. Pleurisy is an inflammation of the membrane covering the lungs and this causes pain on deep breathing, coughing or laughing.

CAUSES Of pneumonia, usually a bacterial infection, although viruses, other organisms and even chemicals may occasionally be to blame. Pleurisy usually results from disease within the lung – typically pneumonia.

There are different types of pneumonia: lobar pneumonia is confined to one section or lobe; bronchopneumonia is patchy and widespread. This is the type most commonly seen in children and old people.

PRESCRIPTION DRUGS

Treatment will vary according to the cause. The main concerns are to expel the secretions from the chest and treat the cause of the inflammation.

Mucolytics, bronchodilators, cough suppressants: *see* ***cough,*** *page 68.*

Antibiotics will only work in cases of bacterial pneumonia; they are ineffective against viruses. The choice of antibiotic will depend on many factors, including: whether the patient has an allergy; whether kidney or liver damage is present; the severity of the illness; whether the patient could be pregant; the type of bacteria most likely to be causing the infection; whether the patient has had an antibiotic recently. If the patient is very ill, more than one antibiotic may be used in combination, and these may be given by injection. Some antibiotics are inactivated by food and have to be taken between meals. The antibiotic may be changed during the course of treatment if the patient does not appear to be responding or if phlegm specimens show that the organism responsible is resistant to the drug. Treatment typically lasts between five and ten days, but duration does depend on the nature of the infection.

How they work: by killing the bacteria responsible for the infection, or by stopping the bacteria from multiplying, thus relying on the body's own defences to complete the elimination. The problem with antibiotics is that bacteria can develop resistance to them, and this happens, typically, when treatment is stopped before all the bacteria have been killed. It may well be worse to take half a course of antibiotics than none at all – the bacteria left behind being more difficult to eliminate. This is also the reason why a different antibiotic is likely to be used if the patient is ill again after a short interval – typically less than a month.

Analgesics: aspirin and paracetamol will ease the pain of pleurisy and help to lower the fever. *See **common cold**, page 134.*

In addition to the drug treatment, there are two other recourses: oxygen to help patients who are finding breathing difficult; and physiotherapy to help loosen secretions and encourage coughing. Thus cough suppressants are rarely used in the early stages.

OVER-THE-COUNTER TREATMENTS
Diagnosis of pneumonia and pleurisy are usually made by a doctor after examination of the chest, and often with the help of an X-ray. Self-treatment is inappropriate and potentially dangerous.

QUESTIONS TO ASK THE DOCTOR
■ How long will the treatment take to work?
■ How long should I take the medicine?
■ What will happen if I stop taking the medicine?
■ Is permanent lung damage likely?

SIDE EFFECTS
Mucolytics, bronchodilators, cough suppressants: *see **cough**, page 68.*

Antibiotics can cause nausea, vomiting, diarrhoea and lethergy; also allergies, which are usually present as a rash, and should be reported to the doctor immediately. Some antibiotics can activate thrush in babies, or in the vagina. Tetracyclines cause staining of developing teeth, and should not be given to children under 12 years or to pregnant or breastfeeding women. Some antibiotics, particularly those given by injection for serious infections, may cause further side effects: all developments should be discussed with the doctor.

Paracetamol has no common side effects when taken in in the correct dose; *see **pain**, page 106,* as also for aspirin's side effects.

SELF-MANAGEMENT
Not all patients with pneumonia or pleurisy need to be admitted to hospital. It is important for the patient to drink plenty of fluids as dehydration can make secretions thicker and more difficult to cough up. Pain in the chest should be controlled with analgesics, so that it does not inhibit coughing, which must be encouraged.

PATIENT'S EXPERIENCE
"My baby of six months had a cough with a fever and she was very restless. She seemed to be breathing rather fast. I took her to the doctor, who listened to her chest and then asked me to take her for an X-ray. This showed a patchy pneumonia on both sides of the chest. She was admitted to hospital where she was given antibiotics by mouth and also physiotherapy to help clear the chest infection. After three days her temperature had settled and she was drinking well again. The doctor said that she could go home but that she must continue the antibiotics. After a week he repeated the X-ray which showed that the infection had cleared. He then stopped the antibiotics; she has been fine ever since."

Anti-tuberculous antibiotics

WHAT IS TUBERCULOSIS?

– Infection with the tuberculosis (TB) bacillus. In the great majority of cases it is only the lungs which are involved, but TB may also infect lymph nodes, kidneys, bowel and brain. Early symptoms include lack of energy and loss of appetite. Later a cough develops and yellow phlegm is produced. Weight loss, a slight temperature and severe nocturnal sweating are common. If untreated, symptoms worsen progressively, weight loss becomes very marked and after some months the disease ends in death from 'consumption'. That, at any rate, is how our grandparents saw TB; it is, however, a disease of the past. Treatment with modern antibiotics is almost always effective, providing it starts at an early stage. The most serious form of tuberculosis affects the membranes around the brain (tuberculous meningitis). This is hard to treat and often ends in coma and death, but is fortunately rare in western countries.

CAUSES Infection occurs most often by inhaling droplets of moisture containing live bacilli coughed into the air by an infected person. Catching TB from infected cow's milk remains, even in developed countries, a real, if rare possibility. Most people who catch TB have been heavily exposed, for example by living with or working closely with an infected person. Others catch it because they have a lowered resistance to infection; this can be the result of diseases such as cancer, alcoholism, and long-term treatment with steroids.

PRESCRIPTION DRUGS

Anti-tuberculous antibiotics are specific for TB and rarely used for other infections. Often two or more are combined in a single tablet. Rifampicin, isoniazid, ethambutol and pyrazinamide are taken as tablets. Streptomycin is given by injection into a muscle.

How they work: by killing the TB bacilli. TB responds only slowly to the drugs and it can be weeks before the symptoms improve. If only one antibiotic is used, the TB bacillus will become resistant. The antibiotic is then ineffective and all the symptoms will return. Thus, two, three or sometimes four antibiotics are used simultaneously. However, although the symptoms may disappear within a month, this does not mean that the disease is cured. There are often a few bacilli left dormant which will grow and cause further disease if the treatment is stopped too soon. Most courses of treatment last at least six months and severe cases may need 18 months.

Pyridoxine (Vitamin B6) may help prevent side effects from izoniazid (see below).

QUESTIONS TO ASK YOUR DOCTOR
- How long should I take the antibiotics?
- How soon will I start to feel better?
- What side effects should I watch out for?
- What happens if I am allergic to the antibiotics?
- Will the drugs react with any others I am taking?
- When will I be non-infectious?

SIDE EFFECTS
Indigestion is common with these **antibiotics;** it may pass off after a few days. If it does not, the antibiotic will be changed. Itchy skin rashes may occur. Rifampicin makes the urine appear a reddish-orange colour. Sometimes the tears are also coloured and soft contact lenses may become stained.

Some side effects are more serious and should be reported to a doctor straight away. Rifampicin, isoniazid and pyrazinamide can affect the liver: usually this is only noticed in blood tests, but in a few cases, jaundice may develop. Isoniazid can cause the hands and feet to tingle and to become numb. Ethambutol can blur the vision, especially when reading, or distort colour vision. With all these reactions the doctor will need to decide which drug is responsible; the symptoms will recover if the drug is stopped immediately.

Additive effects on other drugs: rifampicin causes the liver to work faster, which means that medicines being taken for diabetes, blood clotting problems, heart problems and for oral contraception will be less effective and the dose may need adjusting; or the patient may need a change of drugs.

SELF-MANAGEMENT
Apart from the antibiotics, there are no effective treatments for TB. You can help ensure that the treatment is successful by:

■Taking all tablets as prescribed *each day* for the *whole of the course.* Don't miss a day's tablets because you are feeling better. This may allow the TB to become resistant.

■Eat a varied diet, including fresh vegetables, to help regain the weight you have lost. Appetite improves with treatment.

■ Drink as little alcohol as possible. Don't smoke.

■ Report any side effects to your doctor as soon as possible so that he can change the antibiotics.

TO AVOID PASSING ON TB
Don't socialize, or go to work until your doctor says it is safe. In particular, avoid close contact with children. These precautions are, however, usually only necessary in the first month of treatment. You can act normally with your own family, but do encourage them to attend hospital for a TB check.

Problems of the central nervous system

The brain is the central clearing house for all the messages that come to it, from the eyes, ears and other special sense organs, and from the many nerves which take orders to and receive messages from every part of the body. The way the brain has developed in humans differentiates us in fundamental ways from the rest of the animal kingdom – but brain function is still poorly understood.

ANXIETY	**84-87**
STRESS	**88-89**
FATIGUE	**90-91**
INSOMNIA	**92-93**
ALCOHOLISM	**94-95**
DIZZINESS	**96-97**
HEADACHE	**98-99**
MIGRAINE	**100-101**
DRUG MISUSE	**102-105**
PAIN	**106-109**
EPILEPSY	**110-113**
PARKINSONISM	**114-115**
DEPRESSION	**116-119**
SCHIZOPHRENIA *and other psychoses*	**120-123**
SENILE DEMENTIA, *including Alzheimer's disease*	**124-127**
MULTIPLE SCLEROSIS	**128-129**
ANAESTHETICS	**130-131**

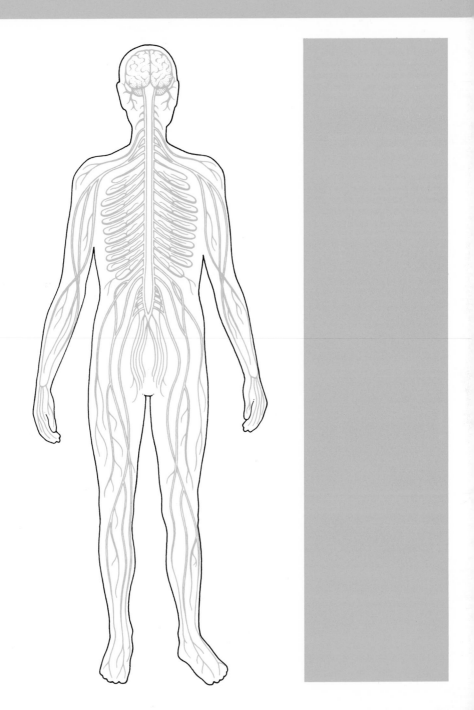

Benzodiazepines, beta-blockers

WHAT IS ANXIETY?

Fear, ranging from a vague sense that something unpleasant might happen, to an overwhelming attack of panic. Patients suffering from anxiety say they feel nervous, tense, uneasy, agitated, edgy and apprehensive; they are often full-time worriers. Their physical symptoms include a dry mouth, choking feelings, tense muscles, a tight or painful chest, rapid pounding of the heart, breathing difficulty, sweating, dizziness, light-headedness, shaking and a strange sensation of distance from the world. Many people do not realize that these symptoms are caused by anxiety and may think that a thumping heart means they are about to have a heart attack, or that dizziness or light-headedness are signs of a brain tumour. This makes them feel even more anxious.

CAUSES The commonest cause of anxiety is stress. One of the most stressful experiences of all is the death of someone close, but problems in marriage, unemployment, poverty, poor housing and growing older can also play havoc. The support of family and friends is crucial for emotional well-being, and those who do not have this support are much more likely to become anxious.

PRESCRIPTION DRUGS

Benzodiazepines: commonly called tranquillizers. They offer relief from anxiety in the first six weeks of a course of treatment but after that there will be no marked changes: the drugs will maintain the level of improvement, but will not increase it. The longer the drugs are taken regularly, the less effective they become.
How they work: by acting on the brain to calm the patient down. Some are fast-acting, some slow-acting. Some are short-acting and some long-acting. Lorazepam takes effect more quickly than diazepam and chlordiazepoxide, and is often prescribed for panic attacks. Another difference between the various tranquillizers is how long they continue to have an effect once they begin to work. Lorazepam is short-acting and disappears from the body fairly quickly.
Beta-blockers: These are not tranquillizers, but can reduce the physical symptoms of anxiety such as shaking and palpitations.
How they work: *see* **hypertension,** *page 48.*

OVER-THE-COUNTER TREATMENTS
None.

QUESTONS TO ASK THE DOCTOR
- How long should I take them?
- Can I drink alcohol or take other pills at the same time as the tranquillizers?
- If I become pregnant, will the drugs affect my baby?
- Can I take the pills only when I feel I need them?

There is a real risk of dependence on tranquillizers: see SIDE EFFECTS.

IS THERE AN ALTERNATIVE TO TRANQUILLIZERS?
If you do not take tranquillizers, there is every chance that your anxiety will decrease by itself within a few weeks. You will then attribute your improvement not to the pills, but to your own efforts; the chance of dependence on tranquillizers is put at one remove. If you are too severely anxious to cope unassisted, tranquillizers *can* be useful in breaking the vicious circle long enough for you to change your circumstances.

SIDE EFFECTS
The most common side effects of **benzodiazepines** are drowsiness and lethargy during the first two weeks of acourse of pills. Concentration and memory may also be affected, so it is advisable to put off important tasks or decisions, driving, or working with mechanical or dangerous machinery.

The most serious risk is dependence bordering on true addiction. One in every three people who take tranquillizers continuously for more than six months will experience unpleasant withdrawl symptoms when the pills are stopped. These include: anxiety and insomnia – the very symptoms the drugs were prescribed to cure; panic attacks; poor memory and concentration; lack of energy. Often, people going through withdrawal feel as if they have flu. Some lose their appetite, feel nauseous, perhaps actually vomiting; others suffer severe hunger. Constipation, diarrhoea, headaches, muscle aches and pains often develop. Muscles can even twitch and jerk quite dramatically. Blurred or double vision, and acute sensitivity or numbness can also play a part of withdrawal. Bright lights and loud noises can become unbearable, and sometimes unusual smells and tastes are noticed. Withdrawal symptoms will not occur immediately after stopping the tablets; it is usually a couple of days or even a week before symptoms develop. Symptoms are often at their worst after a week without drugs and can disappear within a month, but they may persist for up to a year.

Beta-blockers: *see* **hypertension**, *page 48.*

DO SOMETHING DIFFERENT

Take your mind off your anxiety by doing something active. Here are some suggestions:

- Make a cup of tea.
- Telephone a friend.
- Count backwards from 100 to 1.
- Read a magazine.
- Knit or sew.
- Sing or dance to music.
- Take a walk.
- Do some gardening.
- Go for a run.
- Have a bath.

You may find it difficult to distract yourself at first, but with practice it will become much easier. Try to concentrate on what you are doing, rather than on what you feel.

Once you have completed the sequence one to nine, keep your eyes closed and keep breathing slowly and deeply. Let your whole body become more and more deeply relaxed for a few minutes longer without first tensing your muscles. Count silently to three and open your eyes.

SELF-MANAGEMENT

Relaxation techniques really can help. When you feel anxious, sit in a comfortable chair, or lie down, and close your eyes. Begin to breathe slowly and deeply and keep this rhythmic breathing going thoughout the relaxation session. Go through each of the muscle groups below, one at a time. Tense the muscles for five seconds and then relax them for 20 seconds. Follow the order given.

1 Curl your toes and press your feet down.
2 Tense your thighs, straighten your knees and make your legs stiff.
3 Make your buttocks tight.
4 Tense your stomach.
5 Clench your fists.
6 Bend your elbows and tense your arms.
7 Hunch your shoulders.
8 Press your head back into a cushion to tense your neck muscles.
9 Clench your jaws, frown and screw up your eyes.

To relax each muscle group effectively you need to talk yourself through both the tension and relaxation phases. Try the following silent self-instructions:

Tense up

- Tense the muscles slightly – don't strain them.
- Hold it.
- Feel the tension in the muscles.
- Notice where the tightness is.
- Keep the muscles tense.
- Concentrate on the tension.

Relax

- Feel the tension leave the muscles.
- Feel them grow more and more relaxed.
- Feel them become heavier and heavier.
- Feel the warmth flow through them.
- Feel the tension drain away.
- Let all the tension go.
- Feel warm and heavy.
- Say words like 'calm' and 'relax' silently.
- Feel more and more relaxed.
- Let the feeling increase.

TRANQUILLIZER WITHDRAWAL PROGRAMME
Preparing to cut down

Once you have decided to give the withdrawal programme a try, your first step should be to write down your reasons for making that decision. Looking back at these reasons will help you later on. List them in order of importance.

Now write down the order in which you are going to cut down your tablets. Begin with the tablet you could most easily do without, and end with the most difficult.

Cutting down in stages
Cut down in stages, beginning with the part of the day during which you need the tablets least, and working up to the time when you need them most. If, for example, you take tablets four times a day, cut them down in 8 stages:

Stage 1
Cut out half of your least important tablet.
Stage 2
Cut out the other half.
Stage 3
Cut out half of your second least important tablet.
Stage 4
Cut out the other half.
Stage 5
Cut out half of your second most important tablet.
Stage 6
Cut out the other half.
Stage 7
Cut out half of your most important tablet.
Stage 8
Cut out the other half.

If you find it impossible to cut down in this way, set yourself a maximum limit of tablets that you will take each day and keep to this limit until you feel ready to reduce to a lower limit.

Cutting down at your own pace
The more gradually you reduce your tablets, the less chance there is of withdrawal symptoms and the less severe they are likely to be. As withdrawal symptoms can take some time to develop, you should remain at each stage for at least one week. It is likely that you will need to remain at some stages for several weeks before you feel ready to move on, particularly as you near the end. It is not unusual to take several months to come off the tablets altogether, and some people need a year or more.

MONITORING YOUR ANXIETY
As soon as you begin to feel anxious, write down in a notebook:

- The time of day.
- Where you are.
- What you are doing.
- Who you are with.
- How you feel.

This record will enable you to pinpoint the circumstances which are likely to make you anxious. Use relaxation exercises to prepare yourself the next time they crop up. You may not be able to get rid of feelings of anxiety altogether; but you may well find you can keep them under some control.

NAMES YOU WILL HEAR
For benzodiazepines (tranquillizers) *see*
anxiety, *page 84;* for beta-blockers
see **angina,** *page 46.*

WHAT IS STRESS?

'Stress disorder' is an increasingly common diagnosis in general practice. Stress is used here in the sense of tension, or psychological pressure. People vary in the degree of stress they can tolerate before they develop problems in coping. Sometimes it is difficult to recognize the signs of stress in oneself; for many, coping with stress is a matter of pride and the thought of being labelled as unable to cope is unwelcome. Some families seem to condition people to 'go it alone'; others encourage children and others to seek support and to recognize early stress symptoms. Stress disorders, like tension states (see anxiety, page 84), may present in the form of symptoms which can also be caused by infection – sore throats, diarrhoea and cystitis-like symptoms are common exmples. This can cause much confusion in the consulting room.

CAUSES Stressful lifestyles involving long hours of work in crowded environments at high pressure are associated with many physical diseases or conditions such as high blood pressure, stomach and duodenal ulcers, migraine, eczema and dermatitis, heart attack and cancer. The underlying cause is presumably a continual drive on the body's internal mechanisms. The commong stress disorders constitute an early-warning system: your body is telling you to let off the pressure or suffer the consequences.

PRESCRIPTION DRUGS

Many stress-related symptoms can be helped by medication, but if stress is the cause, then the symptoms will not be completely cured until you have worked on reducing the stress.

Propranolol, a beta-blocker, will reduce tremor (shaking hands or legs) and butterflies in the stomach before an exam, but it will not stop the same symptoms next time.

Stress-induced heartburn or indigestion can be treated in the same way as ordinary heartburn or peptic ulcer (*see pages 20 and 24*), but these will resolve quicker if drug treatment is combined with stress reduction in your lifestyle. The same is true of tension headaches or back pain.

Hypertension, migraine, asthma and eczema will react in the same way, requiring more of the usual medication at times of stress.

Many people with stress-related disorders are doubtful about taking tranquillizers as such; they don't want to be slowed down. This is a reassuring sign the times.

OVER-THE-COUNTER TREATMENTS
Symptomatic treatment can be used, but it will not solve all the problems of stress disorders. Painkillers and antacids are the main over-the-counter remedies. It may be worth trying homeopathic or herbal remedies too as they have no side effects.

QUESTIONS TO ASK THE DOCTOR
■ Do you think my symptoms are caused by stress?
■ What if I can't see that my lifestyle is stressful?
■ Do you think I would benefit from tranquillizers?

SIDE EFFECTS
One major problem with **tranquillizers** is their sedative effect (see **anxiety,** page 84). They are even more sedative when combined with alcohol or antihistamines (see **hay fever,** page 260). In addition, they create dependence: withdrawal symptoms make it difficult to come off them once you are 'hooked'. Getting hooked is tragically easy and can happen within a matter of a few weeks. Both the medical profession and the lay public are becoming wary of tranquillizers.
Propranolol and other beta-blockers are not particularly sedative, nor are they addictive. In general they have few side effects as long as you are not asthmatic or diabetic and there is no tendency to asthma in your family (see **hypertension,** page 48).

SELF-HELP
(See also **anxiety,** page 84; **irritable bowel syndrome,** page 32; **insomnia,** page 92).
■ Ideally, self-help groups and health workers should collaborate to make non-drug treatments such as yoga, relaxation classes, books and tapes widely available. These, combined with modifying one's lifestyle to give a balance of activity, stimulation, work, exercise, rest and play are sound long-term measures.
■ Once you have identified and tackled a stress-related disorder, don't be surprised if it recurs some time later. Get back into your chosen routine and try to eliminate the new source of stress. It takes practice to become a cool calm personality.
■ Be aware that alcohol is the time-honoured tranquillizer, and this is what makes it dangerous. Stress does not go away because you have drunk yourself under the table. Above all alcohol should not be combined with prescribed tranquillizers or antihistamines.

PATIENT'S EXPERIENCE
"I went through a six-month period of having to go to the doctor's surgery practically every week. If it wasn't my eczema getting worse, it was heartburn, then cystitis, then thrush, then headaches. I had 12 different prescriptions in three months. Finally I had this aching throat – I thought I must have got a chicken bone stuck in my gullet. This time the doctor called me back for a long appointment and pointed out how I kept coming running in with a new symptom. I broke down and cried – I just felt overwhelmed by it all. I began to see how I'd been trying to compensate for my awful marriage by working 24 hours a day – I was living on aspirin and coffee by that time. To cut a long story short, it really helped to see what it was all about. I found I could cope better once I stopped drinking coffee and tea and started going to a sauna after work, doing the relaxation exercises I'd been taught there. I never even contemplated using tranquillizers – that would be a living death to me."

DOCTOR'S EXPERIENCE
"It's relatively easy to help people who come in and say they are under stress and ask what they should do about it. Easy to say, not so easy to do, as I've found myself – it depends on the level of motivation. Often, however, I can spot a stress disorder miles away, but can't get the patient to recognize it for what it is. Stress, they say, what stress? It's as if the workaholic within them really resists making a connection between, say, seven-day working weeks and nervous indigestion. Everyone recognizes 'pre-exam diarrhoea' but it seems much more difficult to accept that the same mechanism can operate continuously."

NAMES YOU WILL HEAR
Stimulants
Chemical name: caffeine; **trade name:** Proplus. **Chemical name:** dexamphetamine; **trade names:** Dexedrine, Durophet. **Chemical name:** cocaine; **trade name:** none. Fecamfamin and prolintane are ingredients of various stimulant preparations and tend not to be sold separately.

Tonics
Prescription-only tonics may contain strychnine and vitamins or minerals; over-the-counter preparations may contain bitters (eg alkaline gentian mixture), plus vitamins, iron, caffeine and minerals.

WHAT IS FATIGUE?

The sensation of being tired. This is normal, of course, after a hectic day looking after young children or after exercise or a late night. It is when you have the same feeling of being worn out day and night, regardless of how much you are actually doing during the day, that makes you worry about fatigue as a symptom. It may well be associated with other symptoms such as headaches and sore throats, or a general feeling of being run down. It may even be difficult to get to sleep, once overtired, and this completes a vicious circle.

CAUSES Normal tiredness apart, fatigue can have a host of medical causes. Viral illnesses such as 'flu or glandular fever may be followed by months of general malaise and fatigue – the 'post-viral syndrome'. Bacterial infections such as pneumonia and urinary tract infections can also lead to fatigue which generally resolves once the treatment is over. Tension, anxiety and depression, or just continuing difficulties in your personal life, can easily lead to continuing fatigue.

Anaemia, pregnancy and **hypothyroidism** are also common causes of fatigue (*see pages 224, 184, 166*).

There are also many drugs which cause fatigue – see margin. Less common conditions in which fatigue is a major symptom include **tuberculosis** *(see page 80)*, **multiple sclerosis** *(see page 128)*, **cancers** *(see pages 200-213)*.

PRESCRIPTION DRUGS

Tonics used to be a mainstay of prescribing for people suffering from fatigue. It is now recognized that none of the ingredients (*see* **NAMES YOU WILL HEAR**) could possibly have a real chemical effect on tiredness; if they do 'work' at all, it is through psychological suggestion (the placebo effect) which of course can be a powerful force, but is nothing to do with the medicine itself. Tonics are now prescribed in limited quantities for the older generation who have grown up believing in them.

If tiredness is caused by depression, then the appropriate prescription drug is one of the less sedative antidepressants like imipramine (*see **depression**, page 116*). This takes several weeks to work properly, but there may be improvement within seven days.

Amphetamine is rarely prescribed by doctors because of the danger of dependence and long-term side effects. It is prescribed in cases of narcolepsy, usually under supervision by a neurologist. Cocaine is also a stimulant but its medical use is also strictly controlled.

OVER-THE-COUNER TREATMENTS
Tonics: see **PRESCRIPTION DRUGS.**

Vitamins are often advertised for their pick-me-up effects and bought by an unsuspecting public. They are unlikely to have any chemical effect unless there is a deficiency which can usually be detected by a medical examination or a blood test. Again, when they do 'work' in the absence of evidence of a deficiency state, it is presumably by a placebo effect (*see above*).

Caffeine is widely consumed in tea (40 mg per cup), coffee (100-150 mg per cup) and 'cola' drink (20-30 mg per glass). It certainly has a short-term effect in countering fatigue in most people (not all) and is also sold over the counter as tablets of 50 mg useful in long-distance driving.

QUESTIONS TO ASK THE DOCTOR
■ Can you explain why I feel so tired all the time?
■ Have I had all the necessary tests for medical causes?
■ Is there any point in taking vitamins?
■ Would a change of scene help?

SIDE EFFECTS
Caffeine in large quantities produces irritability and interferes with sleep, although some people are more sensitive to it than others.

Amphetamine use induces dependence to a variable degree. This is one major reason for limiting its use; another is that severe psychotic episodes similar to schizophrenic breakdowns can occur long after stopping the drug. Cocaine can also induce dependence.

SELF-HELP
■ Sit down and think about your symptoms. Is your tiredness related to stress, work, bringing up small children, poor sleep? Has it come on gradually or suddenly, out of the blue? Is your body giving you an important message to slow down, or are you in fact ill? Is there anything else wrong – in your body or in your lifestyle? All this information will be useful to your doctor if you do seek medical help.

■ Get used to the idea that apart from cups of coffee, there are no magic potions to cure fatigue. If it isn't caused by a medical condition, then the best you can do is to try readjusting your timetable to give a combination of rest, mental stimulus and exercise.

See also **insomnia,** *page 92,* **anaemias,** *page 224 and* **anxiety,** *page 84.*

DRUGS WHICH CAN CAUSE FATIGUE
Antihistamines (see **hay fever,** *page 260); **sedatives** and* **tranquillisers** *(see anxiety, page 84);* **antidepressants** *(see* **depression,** *page 116);* **anticonvulsants** *(see* **epilepsy,** *page 110) and even some antibiotics.*

WHAT IS INSOMNIA?

Probably the most reliable definition is persistent sleeplessness. It really is a common problem: in any one year up to 30 per cent of the population of a developed country will seek help for insomnia. Sleep needs vary a great deal; older people need less.

CAUSES are numerous, indeed more than one factor may be involved at any given time. The most important causes are: anxiety; depression; medical conditions causing pain, indigestion, constipation, cough, breathlessness, itching, fever; environmental factors including bedroom comfort and neighbourhood noise; daytime naps – not a true cause as the person who sleeps during the day will need less sleep at night; certain drinks including tea and coffee (which are stimulants), alcohol (which helps put you to sleep, but tends to disrupt sleep later in the night); excessive food or fluid intake before bedtime; menopausal symptoms such as hot flushes and excessive sweating.

PRESCRIPTION DRUGS

Sleeping pills – hypnotics – are only really useful for short-term relief of insomnia. The cause or causes of the sleeplessness should always be sought and the thrust of attention brought to bear on these.

Benzodiazepines, also called minor tranquillizers, constitute the bulk of sleeping tablets. A number of types are available, the essential differences between them being their duration of action: nitrazepam, for example, is long-acting (16 hours) whereas triazolam is short-acting (4 hours). They should only be prescribed for short-term treatment – no more than a few weeks.
How they work: In low dosage these drugs have a calming effect, and in high dosage a sleep-inducing effect. In common with all hypnotics, they affect the part of the brain controlling wakefulness. How exactly this is achieved is not fully understood.

A number of **antihistamines** have marked sedative properties and are used to exploit this effect, especially in children. Results vary from child to child.
How they work: by acting on the brain.
Chloral derivatives, principally chloral hydrate, are sometimes used to treat insomnia in children and the elderly. They are also a relatively safe and effective alternative to benzodiazepines.
How they work: by acting on the part of the brain which controls wakefulness.

Chlormethiazole is occasionally used, primarily in some elderly people.

How it works: by acting on the brain.

Antidepressants are genuinely helpful for insomnia if depression is the cause. Many have useful sedative properties and can prevent early waking (at 4 am or so), which is characteristic of depressive illness.

How they work: see **depression**, page 116.

QUESTIONS TO ASK THE DOCTOR

■ Do I really need sleeping tablets?

■ Will the sleeping tablets leave me 'hung over'?

■ If I wake in the middle of the night, is it all right to take another tablet?

■ Can I increase the dose if the first is ineffective?

■ Will the sleeping tablets interact with any other tables I am taking?

■ How long before bed should I take them?

■ Should I have just a one-week course?

SIDE EFFECTS

Benzodiazepines' sedative effect diminishes with continued use and they are addictive, and users will become dependent on them. They may produce withdrawal effects characterized by insomnia, anxiety, loss of appetite and tremor. The outcome could be worse, in terms of insomnia, than the original problem. See **anxiety**, page 84.

Chloral derivatives may bring about a tolerance-reduced response to the same dose – as can all hypnotics.

All **hypnotics** can impair judgement and increase reaction time, thereby interfering with ability to drive or operate machines. Alcohol should be avoided with all hypnotics because together they can cause a dangerous level of sedation, and coma.

SELF-HELP

■ Avoid daytime naps. ■ Go to bed only when tired. ■ A warm milky drink half an hour before bedtime often helps. ■ Physical exercise during the day often aids relaxation. ■ Try to avoid thinking about getting to sleep or worrying about the day's events. Try to think about pleasant places and memories instead. ■ Avoid stimulant drinks – tea, coffee and so on. If you are unable to fall asleep within half an hour, get up and do something else such as reading. Return to bed only when sleepy. ■ Get up at the same time every day, irrespective of how much sleep you had during the night. ■ Try relaxation techniques – see **anxiety**, page 84.

INSOMNIA IN CHILDREN
If you have long-lasting problems with your child's sleep pattern, it is well worth asking your doctor to refer you to a child psychology service.

BARBITURATES
At one time popular, these are rarely used now because overdose can kill, and because stopping them can cause severe withdrawal symptoms.

COMMON PROBLEMS ARISING FROM ALCOHOLISM

When absorbed, alcohol diffuses throughout the body and is capable of harming almost every organ. The gastro-intestinal tract bears the brunt, as it is through the stomach, bowel and liver that the alcohol must pass to get to the rest of the body. As alcohol consumption has risen over the last 20 years, the amount of disease caused by it and deaths directly attributed to it have risen.

Liver disease: The liver can be damaged without there being any symptoms or obvious signs, indeed problems may only be picked up by blood tests or liver biopsy. Many forms occur: The mildest, such as fatty liver, can be reversed if the patient stops drinking. Others, such as *cirrhosis, page 000,* causes permanent scarring. The damage is permanent, but the liver may improve in function if the patient stops drinking completely.

Stomach disease: Alcohol directly damages the stomach lining, causing inflammation and sometimes bleeding. The patient may retch or vomit, often in the mornings, and also vomit blood.

Damage to the pancreas: Either an acute attack of inflammation of the pancreas (pancreatitis) can occur, or the pancreas gland can be permanently scarred, producing chronic abdominal pain, diabetes and inability to absorb food properly.

Nervous system damage: Nerve damage may give rise to tingling or numbness in the hands and feet and unsteadiness, even when not drunk. Periods of forgetfulness can signify brain damage or vitamin deficiency.
continued opposite

WHAT IS ALCOHOLISM?

The rough-and-ready definition is damage due to alcohol affecting any aspect of an individual's well-being, mental health or social life. Being an alcoholic does not imply that someone has gross physical damage, nor is continually drunk.

There is no absolute level of drinking that always produces damage, just as there is no absolutely safe level of drinking below which damage never results. Typical current recommended levels of safe drinking (UK) are 15 units of alcohol per week for men, and ten per week for women. These levels are set so that it is *unlikely* that below them physical harm will result. They demonstrate that women are more at risk from alcohol than men. A unit of alcohol consumption is equivalent to one half pint of normal strength beer, one single measure of spirits, a standard glass of wine or a standard glass of fortified wine (for example sherry). Each unit contains nine grams of alcohol, and whether the alcoholic drink is mixed with other drinks, or is taken with meals, makes no difference at all to its potential for causing damage.

The fact that some people seem to be able to drink prodigious amounts of alcohol without overt signs of being ill should not be taken as proof that it is safe to drink to this level. Many of these heavy drinkers have damage that can only be recognized by careful People who drink more than the recommended safe amounts, but without evidence of alcohol related problems, are usually described as heavy drinkers; they are advised to reduce intake as a preventive measure. People with actual problems related to drinking should seek help before they develop symptoms of addiction and dependence.

The common symptoms of addiction are: the morning shakes; *delirium tremens* (confusion and hallucinations); confusion when the individual stops drinking. Many other symptoms are, in addition, caused by the alcohol damaging individual parts of the body (see margin).

CAUSES Most experts believe that alcoholism is a social habit out of control. By contrast, many drinkers to think of alcoholism as a disease – which conveniently releases them from responsibility.

There is some evidence to suggest that alcoholism may run in families, but this may be more environmental than genetic. Apart from the added danger of damage in women, it is impossible to determine who, on the individual level, is most at risk from what level of drinking. Certain occupations, including seamen and people in the business of running bars and premises where alcoholic drinks are consumed are, however, associated with increased of alcoholism.

TREATMENT
As there is no specific cause, there is no magic treatment for alcoholism – other than avoiding alcohol. Various drugs are used, however, to help the patient get off alcohol and prevent withdrawal symptoms.

Tranquillizers *(see anxiety, page 84)* are given as short courses for a week or two to prevent the symptoms of withdrawal when alcohol is stopped.

How they work: by calming the patient down and suppressing the central nervous system, giving relief from sweating, anxiety, shaking and hallucinations which are common features of withdrawal from any addictive drug such as alcohol.

Disulfiram can be used to try and prevent the alcoholic starting to drink again.

How it works: by interfering with the normal breakdown of alcohol in the body and allowing the accumulation of a toxic chemical in the body. This makes the patient feel nauseous and vomit if alcohol is taken.

QUESTIONS TO ASK THE DOCTOR
■ Have I any signs of physical damage?
■ Do I need specialized help?

SIDE EFFECTS
Tranquillizers: These are only prescribed during drying out. They may make you drowsy, unsteady and excessively tired, but risk of other long-term problems (see anxiety, page 84) is insignificant given the short duration.

Disulfiram: Very few side effects unless you drink alcohol – see HOW IT WORKS.

SELF-MANAGEMENT
■ If you think you have been drinking too much, but are unsure if you have damaged yourself, talk it over with your doctor. If it seems there are no signs of damage but you want help to limit your drinking, try a self-help group.
■ If you have symptoms of addiction and dependence on alcohol, do not stop drinking suddenly. Preferably see your doctor, but in any case, gradually reduce your daily intake.

continued from opposite
There may also be intellectual impairment.
Bowel damage: gives rise to diarrhoea, and inability to absorb food and vitamins.
Heart damage: There may be palpitations. Breathlessness and swelling of the feet can be caused by alcoholism giving rise to heart failure.

DO YOU HAVE A DRINK PROBLEM?
The following questions are used by some doctors to find out if there is a drink problem:
■ Have you ever felt you should cut down your drinking?
■ Have people ever annoyed you by criticizing your drinking?
■ Have you ever felt bad or guilty about your drinking?
■ Have you ever had a drink first thing in the morning to steady your nerves or to get rid of a hangover?
   Two or more positive answers strongly suggests a drink problem.

AFTER DRYING OUT
Once you are dried out, you may need help either to keep your drinking under control, or to help you abstain altogether. In addition to the self-help groups mentioned above, there are many professional counselling agencies, some based in hospitals, others in the community.

PATIENT'S EXPERIENCE
"I started drinking at university and it has gradually increased over the years. I have lost a few days from work and my wife says I drink too much. Recently, after a heavy bout of drinking, I vomited some blood. This gave me a shock, so I stopped drinking, and felt very nervous and shaky. My doctor said I have an enlarged liver, and had me admitted to hospital. A short course of tranquillizers was prescribed: they made me sleepy, but I stopped shaking. I am now seeing a counsellor and have stopped drinking entirely. I feel much better, but still miss alcohol."

NAMES YOU WILL HEAR

Chemical name: prochlorperazine; **trade names:** Stemetil, Compazine, Anti-Naus, Mitil, Vertigon. **Chemical name:** cinnarizine; **trade name:** Stugeron. **Chemical name:** diazepam; **trade names:** Valium, Alupram, Atensine, Evacalm, Solis, Tensium, Valrelease. **Chemical name:** betahistine dihydrochloride; **trade name:** Serc. **Chemical name:** promethazine; **trade names:** Phenergan, Avomine, Progan, Prothazine, Histantil, Lenazine, Prohist, Profan.

WHAT IS DIZZINESS?

'Dizziness' and 'vertigo' are both terms used to denote a feeling of reeling: the patient senses a rotatory movement either of themselves going round and round, or of the environment rotating ("the room is swinging round"). The sense of balance is lost to some extent; in true vertigo, the patient may fall to one side in particular as a result of the feeling of movement.

CAUSES True vertigo is caused by problems in the sensory apparatus (the vestibular system and labyrinths of the inner ear) concerned with balance and co-ordination of movement. These problems include Meniere's disease, labyrinthitis, arterial and nervous conditions, certain drugs and some infections.

It is diagnosed by positional tests and examination to reveal the presence and direction of eye movements related to posture (nystagmus). It may be accompanied by nausea, and sometimes by changes in hearing – deafness and ringing in the ears (tinnitus). These may be mild in degree, or severe and disabling.

Dizziness of a more general kind, not localized to one side or direction, may be caused by anxiety and hyperventilation (accompanied by nausea and faintness), as when blood pressure is low and standing up produces temporary faintness and dizziness (postural hypotension); or when blood glucose is low (hypoglycaemia, which can be caused by long intervals between meals or irregular meals).

PRESCRIPTION DRUGS

Vestibular sedatives such as phenothiazines can suppress or at any rate diminish the symptoms of vertigo as can **antihistamines** (eg cinnarizine). The latter may be given by mouth or by injection or suppository if vomiting prevents oral intake. They lessen nausea, vomiting and vertigo.

How they work: by acting on the brain.

Tranquillizers such as diazepam may sometimes be used to treat dizziness associated with anxiety.

How they work: see **anxiety,** page 84.

In Meniere's disease, **betahistine dihydrochloride** may help in the early stages, along with the vestibular sedatives mentioned above; later, an operation may be needed if attacks become frequent and disabling.

OVER-THE-COUNTER TREATMENTS

Some of the antihistamines, for example promethazine, are available at chemists and are used in motion sickness/travel sickness (chlorpheniramine, promethazine). In pregnancy, and for all other uses, a doctor should be consulted first. Self-treatment of travel sickness is perfectly appropriate, but not of dizziness; dizzy spells and falls related to dizziness should be investigated by a doctor.

QUESTIONS TO ASK THE DOCTOR
- Is there a known cause for my dizziness?
- How long is the dizziness likely to last?
- How long should I take the tablets?
- Will the tablets make me sleepy?
- Is it safe to take the tablets if I get pregnant?

SIDE EFFECTS
Phenothiazines, although very effective, do have side effects especially if taken over long periods continuously; watch for involuntary movements. *See* **schizophrenia,** *page 120.* **Antihistamines** also commonly produce side effects: a dry mouth, difficulty in urinating, sometimes blurred vision, or temporary impotence in men. None of the drugs should be taken in pregnancy. They have an additive effect with alcohol.

SELF-MANAGEMENT
- Notice carefully whether any particular position of head or neck makes attacks come on or get worse.
- Fatigue may worsen or precipitate symptoms: try to relax; lie down and stay down if necessary until symptoms have abated.
- If you have postural hypotension (a doctor can diagnose this by taking your blood pressure while you are sitting or lying down and again when you stand up), take great care when getting out of bed; make a gradual transition from lying down to standing up.

If you are having repeated falls for no known reason, see your doctor.

Semi-curcular canals

Ampulla

Utriculus

Sacculus

Cochlea

The balance system of the inner ear: *the three semi-circular canals are filled with fluid. Its movements – in response to bodily movements – are detected by extremely sensitive cells within the channels.*

WHAT IS HEADACHE?

– Site, severity, frequency and character vary enormously. Even so, most people can distinguish between an ordinary headache and the rare, atypical one which should be reported to a doctor.

CAUSES Ordinary headaches, from which most people suffer occasionally, are probably caused by small blood vessels dilating or contracting under the control of nerves. These blood vessels are probably on the surface of the membranes surrounding the brain. Alterations in these areas probably account also for tension headache, pre-menstrual headaches and migraines *(see pages 99 and 100).*

Tension headaches are aching, rather than sharp pains, and are localized to muscles in the scalp, cheeks, jaw, temples, and the back of the neck, sometimes with a feeling of a tight band around the head. There is often difficulty getting off to sleep, and sometimes nervous indigestion as well. Often, tension headaches occur in known 'worriers'; but sometimes they are the first sign of stress at work or within the family.

Other causes of headache are problems in the teeth, ears, sinuses *(see* **sinusitis,** *page 262);* the nerves, joints and arteries of the head, neck and face. For example: neuralgic pain is usually a shooting pain in a localized area – this might follow an attack of shingles. Temporal arteritis is a rare cause of headache and only occurs after the age of 50; it is associated with tenderness over the scalp, severe headache and painful throbbing over blood vessels at the temples. A blood test is necessary to confirm the diagnosis. Infections such as meningitis, typhoid and encephalitis are uncommon causes of headache, but should be considered if there is severe headache in someone who is also ill with fever, vomiting, diarrhoea or drowsiness.

A very severe headache ('worst ever') with vomiting or drowsiness may possibly, but not definitely, signal a grave problem: see a doctor immediately.

High blood pressure is not, contrary to popular belief, a common cause of headache.

PRESCRIPTION DRUGS

Analgesics are available both on prescription and over-the- counter. **Aspirin** and **paracetamol** are both effective in headache, and can be combined with **codeine** for extra effectiveness. *See* **migraine,** *page 100* and **pain,** *page 106.*

Tranquillizers are sometimes used for tension headache (*see **anxiety**, page 84*).

Mefenamic acid can be used for headache as well as for period pain, *see page 190.*

Because headache is usually a recurrent problem, drugs which are potentially addictive, such as tranquillizers and opiate-related drugs, should be avoided in favour of simple pain killers.

Occasionally, antibiotics, anti-epileptic drugs such as carbamazepine, antidepressants, or steroids may be used to treat the underlying cause of the rarer forms of headache.

OVER-THE-COUNTER TREATMENTS

Aspirin maybe a stronger remedy than paracetamol, which has fewer side effects. *See **common cold**, page 134* and ***pain**, page 106.* Children under 12 must be given paracetamol rather than aspirin – *see page 106.* Remedies containing codeine (beware constipation), and caffeine are also available; *see **pain**, page 106.* Remedies containing anti-nausea drugs are usually reserved for migraine.

QUESTIONS TO ASK THE DOCTOR

■ What sort of headache have I got?
■ How long should I take the tablets?
■ Should I come back for a further check-up if it doesn't improve?

SIDE EFFECTS

Paracetamol is very safe up to eight tablets a day: side effects are extremely rare, except in people with kidney or liver disease. **Aspirin:** Reduce dose, or take it with milk or antacids, if you get indigestion or heartburn, as it increases stomach acidity. Ringing in the ears is a sign that the dose should be reduced. **Codeine:** Constipation can be kept to a minimum by drinking plenty of water and increasing the fibre content of the diet.

The more powerful painkillers sometimes cause drowsiness and 'wooziness'.

SELF-MANAGEMENT/SELF-HELP

*See section on **stress**, page 88* and on ***anxiety**, page 84.* Any method of relaxing/distracting yourself from everyday problems will help a tension headache – you will have noticed how these go away when you are busy doing something you enjoy. Exercise, rest and diet can all help. The relaxation technique described on page 86 is well worth trying.

PATIENT'S EXPERIENCE
"I know some people hate to take tablets at all, but I find that taking a couple of paracetamol as soon as I notice a headache coming on seems to stop it right away – and then I can cope better."

DOCTOR'S EXPERIENCE
"People worry that headaches mean they have high blood pressure, or even a brain tumour. This isn't so. The rare, serious kinds of headache are completely different from run-of-the-mill headaches – they're much more severe and disabling."

Simple analgesics, ergotamine, propranolol, pizitofen, methysergide

WHAT IS MIGRAINE?

– An intermittently recurring headache usually affecting only one side of the head at a time. It is often preceded by visual disturbances (flashing lights, jagged, bright or coloured lines, partial loss of vision) and accompanied by nausea and vomiting. However, many migraine sufferers do not experience the warning symptoms, and the pain can affect both sides of the head.

The problem may affect anyone, but it is rare before the age of 15 or 16. It troubles people mainly in their 20s and 30s, and tends to become less severe with age. Attacks rarely occur for the first time in people over the age of 50. It does not only afflict 'intelligent' individuals; it does tend to run in families.

Don't assume that all severe headaches are migraine. Non-migraine headaches are not preceded by visual disturbances, or accompanied by nausea and vomiting *(see **headache**, page 98)*.

CAUSES The basic biochemical trigger is not known, but many precipitating factors are well recognized: for example, a period of hard work followed by relaxation (weekend migraine); stress; body changes prior to menstruation; certain foods˙ (eg fish, chocolate, cheese); alcohol; oral contraceptives; hunger.

It is possible that the symptoms preceding the headache result from a transient decrease in blood supply to areas of the brain. The headache may be due to a subsequent widening of blood vessels in the scalp.

TREATMENT

In an acute attack: As soon as possible after noticing the warning features of an attack, take either **soluble aspirin** (three tablets of 300 mg each) or **paracetamol** (three tablets of 500 mg each) in a glass of milk or water. Taking pain-killing tablets in this way, before the headache develops, prevents a full-blown migraine attack in many people. It is important to take the tablets as soon as possible because during an attack the stomach empties more slowly than usual, only a small dose of the drug being absorbed.

How they work: *see **pain**, page 106; **headache**, page 98.*

The pain-relieving effect of aspirin or paracetamol may be increased by taking **metoclopramide** in addition.

How it works: by making the stomach empty quicker than usual.

If this combination therapy is ineffective, try **ergotamine** 2 mg – but don't take more than 6 mg (three tablets) in one week.

How it works: Ergotamine is a powerful constrictor of blood vessels. See **SIDE EFFECTS.**

Preventive measures: If the migraine attacks are frequent – say more than one a week – regular long-term treatment with **propranolol** may be effective.

How it works: not fully understood, but the drug does affect blood vessels.

Other effective prophylactic drugs are **pizitofen** (doses from 1.5 mg at night up to 1.5 mg four times a day) or **methysergide** (initially 0.5 mg as a test dose increasing to a maximum of 2 mg three times a day).

How they work: by antagonizing some of the chemicals produced in excess during a migraine attack. Methysergide should be used only as a last resort.

OVER-THE-COUNTER TREATMENTS

Aspirin and **paracetamol:** The choice is a matter of personal preference: see **pain,** page 106 and **common cold,** page 134.

Apart from these simple analgesics, there are of course dozens of proprietary combinations available for migraine: most of them include combinations of some of the drugs mentioned above. The large number of products available testifies, sadly, to the fact that there is no 100 per cent effective treatment for migraine. Sufferers should be able to reduce attacks to one a month with the help of a doctor and the drugs mentioned under TREATMENT.

A real drawback of the combination products is that they often do not contain full-strength doses of the most important agents.

SIDE EFFECTS

Aspirin and **paracetamol:** see **pain,** page 106.

Metoclopramide should not be taken during the first three months of pregnancy, and preferably not at all during pregnancy, to avoid any possibility of risk to the foetus. It should not be taken with certain tranquillizers as it has an additive effect: consult your doctor.

Ergotamine and **methysergide** should not be taken during pregnancy or while breast-feeding; or by patients with coronary artery disease, high blood pressure or poor blood supply to the brain or legs. Exceeding the stated dose can cause permanent damage to the circulation.

Propranolol should not be taken by asthmatics or those with wheezy bronchitis: it aggravates these conditions.

Pizitofen should not be taken during pregnancy or while breast-feeding. It may cause weight gain due to its effect of increasing the appetite.

NAMES YOU WILL HEAR

Opiates
Chemical name: morphine; **trade names:** Nepenthe, MST Continus, Duromorph, Cyclimorph. **Chemical name:** diamorphine; **common name:** heroin; usually prescribed by chemical name. **Chemical name:** pethidine, meperidine; **trade names:** Pethilorfan, Pamergan, Pethoid, Demerol, Demerldine; usually prescribed by chemical names. **Chemical name:** methadone; **trade name:** Physeptone. **Chemical name:** dipipanone; **trade names:** Diconal, Wellconal. **Chemical name:** dihydrocodeine; **trade names:** DF 118, Aust Fortruss, Paracodin, Rikodeine, Tuscodin. *See also **pain**, page 106.*

Stimulants
Chemical name: dexamphetamine; **trade names:** Dexedrine, Durophet. **Chemical name:** diethylproprion; **trade names:** Apisate, Tenuate Dospan, Dietec, D.I.P., Nobensine- 75, Regibon. *See also **fatigue**, page 90.*

Anti-psychotic drugs
Drugs marked * are available as longer lasting depot injections. **Chemical name:** chlorpromazine: **trade names:** Largactil, Dozine, Chloractil, Procalm, Promacid, Protran, Chlorprom, Chlor-Promanyl, Klorazin. **Chemical name:** trifluoperazine; **trade name:** Stelazine. **Chemical name:** thioridazine; **trade names:** Melleril, Novoridazine, Thioril. **Chemical name:** haloperidol*; **trade names:** Serenace, Haldol. **Chemical name:** fluphenazine*; **trade names:** Modecate, Moditen, Anatensol. **Chemical name:** flupenthixol*; **trade names:** Depixol, Fluanxol.

TERMS YOU WILL HEAR

Tolerance
The body will get used to certain drugs, making physical adaptations to compensate for their presence. Thus if the dose has to be increased to maintain the effect, the body is said to have developed tolerance to a drug.

WHAT IS DRUG MISUSE?
– Strictly speaking, taking drugs for non-medical reasons, for example curiosity, because friends take them, or to induce an altered state of being. The drugs are usually obtained illicitly, but some prescribed drugs are also misused. The principal drug types involved are: opiates, stimulants, hallucinogenic drugs and cannabis.

CAUSES Either 'accidental' (a young person is introduced to an addictive drug for commercial gain by the supplier) or an underlying psychological problem. For many, the sense of belonging to a group which takes drugs, with its secrecy and deception, are more important props than the drug itself.

OPIATE MISUSE
Heroin, morphine, opium, pethidine, methadone and **dipapanone** are used medically, in controlled doses, as strong painkillers. When taken non-medically, they induce a euphoric sense of well-being and of unconcern about practical necessities. They are smoked, sniffed, taken by mouth or injected. At first they often cause nausea, sickness, and drowsiness. The dangers are: taking too much – overdose can cause unconsciousness or death, especially if mixed with alcohol or tranquillizers; addiction – see below; health hazards associated with injecting – see below.

Opiate addiction is not invariably the result of opiate misuse, but it is impossible to predict who will become addicted. Anyone dabbling is at risk. Taking opiates can be an intense experience, and it is easy to try them again . . . and again . . . then find you need more to gain the same effect; within a few months, often much sooner, the user is addicted. Smoking opiates can lead to addiction, just as injecting them. An addict takes opiates to ward off withdrawal symptoms as much as for pleasure.

TREATMENT
– Almost always involves counselling to help the addict understand his or her underlying problems. The hardest part is often making the decision it really is time to stop. Different clinics have different approaches, but there are three basic lines of treatment:

Detoxification: The addict stops taking illicit drugs and medicines are prescribed as necessary to help with the withdrawal symptoms on a one-to-two-week basis. A typical regime for the heroin addict could be hypnotics for insomnia plus codeine phosphate for diarrhoea. In case of opiate addiction, the illicit drug may be prescribed in reducing doses.

Short-term prescription over several months. The addict is switched from illicit to prescribed opiates; then the prescribed dose is slowly reduced to minimize withdrawal symptoms. The idea is to provide a legal supply of drugs to free the addict from the hassle of the black market; and to provide time in which to sort out problems before withdrawing.

Maintenance prescription: the opiate is prescribed indefinitely until the addict wants to stop. This line is out of favour with most doctors now.

Prescribed opiates are 100 per cent pure and in known quantities. By contrast, illicit opiates are contaminated with additives, and the amount of drug in any weight sold may vary. Some opiates, for example, methadone, are long-lasting and only need to be taken once a day, while others, such as heroin, last only six to eight hours. The trend is to give addicts longer-acting drugs such as methadone as thick linctus which cannot be injected.

SIDE EFFECTS

All **opiates,** prescribed or illicit, can cause constipation, nausea, difficulty in passing urine, depression and loss of interest in sex. They are sedative: an overdose can cause coma or death, especially if mixed with alcohol or tranquillizers. There can be withdrawal symptoms if they are stopped suddenly.

SELF-MANAGEMENT

Remember: most people who give up drugs do so of their own accord at home. There is more to coming off – and staying off – opiates than going through withdrawal symptoms. Think why you take opiates: To relieve anxiety? To be part of a group? Because you are bored? To forget about problems at home or work? How will you manage without them?

To stop taking opiates:
■ Steadily reduce the amount taken to as little as possible. ■ Get rid of any surplus drugs. ■ Plan when you will stop – you will need to be somewhere you feel comfortable and safe, away from other drug users. ■ Try to enlist the help of your family doctor and the support of a friend or relative who does not take drugs. Withdrawing is like having a dose of 'flu – you may feel feverish, have aches and pains, a runny nose, diar-

NOTIFICATION
In the UK any doctor who attends an addict, or someone who is suspected of addiction to certain opiates or cocaine, must notify details of the patient to the Home Office Addicts Index. The Index is confidential and has two main purposes: **1** A count of the number of addicts in the country each year. **2** An information service on addicts: for example, to check whether someone being treated is also seeing another doctor for drugs.

The police do not have access to the Index.

INJECTING DRUGS

Drugs bought illicitly are rarely pure; the additives can be highly toxic to the veins.

Injecting drugs produces rapid effects, so it is easy to overdose. There is also a considerable risk of infection: bacteria from the skin and fingers can cause abscesses, inflamed veins or septicaemia. These may need treatment with antibiotics – seek medical attention.

Infections can also be caught from other drug users' blood if needles or syringes are shared: *see AIDS, page 214.*

So, avoid injecting drugs. Taking them by mouth, or smoking them, is safer. If you must inject drugs, do it safely:
■ Use sterile equipment and water.
■ Never share needles, syringes or mixing bowls.
■ Keep equipment somewhere clean and dry, for example, in a container or the fridge.
■ To sterilize equipment: Wash your hands, then rinse syringes, needle and bowl with clean water before boiling them in water for five minutes. Use them as they cool down. Mix drugs only with cooled boiled water.

AFTER WITHDRAWAL

■ You will feel good about yourself, but beware: as time goes on, you may start to feel flat, and wonder whether it was worth it. This is the time you will need support and encouragement to put into practice alternative ways of coping with problems. ■ If you relapse after coming off, don't get disheartened; at least you have made a start. Think over what went wrong, and try to plan your next attempt more carefully. With time, being off drugs will just seem normal.

rhoea and find it difficult to concentrate or sleep well. Expect three to five bad days, starting 24-48 hours after you stop; after that things will improve. Look after yourself – even spoil yourself. Get in easily prepared food and drinks, and plan interesting activities to take your mind off yourself. Once you are over the first two weeks, you should be physically well again; restlessness and difficulty sleeping may last longer, but they will stop. Avoid drug-users. Be careful with alcohol and tranquillizers – don't switch one addiction for another.

CANNABIS MISUSE

Cannabis is usually smoked. The typical effect is feeling relaxed or 'high'. It can induce altered sensations so that music appears to sound differently or time to pass more slowly. Feelings of being unreal or anxious are not uncommon. Spatial judgement is impaired; driving or operating machinery is hazardous.

This is probably the safest of the illicit drugs, but regular or heavy use is risky. Some use it to escape problems, which may intensify them in the long run. It can cause psychotic illness, manifested, typically, by excitement, confusion, aggression and delusional ideas. The symptoms usually settle down in a few days if cannabis is stopped. There are not usually withdrawal symptoms when stopping cannabis.

HALLUCINOGENIC DRUG MISUSE

The key drugs in this category are **LSD** and **'magic mushrooms'**, usually taken by mouth or eaten; effects – the 'trip' – start in 20 minutes to two hours, and can last several hours. Experiences are variable, from the wonderful to the disturbing. During a typical trip, the world is seen, heard, smelt and felt much more intensely than usual. Sensations can be distorted, and symbolic significances can be seen in everyday events, so that the experience seems mystical. Dangers include the bad trip – disturbing, nightmare-like experiences which seem to go on forever; abdominal pains; feeling unwell; irrational or impulsive behaviour.

SELF-MANAGEMENT

If you must take hallucinogenics, have other people around who are not under their influence.

The effects usually wear off in 12 hours. If someone has a bad trip, stay with them, take them somewhere peaceful, reassure them it will soon be over, that it is a drug effect, no more, no less, and that they are not going mad. Seek medical help if the drug user is acting dangerously.

STIMULANT MISUSE

Cocaine is usually sniffed as a powder; **amphetamines** are sniffed, injected or taken as tablets. Diet pills may also be misused. The main effects are to induce a sense of well-being, to reduce fatigue and to reduce appetite. Small doses can cause insomnia, irritability, over-talkativeness and paranoid suspicions. Stomach pains, palpitations and repetitive thinking occur. Individuals vary widely in the amounts they can take without complications. Some can take amphetamine occasionally to stay awake, perhaps for exams or a party, without apparent harm. But there is always the risk that the sense of well-being is so attractive that the user will want to experience it again and again.

SIDE EFFECTS

If **stimulants** are taken regularly, tolerance develops, and the edginess and insomnia get worse. As the drug wears off, it is common to feel depressed and tired – symptoms which provide an excuse to take more.

Amphetemine or cocaine can also cause psychotic illness similar to schizophrenia *(see page 120)*, though short-lived by comparison. This tends to be the result of heavy or regular use, but some people are ultra-sensitive to these drugs. Taking **cannabis** or **LSD** at the same time can increase the risk. Short admission to psychiatric hospital may be the only answer for serious cases of stimulant-induced psychotic illness. Clear-cut physical withdrawal is not possible with stimulants. The problem is more psychologcal than physical. It can be difficult to know that you are addicted.

QUESTIONS TO ASK THE DOCTOR

■ Can I talk to you in confidence about illicit drugs?
■ Can I come off drugs at home?
■ If I get pregnant will the drugs affect the baby?
■ Will you help me explain to my family?

SELF-MANAGEMENT

■ If you feel tired and in low spirits when you stop amphetamine or cocaine, reassure yourself this will pass in a few days. Think of it as repaying the debt for the extra energy and high spirits conferred by the stimulant.
■ Seek the support of someone not involved with drugs. ■ Analyse why you started taking the stimulant, and why you have taken it so often.

DOCTORS' EXPERIENCES

"I never thought she could be taking heroin, she didn't seem at all like a junkie. I believed what she said. Perhaps I could have done more for her."

"There weren't any drug addicts in this area until a short while ago. The first one came in February and I gave him some methadone to tide him over withdrawal. He couldn't seem to do without it though, so I kept him on a small dose. Then he passed the word round to his mates that I was a soft touch, and I was inundated. I don't give them anything now."

"Her boyfriend said to me that we might as well give her a prescription (for methadone) for life, as she was only tolerable when she was on something, and if she didn't get a prescription she was paranoid about the police. He's probably right, but that's not how this clinic operates."

"I can't trust drug-takers at all. They're very difficult to help. I believe that if they want to stop they have to do it themselves."

Simple analgesics

WHAT IS PAIN?

– An unpleasant sensory and emotional experience associated with actual or potential tissue damage, or described in terms of such damage. This definition recognizes the psychological factors which can affect pain tolerance and threshold, differentiating pain from the five senses of taste, smell, vision, hearing and taste.

A large proportion of consultations with a doctor are made because of pain. Obviously the doctor will try and identify the cause of the pain, and treat this, whereupon the pain will go. He may give something for the pain itself, or the underlying condition; sometimes both can be treated with the same drug, for example, an anti-inflammatory agent – indeed most simple painkillers have this property.

These two pages deal with minor pain and its relief, the next two with stronger painkillers.

Pain relating to specific areas of the body is dealt with under separate headings. *See* for example **headache**, *page 98,* **period problems**, *page 190,* **strains and sprains**, *page 234,* **migraine**, *page 100,* **ear infections**, *page 256,* **cancer**, *pages 202-13* and **sunburn**, *page 278.*

PRESCRIPTION DRUGS

Simple analgesics are usually given by mouth as tablets, but can be given as suppositories, or rarely by direct application as lotions or creams to the skin. They are often combined with other medications. Many types are available, but none has consistently been proved best.
How they work: by blocking the inflammation caused by injury. Damaged tissues release prostaglandins, substances which irritate nerve endings thereby causing pain. Analgesics inhibit the formation of prostaglandins, reducing inflammation and pain.

OVER-THE-COUNTER TREATMENTS

These will contain aspirin, ibuprofen or paracetamol, often in combination with other substances, which do not normally offer any advantage. Aspirin is so widely available because people are used to it: many of the alternatives are in fact safer. Aspirin is a potent drug, with significant side effects; paracetamol is milder, with fewer side effects. Choice is often a matter of habit, and is learned from parents or others during childhood. Auto-suggestion does have a role in relieving pain too. These drugs have an excellent effect in relieving minor pains which do not require a doctor's attention. But if pain persists, or side effects occur, see a doctor soon.

QUESTIONS TO ASK THE DOCTOR

■ Are there any special risks for me in taking simple pain- killers?
■ Is there a tablet available that I can take less often?
■ Should I carry on with my daily routine despite the pain, or do I need to rest?

SIDE EFFECTS

Aspirin: nausea, indigestion, dizziness, ringing in the ears. If there is bleeding, asthma, skin rashes, confusion, stop taking it and see a doctor. Aspirin may also cause liver or kidney damage with prolonged use. Unless the circumstances are exceptional, it must not be used in people with a history of stomach ulcers, bleeding problems, severe indigestion, asthma, liver or kidney disease, severe allergies, pregnancy, lactating mothers or children under 12. In the latter, evidence suggests that it may a factor in Reye's Syndrome, a rare but serious form of liver failure.

Special problems: indomethacin causes headache; phenylbutazone and oxphenbutazone are associated with bleeding and blood disorders. Phenylbutazone is only used to treat ankylosing spondylitis in UK *(see page 248)*. Acupan is an alternative with less gastric side effects.

Paracetamol's side effects are rare and mild. **Minor:** skin rashes, allergies. **Major and very rare:** liver or kidney damage, usually only in acute or chronic overdose. It is safe in pregnancy.

SELF-MANAGEMENT

■ Local measures: bruises, sports injuries – cold compresses; torn muscles or stiffness – local heat (lamp, rubs, hot water bottles); massage to stimulate blood flow and relax tense muscles.
■ Exercise: gentle to start with, then building up can help minor injuries and nagging ailments: surrounding muscles are strengthened, ligaments stretched, blood flow and healing stimulated.
■ Keep a supply of simple analgesics handy; they should be a type which you know from experience don't upset you. If the condition is long-term, take them in time to prevent the pain breaking through.
■ Rest helps after an acute injury; *see **strains and sprains**, page 234.*
■ If the pain is prolonged, consider safe 'alternative' techniques like acupressure or transcutaneous nerve stimulation. Consult your doctor or Community Health Council for sources of help.

NSAIDs

Chemical name: azapropazone; trade names: Rheumox, Prolix. Chemical name: benzydamine; trade names: Difflam Cream or Rinse, Tantum. Chemical name: bufexamac; trade names: Parfenac Cream, Paraderm, Norfemac, Audax Eardrops. Chemical name: choline salicylate; trade names: Bonjela or Teejel Mouth Gels, Arthropan. Chemical name: diclofenac; trade name: Voltarol. Chemical name: diflunisal; trade name: Dolobid. Chemical name: fenbufen; trade names: Lederfen, Cinopal. Chemical name: fenoprofen; trade names: Fenopron, Progesic. Chemical name: flufenamic acid; trade names: Meralen, Arlef. Chemical name: flurbiprofen; trade name: Froben. Chemical name: ibuprofen; trade names: Apsifen, Brufen, Ebufac, Fenbid, Ibuslo, Ibumetin, Lidifen, Motrin, Nurophen, Paxofen. Chemical name: indomethacin; trade names: Artracin, Imbrilon, Indocid, Indoflex, Indolar, Indomod, Mobilan, Rheumacin, Arthrexin. Chemical name: indoprofen; trade name: Flosint. Chemical name: ketoprofen; trade names: Alrheumat, Orudis, Oruvail. Chemical name: mefenamic acid; trade names: Ponstan, Ponstan Forte Chemical name: methyl salicylate ointments, creams; trade names: Oil of Wintergreen, Balmosa, Bengué's Balsam, Dubam. Chemical name: naproxen sodium; trade names: Naprosyn, Synflex, Laraflex. Chemical name: nefopam; trade name: Acupan. Chemical name: oxphenbutazone; trade names: Tandacote, Tandalgesic, Tanderil, Oxbutazone, Tandearil, Artzone, Buteril, Fibutrox, Otone. Chemical name: phenylbutazone; trade names: Butacote, Butazolidine, Butazone, Parazolidin, Tibutazone, Butacal, Butalan, Butarex, Butoroid, Butoz, Buzon, Algoverine, Butagesic, Intrabutazone, Malgesic, Nadozone, Neo-Zoline, Phenbutazone, Butrex, Panazone. Chemical name: phenazone; trade names: Auralgicin, Auraltone, Sedonan. Chemical name:

Continued on page 108

phenazopyridine; **trade names:**
Pyridium, Phenazo, Azodine. **Chemical
name:** piroxicam; **trade name:**
Feldene. **Chemical name:** salsalate;
trade name: Disalcid. **Chemical
name:** sodium salicylate; **trade
names:** Entrosalyl, Ancosal, Ensalate,
Rhumax. **Chemical name:** sulindac;
trade name: Clinoril. **Chemical name:**
tolmetin; **trade names:** Tolectin,
Tolectin DS. **Chemical name:**
suprofen; **trade name:** Suprol.
Chemical name: morazone; **trade
name:** Delimon. **Chemical name:**
tiaprofenic acid; **trade name:** Surgam.
Chemical name: etodolac; **trade
names:** Ramodar, Lodine. **Chemical
name:** aloxiprin; **trade name:** Palaprin.

Class 1
Chemical name: morphine; **trade
names:** Nepenthe, MST Continus,
Duromorph, Cyclimorph, Haustus
Linct., Brompton Cocktail. **Chemical
name:** diamorphine; **common name:**
heroin; usually prescribed by chemical
name. **Chemical name:** opium; **trade
names:** prescribed by chemical name.
Chemical name: papaveretum; **trade
name:** Omnopon. **Chemical name:**
oxymorphone; **trade names:**
Hydroxymorphone, Dilaudid,
Numorphan. **Chemical name:**
pethidine, meperedine; **trade names:**
Pethilorfan, Pamergan, Pethoid,
Demerol, Demer-Idine; usually
prescribed by chemical name.
Chemical name: anileridine; **trade
name:** Leritine. **Chemical name:**
dextromoramide; **trade name:**
Palfium. **Chemical name:** dipipanone;
trade name: Diconal. **Chemical name:**
oxycodone; **trade names:** Endone,
Proladone, Supeudol. **Chemical name:**
phenazocine; **trade name:** Narphen.
Chemical name: lerorphanol; **trade
names:** Dromoran, Levodromoran.
Chemical name: methadone; **trade
name:** Physeptone. **Chemical name:**
dextropropoxyphene; **trade names:**
Propoxyphene, Cosalgesic, Co-
Proxamol, Dextrogesic, Distalgesic,
Dolasan, Doloxene, Napsalgesic,
Paxalgesic, Algaphan, Algodex,
Darvon-N, Depronal SA.

SEVERE PAIN
Pain can be classified as follows:

Acute – minor: headache, period pains, sunburn and
minor injuries/strains and sprains. *See pages 98, 190,
274 and 234.*
    – major: heart attack, post-operative, labour,
kidney or gall stones; may need medical treatment with
potent drugs.
Chronic – trauma: low back, fractures, crush injuries.
                infection: after shingles.
                degenerative: arthritis, gout.
                vascular: arteriosclerosis, migraine.
                neurological: trigeminal neuralgia.
                cancer: tumours, secondary deposits.
                psychological: anxiety, tension,
                stress, depression.

    As pain may be acute or chronic, minor or severe, in-
termittent or continuous, many different treatments are
available. These two pages deal with drugs commonly
used for moderate to severe pain, including that caused
by cancer.

PRESCRIPTION DRUGS
Class 1: morphine or **morphine-like narcotics.** These are the
most potent, and are either naturally occurring for example opium, or synthetic, for example methadone.
Class 2: narcotic derivatives. Not as potent as Class 1, and
less likely to produce addiction and major side effects.
Class 3: antagonist drugs. Also less addictive, but may be
quite strong. They produce minor side effects in quite a
large number of people.
    Unless the pain is expected to be very severe (for ex-
ample after major surgery or a heart attack), the doctor
will usually start with Class 2 drugs (for example codeine, dihydrocodeine, dextropropoxyphene). If the
pain persists, stronger drugs may be used, often
tailored to the expected duration of pain. Of these, dextromoramide is potent and short-acting; morphine,
pethidine and methadone are medium term; M.S.T.,
oxycodone and buprenorphine are long-acting. They
can be given orally, or, if swallowing is a problem,
under the tongue, rectally, intramuscularly or intravenously, subcutaneously or by epidural infusion.
Some anaesthetic agents can be inhaled – *see
anaesthetics, page 130.* The drugs *must* be given at
regular intervals, according to their length of action, if
the pain is expected to persist. Dose is gauged in-

dividually for the particular pain. The correct dose is that which stops the pain.

OVER-THE-COUNTER TREATMENTS
Not available, except for some small (usually insignificant) amounts found in combination with aspirin or paracetamol.

QUESTIONS TO ASK THE DOCTOR
■ What are the side effects?
■ How long can I take them without risk of addiction, and how often?
■ Will I be able to stop them easily?
■ Can I take more if the dose is ineffective (particularly with cancer)?
■ What can I do/What should I avoid? Driving? Drinking? Work?

SIDE EFFECTS
Narcotics: constipation. Laxatives are essential if narcotics are given for more than two days; nausea and vomiting, drowsiness. These last two usually settle after one week. Confusion, nightmares, sweating, flushing, dizziness due to low blood pressure, and itching. These effects are rarer, and may settle. Depression of breathing can be dangerous especially in the elderly. Addiction. This last is not regarded as a problem in terminal illness. Narcotic derivatives: very similar to narcotics, but addiction and breathing problems are much rarer.
Buprenorphine: much less addictive than other narcotics. Less constipation, and fewer problems with breathing. Conveniently dissolves under the tongue. Incidence of vomiting, sweating and dizziness higher than with Classes 1 and 2.

MANAGEMENT OF SEVERE PAIN
Very dependent on cause. Self-management strategies may play a part with some types: ask your doctor. Medical treatment is often directed at the cause, and unfortunately this can mean that actual pain is poorly treated. Insist on adequate painkilling drugs in labour, after surgery or a heart attack, and for cancer pain. In chronic non-cancer pain, a high chance of addiction, major side effects, or increase in pain on stopping medicine means that most doctors are rightly reluctant to give all but codeine-type preparations. Even these are better stopped after three months if not fully effective.

Class 2
Chemical name: codeine; **trade names:** Codlin, Paveral. **Chemical name:** codeine combined with aspirin; **trade names:** Anodyne Dellipsoids D4, Hypon, Safapryn-Co, Veganin. **Chemical name:** codeine combined with soluble aspirin; **trade names:** Antoin, Codis, Myolgin. **Chemical name:** codeine combined with paracetamol; **trade names:** Medocodene, Neurodyne, Panadeine Co, Paracodol, Paradeine, Parahypon, Parake, Paralgin, Pardale, Pharmidone, Propain, Solpadeine, Syndol. **Chemical name:** dihydrocodeine; **trade names:** DF 118, Onadex 118, Paramol 118, Rikodeine, Tuscodin, Co-Dydramol, Paracodin, Fortuss. **Chemical name:** hydrocodone; **trade names:** Dicodid, Hycon, Corutol DH, Hycodan, Robidone. **Chemical name:** ethoheptazine; **trade names:** Equagesic, Zactipar, Zactirin.

Class 3
Agonist/antagonists
Chemical name: pentazocine; **trade names:** Fortagesic, Fortral, Talwin, Sosegon. **Chemical name:** meptazinol; **trade name:** Meptid. **Chemical name:** buprenorphine; **trade names:** Temgesic, Buprex. **Chemical name:** butorphanol; **trade name:** Stadol. **Chemical name:** nalbuphine; **trade name:** Nubain.

MANAGEMENT OF CANCER PAIN
The causes of the pain must be identified, and treated accordingly:
– Bone/soft tissue pain: aspirin-like drugs, radiotherapy, calcitonin, rest.
– Pain from organs: Start with codeine, going on to morphine if no effect. Give sufficient doses, by the clock. It is important that the painkillers be given in time to stop the pain "breaking through". If the painkillers are regularly used to *prevent* pain, then a lower dose may well suffice. Nerve blocks or steroids (cortisone) may be needed – Nerve pain: stabbing – anticonvulsants; burning – amitriptyline. May also respond to nerve blocks or radiotherapy.

Anticonvulsants

NAMES YOU WILL HEAR

Chemical name: phenytoin; **trade names:** Epanutin, Dilantin, Dantoin, Toin Unicelles. **Chemical name:** carbamazepine; **trade name:** Tegretol. **Chemical name:** sodium valproate; **trade name:** Epilim. **Chemical name:** ethosuximide; **trade names:** Emeside, Zarontin. **Chemical name:** phenobarbitone; **trade names:** Luminal, Gardenal, Maliasin, Nova-Pheno. **Chemical name:** primidone; **trade names:** Mysoline, Midone, Sertan. **Chemical name:** clonazepam; **trade name:** Rivotril. **Chemical name:** Clobazam; **trade name:** Frisium. **Chemical name:** diazepam; **trade names:** Valium, Alupram, Atensine, Evacalm, Solis, Tensium, Valrelease.

WHAT IS EPILEPSY?

– A tendency to have fits, seizures or convulsions: the three terms mean the same.

The condition results from disturbance of normal electrical activity in the brain – something like a short circuit. Normal communication between brain cells is disrupted and a variety of aberrant discharges are produced. There are three main types of fit:

Generalized tonic clonic or 'grand mal' fits: Here the electrical disturbance passes over the whole brain. There is a loss of consciousness; the patient becomes rigid and may cry out. He or she falls to the ground; the limbs jerk as muscles alternately contract and relax. Sometimes the patient loses bladder control or bites the tongue. Recovery follows spontaneously over a few minutes, although dazed or confused state may persist for an hour or two.

'Partial' or 'temporal lobe' fits: These occur when the electrical discharge is confined to one part of the brain only – commonly one of the temporal lobes. The patient can be quite unaware of what happens: involuntary movements, loss of speech, confusion or complicated automatic actions all occur. Sometimes the event may be confined to a momentary loss of concentration; occasionally it develops into a generalized tonic-clonic convulsion. 'Partial' fits vary greatly from person to person.

Absence or 'petit mal' **fits:** Found primarily in children, these are short periods of interrupted or clouded consciousness, easily mistaken for day dreaming. The child stops what he/she is doing, remains motionless and stares into space. The episodes last only seconds but they may be frequent throughout the day and disrupt his/her educational performance.

Epilepsy is not inherited in any direct sense apart from a few rare instances. Even if both parents are epileptics, the chance of offspring having fits is only increased very slightly.

In the UK, people with 'grand mal' epilepsy are not allowed to hold a driving licence until they have been free of fits for two years.

Children with epilepsy are usually educated in normal schools. They can take part in most activities except climbing and underwater diving. Epilepsy carries a real stigma which at times can seem almost medieval: people need educating about this condition. If required to fill in a form with a question about fits when applying for a job, be truthful, but if possible return the form to the firm's medical department or officer rather than the personnel department: you may find a more understanding attitude.

Between episodes, the brain usually works normally. Epilepsy can affect every age from infancy to the elderly.

CAUSES There are a large number. It is thought that the most common is previous brain damage. This may be a consequence of a difficult birth, a brain infection, a head injury or even a stroke. Very rarely, it is the first sign of a brain tumour. Many years can elapse from the time of the injury to the onset of epilepsy, which usually takes the form of partial seizures. However, in most cases, no specific cause can be identified.

INVESTIGATIONS

The electroencephalogram (EEG), an amplified measure of the brain's electrical activity, will identify abnormal discharges coming from a scar and can sometimes pick up evidence of low seizure threshhold. Unfortunately, an EEG may be normal in people with epilepsy and abnormal in some others who have never had a fit. Brain scans can detect an area of brain damage which may be responsible for the fits. Occasionally this enables the malfunctioning part to be removed surgically and the epilepsy cured.

PRESCRIPTION DRUGS

Most doctors will not start treatment unless more than one fit has occurred. However, if the original event is clearly witnessed, if the condition runs in the family or if there is a clear-cut brain abnormality on the EEG or brain scan, it may be prudent to prescribe one of the many **anticonvulsant drugs** after the first episode.

There is a considerable overlap in the action of the various drugs listed; initial choice depends on the type of epilepsy and the clinical response, but it is usually between a well-tried drug such as **phenytoin, carbamazepine** or **sodium valproate.** Sometimes the first drug chosen will not suit an individual while an alternative will. There is still, unfortunately, an element of trial and error in these decisions.

Current medical thinking suggests that for most people a single drug in the right dose causes fewer long term problems than a combination, and offers equal or improved benefit. Nevertheless, a few patients seem to require more than one drug. Although many individuals require life-long treatment, the condition can remit and therapy may be slowly withdrawn over a number of

FIRST AID IN AN ATTACK

Generalized tonic-clonic or 'grand mal' fits

What to do:

1 Note the time. **2** Clear a space round the person having the attack and remove sharp objects which might cause injury. **3** Cushion the head, loosen collar and remove spectacles. **4** Remove false teeth if this is easily done (see 3 below). **5** As soon as the attack appears to be settling, turn the patient on their side to aid breathing. **6** At the end of the attack, reassure the patient and talk to them quietly until full recovery takes place. **7** Only get medical help if the attack lasts longer than five minutes or if one fit follows another without consciousness being regained.

What not to do:

1 Don't move the patient while the fit is in progress unless they are in acute danger. **2** Don't restrict movements. **3** Don't force anything between the teeth. **4** Don't give anything to drink. **5** Don't try to rouse the patient.

Partial or 'temporal lobe' fits

The patient may wander around aimlessly with a glazed expression, so accompany them, and gently lead them away from any source of danger. Don't interfere unnecessarily. Afterwards, calm reassurance will be greatly appreciated. Don't try to stop the attack; don't bother to send for an ambulance.

months without recurrence of the fits. The decision to withdraw treatment is a difficult one but the longer the person is seizure-free, the more he/she is likely to remain in permanent remission. This is particularly so for children who develop the disorder in adolescence but have no evidence of brain damage or a family history of epilepsy.

How they work: All the anticonvulsants act on the brain to increase the seizure threshhold and prevent the spread of the abnormal electrical discharge. They are wholly successful in about 80 per cent of patients. A minority, however, will continue to have fits no matter what drug or combination is used – although their frequency may be reduced. This is particularly true of people with brain damage and in those who do not take their medication regularly. There is no doubt that frequent fits can themselves cause brain damage and so perpetuate the disorder. Effective daily treatment is important in preventing this outcome.

OVER-THE COUNTER TREATMENTS

None.

QUESTIONS TO ASK THE DOCTOR

■ What type of epilepsy have I got?
■ Is there any evidence of brain damage?
■ What possible side effects can I expect from my treatment?
■ Will I have to take medication all my life?
■ What should I tell my friends, family and employer?
■ Can I drive?
■ Will I pass on epilepsy to my child? Can my child go to a normal school?

SIDE EFFECTS

At the start of treatment, the dose is gradually increased until the fits come under control, or, if they are infrequent, until a satisfactory blood level is obtained. This is to avoid the dampening effect of the drug on the other electrical activities of the brain which are concerned with alertness, concentration and memory. At high dosage, all the **anticonvulsants** can cause some degree of drowsiness. Some patients become sedated before the beneficial effects are obtained and so must try an alternative preparation.

There are few other predictable side effects of these drugs. **Phenytoin** can cause gum overgrowth, which can be prevented by scrupulous dental hygiene. **Sodium valproate** can produce a tremor. All may rarely cause

Spike disturbance

Normal background activity

damage to the liver or to the bone marrow in susceptible individuals. This is an allergic response, usually occurs within three months of starting treatment, is reversible, and can be anticipated by carefully monitoring the patient's general health.

Anticonvulsants taken during pregnancy: there is a small risk (less than six per cent) that these drugs will affect the foetus. Discuss the problem fully with your doctor. Usually there is no reason why an epileptic should not plan her family normally.

Some of the anticonvulsant drugs, particularly carbamazepine, phenobarbitone and phenytoin, increase the turnover of hormones, and so bigger doses of the oral contraceptive pill may be required than that normally prescribed.

HOW TO PREVENT FITS

■ Take the medication regularly: control of fits is greatly helped by maintaining a consistent level of the drug in the blood and brain. If you have a complicated life or are just forgetful, you should probably be prescribed a drug which can be taken once or, at most, twice a day. If you forget to take your tablets on time, have the dose immediately you remember and follow-up with the next dose at the usual time.

■ Some children only have fits when they develop a high fever. Simple measures such as tepid sponging and giving paracetamol elixir can keep the temperature down. If this is not effective, parents can be taught to administer diazepam into the child's rectum as soon as there are signs of twitching or irritability.

■ Take as little alcohol as possible: it can cause fits. It can also act in concert with medication to make the patient feel drunk very quickly. It may also help you to forget to take your tablets.

■ Fits can be triggered off by stimuli such as flashing lights, loud noises or hunger. Tiredness can also make an individual more susceptible. A healthy, sensible lifestyle is important. Some people find boredom, anxiety, depression or stress make them worse. Keep busy, realistic and positive.

PARKINSONISM

Levodopa, anticholinergics, bromocriptine, amantadine, selegiline

WHAT IS PARKINSONISM?

A disorder affecting the basal ganglia – an area in the brain concerned primarily with co-ordination of voluntary movement. The principal symptoms are shaking (tremor), difficulty starting movement, and slowness when moving; also stiffness or rigidity. Individual patients may have one or more of these symptoms. The condition may affect just one side of the body. It is chronic, and usually requires treatment for life. Although more than half the sufferers are disabled by the disease in time, this is not universal: with medical treatment patients may live full lives for five or ten years, possibly more.

CAUSES Nerve cells containing the neurotransmitter dopamine die at an unusually rapid rate in Parkinsonian patients. This results in an imbalance of nerve signals, and hence the symptoms. In some patients, symptoms of Parkinsonism may be due to the administration of drugs (for example metoclopramide) used to treat other medical problems such as dizziness or vomiting, and which act to block dopamine receptors. Stopping these drugs will usually give improvement. But in most cases the origin is unknown.

PRESCRIPTION DRUGS

Levodopa (L-dopa): often given in combination with another drug (in the same tablet) to prevent breakdown of the L-dopa outside the brain and increase its effect. **How it works:** by increasing the amount of dopamine in the brain.

Anticholinergic drugs counteract the relative excess of the transmitter acetyl choline present as a result of lack of the dopamine-containing neurones. They seem to help the tremor more than the rigidity.

Dopamine agonists: drugs such as **bromocriptine** act directly on dopamine receptors. In theory they are more attractive than L-dopa since they do not require conversion to dopamine. In practice they have not been an outstanding success, primarily because of adverse side effects and lack of specificity – they affect all parts of the brain.

Amantadine is a milder-acting alternative to L-dopa. Sometimes used as an initial treatment, so as to leave the other drugs in reserve. **Selegiline** is used in combination with L-dopa to treat late complications.

The response to treatment is variable. Over 75 per cent of patients respond to drugs. About a third can hope to return virtually to normal; the remainder must expect varying success. A small proportion do not respond to treatment at all, or find the side effects worse than the disease. For these, physiotherapy may sometimes be beneficial.

OVER-THE-COUNTER TREATMENTS
None.

QUESTIONS TO ASK THE DOCTOR
■ Am I taking drugs which might be adding to my symptoms?
■ Should I take a full dose to start with, or increase to the dose you prescribe over a few days?
■ How long should I take what you are prescribing?
■ Should I look for any particular side effect?
■ Should I increase the dose if the drugs don't work?
■ Are there any physiotherapy exercises you can recommend?

SIDE EFFECTS
Nausea may occur when starting **L-dopa.** This can be reduced by taking tablets with meals and by gradually increasing the dose to an optimum level. Odd uncontrolled movements, particularly of the face or limbs, indicate overdosage. **Anticholinergics** may cause dry mouth, difficulty in focusing, difficulty passing urine and constipation. *See also **asthma**, page 74.*
Bromocriptine may cause nausea, dizziness and confusion.
   L-dopa also carries some more serious, though rare side effects including dizziness on standing, a tendency to fall, constipation, difficulty with memory and occasionally hallucinations. Adjustment of dose (in consultation with a doctor) may be helpful in either case.

SELF-MANAGEMENT, SELF-HELP
■ Symptoms are helped by taking the medication regularly. If symptoms are bad first thing in the morning, consider taking pills in bed before getting up to get a 'booster effect' for dressing and washing.
■ Many sufferers tire by the end of the day, so consider planning your day around times of peak drug effect.
■ Try simple aids such as 'Velcro' fasteners instead of buttons, a higher chair and a stick for walking.
■ Don't stop anti-cholinergic drugs suddenly as this may cause 'freezing up' or severely restricted movement.
■ Accept that other illness experienced while on these drugs may upset response to treatment and stabilization may take some days.

Tricyclic antidepressants
Chemical name: imipramine; trade names: Tofranil, Imiprim, Tramil, Melipramine, Prodepress, Simipra, Impril, Novopramine, Panpramine. **Chemical name:** amitriptyline; **trade names:** Tryptizol, Lentizol, Domical, Elavil, Laroxyl, Tryptanol, Saroten, Amiline, Deprex, Levate, Meravil, Novotriptyn, Amilent, Trepiline, Tryptanol. **Chemical name:** desipramine; **trade names:** Pertofran, Norpramin, Pertofrane. **Chemical name:** dothiepin; **trade name:** Prothiaden. **Chemical name:** nortriptyline; **trade names:** Allegron, Aventyl, Nortab, Nortrilin.

Atypical (novel) antidepressants
Chemical name: mianserin; **trade names:** Solvidon, Norval, Tolvon, Lantanon. **Chemical name:** maprotilene; **trade name:** Ludiomil. **Chemical name:** trazodone; **trade names:** Molipaxin, Desyrel.

Monoamine oxidase inhibitors (MAOIs)
Chemical name: phenelzine; **trade name:** Nardil. **Chemical name:** tranylcypromine; **trade name:** Parnate.

Lithium salts
Chemical name: lithium carbonate; **trade names:** Camcolit, Priadel, Liskonum, Phasal, Lithicarb, Manialith, Carbolith, Lithane, Lithizine, Lentolith, Quilonum Retard. **Chemical name:** lithium citrate; **trade name:** Litarex.

WHAT IS DEPRESSION

The term is used in two different ways: **1** to signify a *symptom* – a patient's report of the subjective experience of low mood; **2** to describe an *illness* in which, apart from low mood, a group of symptoms occur together. While the symptom of depression is a common experience to everybody and in itself does not require treatment, depressive illness is a distressing and dangerous, and usually requires medical attention.

The characteristic symptoms of depressive illness are depressed mood (feeling 'blue', 'under the weather', being 'fed up', sad or gloomy), weepiness, difficulty in concentration, loss of interest in one's work, hobbies and family, a feeling of hopelessness, low self-esteem, loss of appetite for food and sex, disturbed sleep. If the symptoms persist, the patient loses weight as a result of poor appetite and reduced eating. In severe forms, the patient may blame him- or herself for mistakes, wrong-doings or even crimes not committed; suicide may be contemplated.

Depression is typically an episodic illness; an episode usually lasts for a few weeks or months. Although most patients would recover eventually without treatment, treatment is often necessary to shorten the depressive episode or to prevent a recurrence.

CAUSES An episode of depression may be the result of some adverse event (usually a significant loss, such as death) in the patient's life (reactive depression). Depression may also be secondary to some hormonal change (for example post-natal depression) or to some disease of the brain or body (for example depression in dementia or in a patient suffering from a brain tumour). In some patients, however, the symptoms may appear for no apparent reason (endogenous depression). Endogenous depression often occurs several times in a lifetime (recurrent depression). In some patients suffering from recurrent depression, episodes of depression alternate with episodes of complete well-being (unipolar depression). In some patients, however, episodes of depression may alternate with episodes of elation and over-activity (mania) and with episodes of normal mood: manic depressive illness, manic depression or bipolar depression. Endogenous depression might be due to some malfunction of brain chemistry, and it may be inherited.

PRESCRIPTION DRUGS

Antidepressants: these are frequently prescribed either by the family doctor or the psychiatrist. There are three major groups in current use: **1** tricyclic antidepressants; **2** novel (or atypical) antidepressants; **3** monoamine oxidase inhibitors (MAOIs). All are taken in tablet or capsule form. Most can be taken in one daily dose.

How they work: It is believed that antidepressant drugs act by modifying the effects of certain natural chemicals ('monoamines') in the brain. Since monoamines also occur outside the brain, for example in the gut, blood vessels and glands, antidepressants can have undesired side effects. *See page 118.*

These drugs do not have an immediate effect: it may take two or three weeks before the patient experiences significant improvement. The **tricyclic antidepressants** are the most commonly used, and their effectiveness in depressive illness is well established. The novel or **atypical antidepressants** are chemically different from the tricyclics. Their initial advantage was that they had fewer effects outside the brain, and thus fewer side effects; however recent experience has shown that severe side effects can occur. The **monoamine oxidase inhibitors** are usually prescribed when the other two classes of drugs do not work.

Lithium: Patients suffering from recurrent episodes of depression, either of the unipolar or bipolar kind, can benefit from long-term maintenance treatment with a lithium. If a patient is responsive to lithium, further episodes of depression and/or mania will not occur, or will occur less frequently or in a much milder form. Lithium is usually supplied in tablet form, and can be taken once daily at bedtime.

How it works: Lithium salts are common to the crust of the earth, but normally do not occur in the body. However, lithium, a simple element, is similar to sodium, an important constituent of body fluids. Lithium can to some extent be a substitute for sodium in the body, and this may result in the stabilization of mood. It is not known how this effect is brought about. Lithium is usually prescribed by a psychiatrist, and the patient taking it needs follow-up, with regular checks of the amount of lithium in the blood.

OVER-THE-COUNTER TREATMENTS
No established antidepressants are sold without a prescription.

QUESTIONS TO ASK THE DOCTOR
■ How long should I take the antidepressant/lithium?
■ How long will it take before the drug works?

117

■ Can I drink alcohol or take other pills as well?
■ Is there anything I should avoid eating while taking the tablets?
■ Can I drive a car while on this medication?
■ Will the tablets affect my work?
■ What happens if I cannot tolerate the antidepressant/lithium? Is there an alternative?
■ May I become pregnant while on the drug?

SIDE EFFECTS

Antidepressants are usually prescribed for several months. The beneficial effects usually develop gradually during the first few weeks of treatment: very often the patient does not experience much improvement during the first week. Some of the side effects, on the other hand, appear at the beginning of treatment, and many of them may subside after a few weeks. It is therefore important that the patient does not give up the antidepressant on the grounds that it does not work and causes unpleasant side effects. If the patient perseveres, the depression should gradually lift, and the side effects will become less and less troublesome. After the depression has lifted, most doctors prefer their patients to continue with the medication for six to eight months: it has been shown that continued medication reduces the risk of relapse.

The most common side effects of the **tricyclic antidepressants** are dry mouth, blurred vision, constipation, occasionally difficulties in passing urine, dizziness and drowsiness. Some patients may complain of increased sweating or slight shakiness of the hands. Patients with a history of heart disease need careful monitoring. At the start of treatment with all these drug types your doctor will advise you on the safety of driving a car or operating machinery. The novel or **atypical antidepressants** are less likely to produce some of these side effects; with some of the drugs (eg trazodone) drowsiness and dizziness may occur.

The **monoamine oxidase** inhibitors usually cause a drop in blood pressure resulting in dizziness: this symptom normally dissipates with time. Patients taking these drugs should avoid certain foods, in particular cheese, Marmite and red wine: they can result in a dangerous increase in blood pressure. Patients are given a card listing all foods to avoid. They must avoid *all* other drugs or medicines, even ones bought at the chemist, unless these have been cleared with the doctor.
Lithium salts have to be taken over many years for the prevention of the recurrence of depression. Side effects

include nausea, diarrhoea, shakiness of the hands, increased thirst and passing more than the usual quantity of urine. These side effects are usually mild if the level of lithium in the blood is not too high. Patients on lithium salts have to drink adequate amounts of water (usually three pints per day), especially if there is an excessive loss of fluid (for example as a result of diarrhoea or hot weather). Consequences of a wrongly adjusted dose are serious, including convulsions.

SELF-MANAGEMENT

As adverse events in one's life can lead to depression it is important to learn how to cope with stress.

■ Try to share your distress with someone close to you: sharing *can* relieve anxiety and distress; 'bottling things up' *can* increase the anguish.

■ Do not medicate yourself: do not use alcohol or other people's sedatives. These drugs do not solve problems and they can lead to serious complications.

■ If your sleep is disturbed, try going for a walk for a couple of hours before bedtime. Avoid tea and coffee, which are stimulants.

■ If symptoms of depression persist, or you cannot cope with your daily life, go and see your doctor. Your doctor will take your complaints seriously: he or she *can* help you decide whether you are suffering from a 'normal' reaction to an adverse event or whether you are suffering from depressive illness.

HELPING A DEPRESSED RELATIVE

Don't underestimate the distress of true depressive illness. While some patients are able to describe their feelings and experiences, others may find it difficult to put their anguish into words. An understanding relative can be crucial in helping the patient.

■ Appreciate that depression is an illness and the patient cannot help some of his feelings, thoughts and behaviour. Do not reproach the patient for being unaffectionate or selfish: the patient is already plagued by feelings of self-blame and guilt. It is no use saying 'Pull yourself together', or 'It is up to you'.

■ Treat the patient as a normal person with understanding and compassion. Try to involve the patient in family activities, but do not apply too much pressure.

■ The patient has a low self-image. Try to emphasize achievements, and give praise as appropriate.

■ The patient may not appreciate what is wrong, and may even refuse to see a doctor. In such a case contact the family doctor yourself; suicide is a risk.

Anti-psychotic drugs, anti-Parkinsonian drugs

WHAT IS SCHIZOPHRENIA?

– A common, and serious mental illness. The symptons vary widely, but fall into two main groups: 1 unusual experiences and 2 loss of drive and interest in life.

Typical unusual experiences are: hallucinations (hearing voices, seeing or feeling things when no one is present); difficulties in thinking clearly; delusions – firmly believing in something which is untrue and out of the ordinary. Paranoid delusions are common, typically the belief that people are against one. These experiences may feel so real to sufferers that they actually respond to them. Patients may talk back to imaginary voices, or try to protect themselves from people they believe wish to harm them. The schizo-phrenic loses the ability to distinguish reality from what is imagined.

The second group of symptoms include: apathy; self-imposed isolation; loss of emotion; difficulties in relating to people.

Symptoms can develop slowly over a period of years, or rapidly, as a reaction to stress. Relatives and friends will probably notice changed, sometimes bizarre behaviour. The outcome of the illness is variable: some have only one episode; others recover from a first episode and have further symptoms when stressed, whilst a proportion never fully recover from the symptoms and are permanently disabled. Not all cases need hospital admission; but some inevitably require institutional care, even against their will, because of self-neglect, or potentially dangerous behaviour.

CAUSES Not known, but a bio-chemical abnormality affecting part of the brain is suspected. The illness can run in families, but the pattern of inheritance is not clear-cut. Theories of family interaction causing schizophrenia promoted in the past are now discounted. Once a person has had schizophrenic symptoms, however, the tendency to relapse can be affected by family attitudes and relationships.

OTHER PSYCHOTIC ILLNESSES

Schizophrenia-like symptoms can develop as a consequence of drug or alcohol misuse, or as a long-term complication of certain types of epilepsy. The drugs commonly implicated are amphetamines and cannabis.

Also in this category are miscellaneous individual psychoses in which an unfounded idea develops out of proportion to reality: for example delusional jealousy; delusions about body size or shape; paranoid beliefs about neighbours.

PRESCRIPTION DRUGS

Schizophrenia and other psychotic illnesses share similar drug treatments; however, management of associated problems such as excessive drinking, marriage problems, drug misuse, isolation and deafness is of course just as important.

Anti-psychotic drugs are used both to treat psychotic episodes and to prevent relapses. There are many types. They can be taken by mouth as tablets or syrup, or by injection. Depot preparations are given as injections to release the drug slowly into the body, one injection lasting several weeks. Anti-psychotic drugs are not addictive, but it is always better to reduce them slowly.
How they work: by acting on certain nervous pathways in the brain. They have a calming action, and they damp down the unusual experiences. Doses needed to treat an acutely disturbed person are usually greater than those needed to prevent a relapse.

Anti-Parkinsonian drugs are used to treat the side-effects of anti-psychotic drugs (see below), not the psychiatric symptoms. As they can have side effects themselves, their use is kept to a minimum. Despite these drawbacks they can be particularly helpful while high doses of anti-psychotic drugs are being given, or for the first few days after a depot injection. They are not addictive.
How they work: by acting on certain nervous pathways in the brain to balance the effect of anti-psychotic drugs on muscle tone and movement.

Anti-depressant drugs: Depression and mood changes are not uncommon in association with schizophrenia, and a course of anti-depressants may well be combined with anti-psychotic drugs. *See **depression**, page 116.*

OVER-THE-COUNTER TREATMENTS
None.

QUESTIONS TO ASK THE DOCTOR
- For how long should I take the drug(s)?
- Should I stop them when I feel better?
- May I just take them when I need them?
- Should I drive?
- What else can I do to help myself?

SIDE EFFECTS
Anti-psychotic drugs have a number of side-effects but there is considerable variation between the different drugs and it is often possible to find one that suits the

HOSTEL STAFF'S EXPERIENCE

"Bill used to just stay in his room, snoozing in bed and he wouldn't do anything. We all thought he was on far too much medication and asked for it to be reduced. When it was cut down he went mad and was up all night talking to himself, shouting obscenities or pacing around the streets. We've got to find a balance for him when he settles down."

IF THE DRUGS DON'T SEEM TO HELP

■ Don't despair. Recovery is often slow and can take months or years, rather than days or weeks. Find 'asylum': somewhere you feel safe and unafraid, where you can cope with any demands made, somewhere that understand what you are going through. Hospitals have traditionally provided such a haven, but so can friends, some lodgings or hostels, cafés, sheltered workshops, day hospitals and so on. Adapting to the effects of the illness, and regaining confidence, take time.

individual even if several produce side effects which are unacceptable.

In the first few days of treatment they tend to cause a dry mouth, blurred vision, constipation and difficulty in passing urine. Fainting is a risk, especially in the elderly. These side effects normally wear off as the body gets used to the drugs.

More seriously, they can increase the tendency to have epileptic fits in those who have had them before, and occasionally in those who have not. They can also cause weight gain, and chlorpromazine, in high doses, makes the skin sensitive to sunlight: a sun-screen *(see page 278)* should be used to prevent burning. Jaundice and damage to blood cells are further serious, but rare, complications.

The most troublesome side effect of the anti-psychotics are on muscle tone and movement. In the first few days of treatment, muscle spasms can occur, typically at the back of the neck, or in the tongue or eye muscle. Restlessness of the limbs may be experienced, too. Most common of all is a slowing of movements and a stiffness in the limbs and face muscles. This drug-induced Parkinson's syndrome starts after some days or weeks of treatment, and fortunately responds to anti-Parkinsonian drugs.

Long-term treatment with anti-psychotics can cause abnormal muscle movements, particularly of the face (tardive dyskinesia). Sucking or chewing movements are typical. They are most likely if high doses of drugs are used over long periods, and may not cease, even if the drugs are stopped

Is treatment worth all this trouble? Families and friends of schizophrenics, with first-hand experience of the miseries of mental illness, usually have few doubts. The side effects are not invariable, and in the short-term, the potential benefits of treatment usually outweigh them. Long-term complications, including tardive dyskinesia, are another matter: careful supervision is essential.

Anti-Parkinsonian drugs cause drowsiness, dry mouth, blurred vision, constipation and difficulty in passing urine, but these tend to pass off in a few days. The elderly may become confused. If taken regularly over a long period, the drugs can increase the risk of tardive dyskinesia developing (see above).

Anti-depressive drugs: *see depression, page 116.*

SELF-MANAGEMENT

Resist the inclination to carry on without professional

advice. Precisely because the experiences can seem so real, it is difficult for the sufferer to gauge the extent of the problem, or the need for help.

To prevent further attacks:
■ Don't fight against the drugs. They do prevent further episodes and they will keep symptoms at bay. Balance the disadvantages in taking them against the risk of a further breakdown. Consider the possible consequences of this at home or work; bear in mind that next time it might have to be admission to hospital. Discuss the options with your doctor or psychiatrist.
■ Try to steer a middle course between becoming isolated or lonely and seeing people who worry or annoy you, or vice-versa.
■ Aim for a middle way also between being stretched by work or responsibilities and giving up routines and responsibilities. Try to keep active and get out of the house at least every day.

Ideas for friends and relatives:
It is difficult to give general advice which will be helpful in specific circumstances, but:
■ Living with someone suffering from schizophrenia can be draining: friends and relatives may need help and support themselves. Remember this is available from self-help groups, and from professionals such as family doctors, psychiatrists, psychiatric nurses or social workers.
■ Remember that negative symptoms such as loss of drive and ability to respond to other people are just as much a part of the illness as the unusual experiences. Don't view apathy as laziness. Encourage the schizophrenic to take part as much as possible, but accept the handicaps and avoid behaving like a school teacher.
■ Don't argue with delusional ideas: it is probably best to accept them and change the subject: ''Well, it may seem as if the TV's affecting you, but anyway it's supper time now.''
■ Getting on with other people, particularly those close to them, can be difficult for schizophrenics. Don't press them; if in doubt, let them be. If you are getting irritated or worried, the schizophrenic will often sense it, and this can make things worse. Can you spend less time together, develop other interests for yourself, or talk about it with an objective outsider?
■ Remember, the drugs are *not* addictive, and they are often used to prevent relapse. Don't press for them to be stopped just because a schizophrenic seems well.

DOCTORS' EXPERIENCES
"If John had stayed in the boarding house with the landlady looking after him, and carried on pottering down to the workshop in the week, he would have been fine without any drugs at all. But when his landlady fell ill he went back home to his parents; they expected too much of him."

"I feel guilty and embarrassed when I talk to patients who have tardive dyskinesia as a result of their drug treatment. It almost makes it worse that they don't seem to either notice or care."

"It's always difficult to decide when to advise coming off anti-psychotic drugs. The statistics about relapse rates and risk factors don't help much with individual patients, and if someone does break down again, they often lose insight into what's happened and don't come for help."

Antidepressants, tranquillizers, hypnotics, vasodilators

NAMES YOU WILL HEAR

Anti-depressants
Chemical name: amitriptyline; **trade names**: Tryptizol, Lentizol, Domical, Elavil, Laroxyl, Tryptanol, Saroten, Amiline, Deprex, Levate, Meravil, Novotriptyn, Amilent, Trepiline. *See also **depression**, page 116.*

Tranquillizers
Chemical name: chlorpromazine hydrochloride; **trade names**: Largactil, Dozine, Chloractil, Procalm, Promacid, Protran, Chlorprom, Chlorpromanyl, Klorazin. *See also **anxiety**, page 84.*

Hypnotics
Chemical name: chloral hydrate; **trade names**: Chloralex, Chloradorm, Chloralix, Dormil, Elix-Nocte.

Vasodilators
Chemical name: co-dergocrine mesylate; **trade name**: Hydergine. Chemical name: cyclandelate; **trade names**: Cyclospasmol, Cyclobral. Chemical name: isoxsuprine hydrochloride; **trade names**: Defencin, Duvadilan, Vasodilan. **Chemical name**: naftidrofuryl oxylate; **trade name**: Praxilene.

WHAT IS SENILE DEMENTIA?

– Loss of mental function to the extent that it causes problems in daily living. It does not involve loss of consciousness, but intellect and memory, especially recent memory, gradually deteriorate. There may also be impaired judgement or impaired abstract thinking (for example difficulty in defining words), personality changes and speech difficulties.

The doctor must be at pains to exclude any other medical cause for these symptoms: drugs, infections, emotional disorders, pain, nutritional deficiencies, eye and ear problems and heart failure can aggravate the symptoms and once these factors have been identified and treated there can be a vast improvement.

CAUSES Usually, degeneration of brain cells. Premature degeneration of brain cells is known as Alzheimer's Disease, but sometimes this label is extended to include brain degeneration in all age groups. What ultimately causes this degeneration in the brain is unknown: it may be a disease process within the brain, or simply an aspect of the normal ageing process.

One cause of brain damage in the elderly is relatively identifiable: poor blood supply to the brain due to chronically narrowed blood vessels. This is often associated with a history of high blood pressure and/or stroke. In some cases there is a mixture of brain degeneration and reduced blood supply.

Senile dementia progresses gradually, although in patients where the disease is caused by narrowed blood vessels, deterioration may be in identifiable steps as new areas of the brain suffer reduced blood flow.

PRESCRIPTION DRUGS

In old people, drugs often have more marked side effects, some of which may result in aggravation of the dementia. Therefore it is important never to use a drug without a definite reason; to use as small a dose as possible; and to avoid using more than one drug.

Antidepressants: Depression is common in old people, especially when mobility is restricted or when eyesight or hearing fail. It may be difficult to distinguish at first between dementia and depression, so expert assessment is worthwhile. Alternative interests should be encouraged, and old people should be made to feel useful even if they can only perform simple tasks. If they live alone, they should be encouraged to go out. These general measures can lessen the need for antidepressants. Drugs used in the treatment of depression are discussed in detail under **depression,** *page 116.* Amitriptyline is the one most commonly used in the old because it has relatively few side effects.

Tranquillizers may be necessary: *see* **anxiety,** *page 84;* but equally, they may not. A few kind and reassuring words can be better than any medicine. The knack is to probe for the cause of the anxiety and treat that. Is the anxiety over an animal left alone at home? Or a minor physical symptom such as constipation? Pinning down the cause can be difficult when the patient is confused and cannot communicate effectively, but it is worth trying.

Hypnotics: Difficulty sleeping is all too common in the elderly. It is normal for older people to need less sleep, and they need reassurance that just a few hours at night may be enough for them, especially if they catnap during the day. *See* **insomnia,** *page 92* for the drugs used. Chloral hydrate is perhaps the most commonly prescribed for the elderly, who seem to suffer less from its side effects than the young.

Vasodilators are controversial drugs in this context. The drugs listed are thought to have a selective effect on blood vessels in the brain – but many doctors mistrust them. Certainly they should only be used when there is good reason to believe that dementia is due to narrowing of blood vessels in the brain. Psychological test results have suggested the drugs give some improvement, but the results in practice so far are inconclusive.

How they work: by dilating the blood vessels in the brain; however, the drug may succeed only in dilating healthy blood vessels, diverting blood away from vessels already narrowed. Symptoms can thus be made worse.

OVER-THE-COUNTER TREATMENTS

No generally available remedies have any significant effect on senile dementia, despite the claims of advertising. Don't be persuaded to spend money on such drugs; if you are tempted, ask your doctor first for advice.

QUESTIONS TO ASK THE DOCTOR

■ What plans can I make for the patient's care?
■ If the patient remains with the family, what outside support can the family get?
■ What about alternative accommodation?

SIDE EFFECTS

Drug reactions and interactions between drugs are much more common in the elderly because:
– Most drugs are broken down in the liver or excreted

PATIENT'S EXPERIENCE

"My husband was fit and active until he was 66. Then he gradually became more forgetful and seemed to lose touch with what was going on around him. At first I paid little attention: most people have some difficulty remembering things as they get older. But soon it became embarrassing. He had retired from a highly responsible job only a year before; but now I could see that he was not capable of working on the committees he was still involved with. I had a private talk with our doctor, who asked to see my husband. The doctor confirmed my suspicions: George was suffering from an early onset of senile dementia. He gave me all the advice he could. For example, we have some good friends, and although I had been embarrassed about George's behaviour, once I had explained the problem to them, they were understanding. Some of the men carried on taking him to the pub or to play bowls as they had done before, although it can't have been easy as he had to be looked after like a child. He was unable to drive on his own; he kept getting lost.

It was difficult for me. He didn't look like an old man. I couldn't leave him alone: he would wander away from the house and as he had no road sense, I was always terrified he would be knocked over by a car.

The doctor was a help, even though there was nothing he could do to treat the condition. He suggested having George admitted to a hospital so that I could get away for a while; but it did not work out because George had become totally dependent on me. Even if my daughter came to look after him for an afternoon, he would keep on asking when I would be home and get very agitated.

Over the next year and a half the strain became too much. It was intolerable being alone with him, yet I was reluctant to go out with him or invite friends around. Eventually, I decided to take up my other daughter's offer of a small separate

Continued on page 127

by the kidneys. Decreased liver and kidney function is common in older people and this means that drugs are not eliminated efficiently. Side effects are therefore more frequent.

– If the patient is confused, he or she may forget having taken a tablet, and take the dose twice.

– The patient may not take the tablets, and the doctor may increase the dose on the grounds that the drug is not working. If the patient then takes the increased dose, there may be side effects.

Antidepressants: *See* **depression,** *page 116.* The mono-amine oxidase group are not usually used in the elderly because of the high risk of side effects.

Tranquillizers: *See* **anxiety,** *page 84.* Tranquillizer drawbacks specific to the elderly include falls – potentially serious because of brittle bones; confusion; depression; memory failure and incontinence. An additional problem is that these side effects may not be recognized as a result of the drugs, but attributed to deteriorating mental function.

Hypnotics can have a reverse effect in the elderly (ie keep them awake) particularly if they are in pain. So, give something for the pain first; when it has eased, use the sleeping tablet. An old person who has had a sleeping tablet is especially likely to have a fall if they try to get up during the night. *See* **insomnia,** *page 92.*

Vasodilators bring a risk of excessive fall in blood pressure. This leads to dizzy spells or fainting, and in the extreme, a reduced blood supply to the brain can be followed by a stroke. Vasodilators can also cause skin rashes, nausea, palpitations and insomnia. They are not usually used in patients who have recently had strokes nor in those with heart disease or severe anaemia.

SELF-MANAGEMENT

■ Patients with memory loss do better if pressure to remember is removed. So, set them up with memory aids: note pads, a notice board, a clock with large digits, an easily read calendar. An established routine also gives a sense of security.

■ Symptoms can suddenly become worse if the old person is moved to unfamiliar surroundings.

■ Symptoms can also suddenly worsen if the patient becomes physically ill, depressed, or has side effects from drugs. Thus any sudden deterioration in mental condition should be investigated by the doctor.

■ Symptoms are often exacerbated by alcohol.

■ Many old people, especially (but not only) those living alone, have a restricted diet. Vitamin deficiencies, anaemia and malnutrition can all aggravate dementia. These factors must be carefully evaluated, and the diet supplemented with vitamins and iron if necessary.

■ Loss of vision or hearing can aggravate symptoms.

■ Remove all unnecessary medicines: confused old people, like children, can accidentally take dangerous overdoses, even of aspirin, iron or paracetamol.

■ The patient should see the doctor regularly for reviews of drugs. Don't allow an old person to have indefinite repeats of prescriptions, even though it is convenient. Symptoms may be due to accumulation of drugs in the body, not progression of the disease.

■ If using tranquillizers and sleeping tablets, guard against falls by making the route to the lavatory as unobstructed as possible, or put a pot or bedpan in an easily accessible position in the bedroom. A night light can help.

■ Living arrangements may have to be adapted so that stairs need not be used.

■ Social support is important. Visits by the doctor, social worker and health visitor will help to define problems in the home and their possible solution.

■ Temporary admission to hospital or nursing home can give family carers a rest or holiday. This change in environment may upset an old person, but their memory for recent events is short. It is essential for care-givers to have a break, otherwise the quality of the care that they can give deteriorates.

■ Recent onset of urinary incontinence should be investigated for the possibility of a bladder infection. Urinary incontinence can be distressing, but gentle persuasion to use absorbent pads inside underwear pays dividends. See **urinary incontinence,** page 188.

■ Old people often prefer life in their own homes to the safe but unhappy existence in an institution. Their point of view should at least be considered in milder cases of dementia.

■ Markedly confused patients can be like young children and the same precautions apply: safety in the kitchen; protection of open fires; locking away medicines; help with crossing roads.

■ Some confused elderly patients may wander away from home. Make sure the patient has their name and address in a pocket or on a bracelet that cannot be removed. Regular exercise may be a solution: the elderly person is less likely to wander if tired.

■ Local support groups *can* be helpful. In Britain there is an Alzheimer's Disease Society.

PATIENT'S EXPERIENCE
Continued from page 125
house on their farm. It means that I am close to the family, and my husband is able to walk more safely and there are things on the farm which interest him. It appears to be working well, but life is still a strain.

Not everyone is so lucky. This move however, does underline the fact that care of the old ought to be shared: if one person tries to do it alone, the quality of care becomes deplorable."

MULTIPLE SCLEROSIS

Steroids, immune suppressors, baclofen, dantrolene, carbamazepine, diazepam

WHAT IS MULTIPLE SCLEROSIS(MS)?

– Damage to the insulating sheath of myelin around nerves – see diagram. As a result, nerve inputs are no longer conducted. In young people, MS tends to come in attacks lasting between weeks and months; each attack follows damage to a group of nerves in one part of the central nervous system. As each attack settles, the symptoms usually improve and full recovery may occur especially after early attacks.

In older people, or young people who have had the disease for some time, MS tends no longer to occur in attacks, but to follow a slowly progressive course.

To make a diagnosis of MS, the clinician needs to have sound evidence for multiple attacks occurring in different parts of the nervous system or occurring at different periods. If a single attack of inflammation or damage has occurred in only one part of the nervous system, there is no basis for a diagnosis – although the patient may go on to develop MS.

CAUSE Ultimately unknown. There is a weak genetic component; people with a certain gene pattern are prone to develop MS, although it rarely occurs in more than one member of a family. There is also an environmental factor, possibly a virus encountered during the first 20 years of life. MS is more common in whites than in coloured people. However, if a coloured person is born in or moves to a temperate climate zone before the age of 15, the risk of developing MS rises; the reverse is also true for whites who move from temperate to hotter climates.

PRESCRIPTION DRUGS

Short courses of **steroids:** these drugs, including prednisolone, dexamethasone or ACTH probably shorten the duration of minor attacks; however, they have no effect on the long-term outcome. Thus most physicians reserve steroids for severe attacks.

Immune suppressors such as azathioprine can benefit patients who experience frequent attacks. Their use is a comparatively recent development, and the object is simply to reduce the frequency of attacks.

How they work: by acting on the immune system, preventing the body from breaking down myelin.

Others alleviate specific symptoms: Impotence, depression, urinary incontinence, constipation, pain and dizziness/vertigo are common at various stages of MS, treatment of which is dealt with on *pages 172, 116, 188, 30, 106 and 96*. Spasticity or increased stiffness in the legs is common and may be helped by baclofen, dentrolene, carbamazepine or diazepam.

OVER-THE-COUNTER TREATMENTS
None.

QUESTIONS TO ASK THE DOCTOR
■ What about my work?
■ Can I carry on being active?

SIDE EFFECTS
Steroids given in short courses for this condition have no serious side effects.

Immune suppressors have considerable side-effects, some serious. Azathioprine can, for example, cause mild gastro-intestinal upset; mouth ulcers and recurrent infections indicate the serious side effect of bone marrow suppression. In practice this should not occur since blood tests will give warning. No patient should start this type of treatment without full discussion of the risks. Any side effects should be reported immediately. **Baclofen** can cause gastro-intestinal upset, drowsiness and faintness. **Dantrolene** can give transient drowsiness, fatigue and diarrhoea; a possibly serious side effect may be liver malfunction and tests should be conducted six weeks after starting treatment. **Carbamazepine** may cause dizziness, drowsiness, gastro-intestinal upset and a rash. For *diazepam, see page 84.*

SELF-MANAGEMENT
Most physicians advise MS patients to avoid saturated fats (mainly animal fats and dairy produce) and to switch to a diet rich in polyunsaturated fats; there is some evidence that this improves myelin repair and thus the long-term outlook. A gluten-free diet or hyperbaric oxygen have had their vogue but there is no evidence that they are of any significant value.

SELF-HELP IN AN ATTACK
It is usually best to rest. The trigger for most attacks is unknown. They are slightly more likely to occur after the birth of a baby, and some follow viral infection such as flu. In general, however, most attacks occur without warning. Most physicians do not discourage their patients from having children.

It is important to remember that 60 per cent of patients are still working ten years after onset. Only 20 per cent will end up in a wheelchair. The outlook is therefore not as bleak as commonly conceived.

Basic nerve structure

Insulation sheath made up of myelin.

Central nerve fibre *which conducts messages:* the axon.

HOME ADAPTATIONS
Home assessment by an occupational therapist can provide a considerable range of aids to improve mobility and increase independence, as well as advice on how to prevent the complications associated with immobility. These are frequently the most important issues in caring for MS patients. Regular gentle exercise is important, and physiotherapy can be of considerable benefit.

ANAESTHETICS

Local, general

NAMES YOU WILL HEAR

Premedication
Chemical name: diazepam; **trade names:** Valium, Alupram, Atensine, Evacalm, Solis, Tensium, Valrelease. Chemical name: lorazepam; **trade names:** Lorazepam, Ativan. **Chemical name:** papaveretum; **trade name:** Omnopon. **Chemical name:** papaveretum and hyoscine; **trade name:** Omnopon and Scopolamine. Chemical name: morphine; **trade names:** Nepenthe, MST Continus, Duromorph, Cyclimorph. **Chemical name:** pethidine, meperedine; **trade names:** Pethilorfan, Pamergan, Pethoid, Demerol, Demer-Idine; the chemical names is usually employed. Chemical name: atropine sulphate; **trade names:** Atropine Sulphate or Atropine Sulfate. **Chemical name:** hyoscine hydrobromide; **trade name:** Scopolamine.

Intravenous induction agents
Chemical name: thiopentone sodium or thiopental sodium; **trade names:** Pentothal, Intravel Sodium. **Chemical name:** methohexitone sodium or sodium methohexital; **trade name:** Brietal. **Chemical name:** midazolam; **trade name:** Hypnovel. **Chemical name:** diazepam; **trade names:** Valium, Alupram, Atensine, Evacalm, Solis, Tensium, Valrelease.

Inhalation agents
Chemical name: halothane; **trade name:** Fluothane. **Chemical name:** enflurane; **trade name:** Ethrane. Chemical name: isoflurane; **trade name:** Forane. **Chemical name:** nitrous oxide; **trade name:** Nitrous Oxide.

Muscle relaxants
Chemical name: suxamethonium chloride; **trade names:** Scoline, Anectine. Chemical name: alcuronium chloride; **trade name:** Alloferin. Chemical name: pancuronium bromide; **trade name:** Pavulon. Chemical name: vecuronium; **trade name:** Norcuron. Chemical name: atracurium besylate; **trade name:** Tracrium.

WHAT ARE ANAESTHETICS?

– The drugs used to produce 'anaesthesia', a state of freedom from pain during surgical operations. Some examinations are also carried out under anaesthesia, for example of the bladder (cystoscopy) and some X-ray procedures. Anaesthesia may be 'general', in which case the patient is unconscious during the procedure, or 'local', when the nerves to the part to be operated on are 'frozen' and the area feels numb and sometimes cannot be moved. The patient may be conscious during a local anaesthetic, or sedated.

PRESCRIPTION DRUGS

Premedication is given by mouth or injection before the patient leaves the ward. Its purpose is to provide relief from anxiety, a measure of sedation, and sometimes loss of memory; it may also cause a dry mouth.

How they work: by acting on various parts of the brain. Drugs which dry the mouth act on the autonomic nervous system – which controls involuntary functions such as digestion.

The **intravenous induction** agents are most commonly given by injection into a vein, usually by the anaesthetist, to induce unconsciousness. If a patient really dislikes injections, or if a suitable vein is difficult to find, an inhalation agent is the alternative.

Modern anaesthesia is not just a single state produced by a single drug, but is comprised of different aspects, provided by different drugs administered during the course of an operation. In addition to unconsciousness, the aim is to provide pain relief, by means of analgesics; and also physical relaxation, by means of muscle relaxants. Using these procedures, an anaesthetist can maintain an unconscious, pain-free patient at a relatively light level of anaesthesia. This means that the patient recovers consciousness more quickly after surgery, and suffers fewer of the adverse effects of deep anaesthesia.

How they work: General anaesthetics depress the brain, producing unconsciousness, but they can also depress other body functions, such as those of heart, lungs and blood vessels and this is why the state of anaesthesia needs to be continually monitored. Local anaesthetics block nerves and stop pain impulses from the surgical operation site from passing along these nerves to reach the brain. The drugs are injected near the nerves, and during the injection, the patient may feel tingling or 'pins and needles', and occasionally, transient pain. These drugs can also be applied to the skin, eyes and linings of body orifices such as the mouth, nose, anus and urethra. Such preparations are used before minor procedures such insertion of a catheter; removal of a foreign body from the eye; insertion of an intravenous drip.

How they work: a complex chemical process involving ion changes across nerve membranes.

OVER-THE-COUNTER-TREATMENTS
The pain of a sore throat or painful haemorrhoids can be relieved by the use of proprietary preparations which contain local anaesthetic as one of the constituents.

QUESTIONS TO ASK THE DOCTOR
These questions are better put to a hospital doctor, rather than to a general practitioner. They are especially important before having an anaesthetic as a day case.
- Will I have a local or a general anaesthetic?
- How long must I not eat or drink before the anaesthetic?
- When will I be able to resume normal activity?
- When will I be able to drive my car?
- Should I stop smoking before the anaesthetic?
- Should I continue to take my usual tablets?

SIDE EFFECTS
Even after a long **general anaesthetic** for major surgery, recovery of consciousness will be quite rapid, although there may be disorientation and drowsiness afterwards. Some, probably a minority, suffer nausea and vomiting – but this is not a major problem of modern anaesthetics. Likewise, some patients feel 'hung-over'; others not at all. After **minor day case surgery,** recovery is usually fast and complete, but there will nevertheless be some who suffer headache, sickness, sore throat and soreness at the site of injection. These are usually mild and short-term. There is also the remote, but real chance that a patient may react adversely to an anaesthetic, and here the consequences can be grave. In practice, this risk is tiny, provided the anaesthetist has the appropriate background information about the patient – see BEFORE GOING INTO HOSPITAL. The range of modern anaesthetics available means that there is a safe one for almost all.

SELF-MANAGEMENT
- You may not be allowed a drink immediately after a general anaesthetic; if you are, take just a few sips. If you feel no nausea, then drink larger amounts.

Analgesics
Chemical name: morphine; **trade names:** Nepenthe, MST Continus, Duromorph, Cyclimorph. **Chemical names:** pethidine, meperedine; **trade names:** Pethilorfan, Pamergan, Pethoid, Demerol, Demer-Idine. Chemical name: fentanyl citrate; **trade names:** Sublimaze, Thalamonal.

Local anaesthetics
Chemical names: lignocaine hydrochloride, lidocaine hydrochloride; **trade names:** Xylotox, Lidothesin, Lignostab, Xylocaine. **Chemical name:** bupivacaine hydrochloride; **trade name:** Marcaine.

PATIENT'S EXPERIENCE
"I had the premedication at breakfast-time and to my astonishment, after a two-hour operation, I was feeling back to normal at lunch time: clear-headed, wide-awake and not even queasy. It was nothing like my last operation ten years ago."

PRE-SURGERY NERVES
If you are especially anxious about an operation, you could have a sleeping tablet the night before the attendance: your family doctor will advise. Don't drive yourself to hospital; allow plenty of time for the journey so that you can arrive calmly. Don't take any alcohol on the evening before going into hospital.

ILLNESS BEFORE ANAESTHESIA
Telephone the hospital if you have an illness within four weeks of admission for a procedure under anaesthesia. This applies to any illness, even a common cold. You will be advised on whether the operation should be postponed.

BEFORE GOING INTO HOSPITAL
Make a note of everything you can remember about illnesses; previous anaesthetics; all drugs you are taking, especially steroids; any allergies to anything, even sticking plaster; any problems which you or any member of your family has had with anaesthesia.

Infections

The body is prone to infections by many different organisms. Sometimes these are viruses which establish themselves inside cells (for example influenza); sometimes they are caused by bacteria and occasionally by parasites. In tropical countries, parasitic diseases are common, but the only one of real concern in developed countries is malaria. This disease is on the increase in the West, due largely to the growth of air travel.

Some infections are dealt with in this book under the part of the body affected rather than here. For example pneumonia, page 78 and cystitis, page 142.

COMMON COLD   134-137

INFLUENZA   138-139

SHINGLES   140-141

CYSTITIS   142-143

STD
(Sexually Transmitted Diseases), 144-147
including syphilis, gonorrhoea, NSU, vaginal discharge, herpes, genital warts (AIDS, see page 214)

MALARIA   148-149

MENINGITIS   150-151

See also: *Pneumonia and pleurisy, page 78; tuberculosis, page 80; middle and external ear infections, page 256; sinusitis, page 262; laryngitis, page 266; red eye and dry eye, page 268; acne, page 274; fungal infections, page 284; scabies and nits, page 286.*

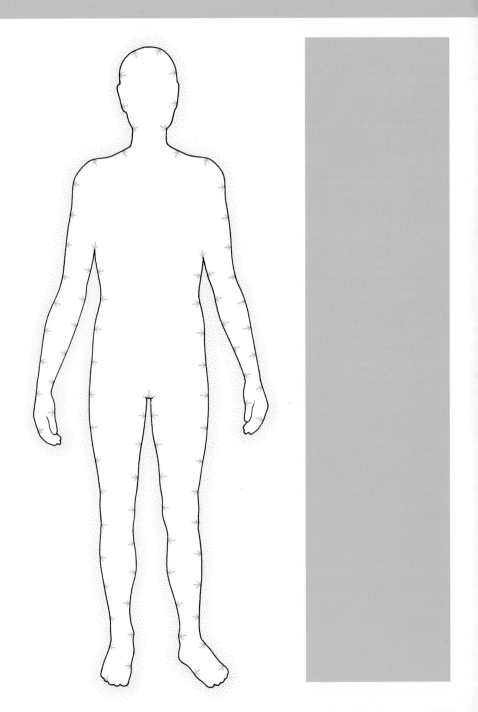

133

WHAT IS A COMMON COLD?

– A viral infection of the nose and throat. The illness begins suddenly with sneezing, a sore throat and a profuse watery discharge from the nose. There may be associated fever and general malaise. These symptoms usually last two or three days. Secondary infection by bacteria may occur, causing sinusitis *(page 262)*, ear infection *(page 256)*, laryngitis *(page 266)*, tonsillitis *(see below)*, or pneumonia *(page 78)*.

CAUSES A number of different viruses are usually responsible. Infection occurs from contact with other people who have the virus, which is spread via moisture droplets, either breathed or sneezed out. Cold weather does not cause colds, but rapid changes in body temperature may make the body more susceptible to viral infection. Overcrowding also favours spread of the virus. Infection by one of the common cold viruses does not give immunity to others.

PRESCRIPTION DRUGS

Antibiotics should not be used at the onset of a cold. In the elderly and the very young, in patients with chronic diseases like asthma, chronic bronchitis or heart disease, there may be a temptation to use antibiotics to prevent the development of bacterial infections which could rapidly result in serious illness. Antibiotics do not, however, shorten the duration of a common cold, as they have no effect on the viruses causing it. Antibiotics are used for the treatment of bacterial sinusitis, ear infection, laryngitis, tonsillitis and pneumonia if they develop during a cold.

How they work: by killing bacteria responsible for infection. *See **pneumonia and pleurisy**, page 78 and **drugs in children**, page 196.*

OVER-THE-COUNTER TREATMENTS

Analgesics/antipyretics such as apirin and paracetamol are useful during a cold; they help to lower the temperature (antipyretic effect) and ease muscle pains and headache (analgesic effect). Their action only lasts four to six hours and they should be repeated regularly if the temperature is high.

How they work: *see pain, page 106.* Children under 12 should be given paracetamol, not aspirin: see **SIDE EFFECTS.** For adults, the choice between the two can be entirely personal. Aspirin may be more effective, both as a painkiller and as an antipyretic; paracetamol is a mild drug, with few side effects. If in doubt, use the one you feel happy with – auto-suggestion has a role to play in pain relief.

Decongestants are meant to dry up the nasal secretions, reduce swelling of the nasal passages, and so unblock the nose.

How they work: by constricting the blood vessels in the nose, thus limiting the secretions and reducing swelling of the membranes in the nose. They are not always effective.

Decongestant nose drops also help to reduce nasal secretions and unblock the nose.

How they work: in the same way as decongestants taken by mouth. Normal saline (salt water) nose drops work by loosening the mucus in the nose, thus helping to unblock the nasal passages.

It is best to choose single-ingredient medicines rather than those with analgesic and decongestant combined. Some ingredients need to be given more frequently than others and the doses in a combination treatment are not always in the right concentration. active ingredient gives more flexibility of timing and dose.

All of these medicines may be used together, and antibiotics can be combined with any of them, too.

QUESTIONS TO ASK THE DOCTOR
■ What will happen if my temperature goes up? How can I get it down?
■ How long will the cold last?
■ How long should I take the medicine(s)?

SIDE EFFECTS
All medicines have side effects so it is important to take only those medicines which are absolutely necessary to relieve significant symptoms and promote recovery. Taking excess drugs for minor illnesses such as the common cold may result in side effects which are worse than the illness.

Antibiotics: *see **pneumonia** and **pleurisy**, page 78.*

Paracetamol has no common side effects when taken in the correct dose, except in patients with severe liver or kidney disease. Because it has an effect on the liver, it is not advisable to take it with alcohol. Skin rashes occur occasionally.

Aspirin can cause nausea, ringing in the ears and even deafness. These effects are not usually seen except in very high doses and will disappear as soon as the drug is stopped. It also causes indigestion due to gastric irritation, which can be minimized by taking the drug after food. Occasionally it causes such severe irritation to the stomach that vomiting or bleeding results. This complication usually occurs on high doses, but some people are more sensitive than others. Aspirin should not be taken with alcohol, as both have this effect on the stomach and the risk of vomiting blood is increased.

Occasionally, a patient has an allergic reaction to aspirin. This manifests itself as a skin rash, and wheezing with difficulty breathing. If this occurs, aspirin should not be taken again. Aspirin should not be given to children under age 12 years, except on instruction by the doctor. Reye's syndrome, a serious disease of brain and liver, has occurred in some children given aspirin for fever. Aspirin should not be taken during pregnancy and should be used with caution in patients with asthma, liver or kidney disease.

Decongestants usually contain two active compounds. One of these acts on the blood vessels in the nose and in other parts of the body; they should not be used in patients with high blood pressure, heart disease, diabetes, thyroid disease nor in patients on some drugs for the treatment of depression. They should not be given to babies under one year since they may cause hyperactivity. Many decongestants also contain antihistamines which cause drowsiness, and should not be taken when driving or working in a potentially dangerous environment. This effect is made worse by drinking alcohol. Do not take decongestants during pregancy: their antihistamine content has been associated with foetal abnormality and they may constrict blood supply to the placenta.

Nose drops can cause irritation to the membranes inside the nose, which in turn may cause more congestion. If used for long periods (two weeks or more), they can cause permanent damage to the sensitive membrane inside the nose. These drugs should not be given to babies (see above). It is safe to give babies normal saline nose drops, but even these are only indicated if there is extreme difficulty in feeding.

SELF-MANAGEMENT
In older children, and in adults, the common cold is usually mild: it is often not necessary to see a doctor.
■ Bed-rest is not essential. This applies equally to children and adults. A day or two spent quietly at home, however, will tend to shorten recovery time.
■ The temperature may be high, and this should be brought down with aspirin or paracetamol (see above), particularly in children under six, in whom there is always a risk of 'febrile convulsions'. Bring the fever

down immediately, even if the doctor has already been called. A cool (not cold) bath is often useful, indeed necessary, if the fever is running high. It lowers the temperature for four to six hours, and may need to be repeated. Patients often feel dramatically better once the temperature has returned to normal, so it is doubly worthwhile treating fever early and effectively. The patient will probably feel more inclined to eat and drink when the temperature is lowered, and vomiting is less likely.

■ The temperature is more likely to go up in the late afternoon and early evening and this should be anticipated. It is better to put a child into a cool bath *before* he or she starts feeling uncomfortable. Repeat the cool bath during the night if necessary: the child will often sleep for a few hours if the temperature is down to normal.

■ Don't hesitate to treat the symptoms of headache and muscle pains with paracetamol or aspirin.

■ Decongestants are useful if the blocked nose is so severe that it interferes with rest.

■ Drink plenty of fluids, particularly water or fruit drinks: a high temperature can lead to dehydration.

■ Food intake is less important than fluid intake, as the illness does not usually last for long. Children, in particular, should be allowed to eat whatever they like.

■ Colds in babies up to about six months are particularly distressing. The blocked nose may interfere with feeding. Ephedrine nose drops are too strong; but normal saline nose drops will liquify the mucus in the nose and usually helps to unblock it. If this does not work, a baby can be given milk with a spoon for a while. Breast feeding should be continued whenever possible. If the mother has some resistance to the infecting virus, antibodies from the mother's milk will pass on some resistance to the baby and help speed recovery. Clear fluid should also be offered as well as milk, especially if the temperature is high: again, the object is to prevent dehydration.

Controlling the temperature is very important. A baby with a cold should be dressed in cool, loose clothing, a vest and nappy are usually all that is necessary. Paracetamol should be given in the correct dose for age and frequent cool baths may be necessary. Cooling a baby in this way is not dangerous; but a high temperature left untreated can be serious because of the risk of convulsions.

■ The patient should start feeling better after two or three days. If recovery is delayed, consult a doctor.

TONSILLITIS
– Can be confused with the common cold. It is an infection of the tonsil glands, which guard the entrance to the gullet at the back of the mouth. There is usually a sore throat and it may be painful to swallow. A gargle with salty water (one teaspoonful per pint) or with dilute aspirin solution is often the best treatment, although in severe cases a doctor may have to prescribe an antibiotic.

WHAT IS INFLUENZA?

– An acute, highly infectious disease which tends to occur in epidemics. The symptoms are those of a general illness, and include fever, headache and muscle pains, with or without nausea and vomiting. Sneezing, sore throat and a profuse watery discharge from the nose can also occur, as in the common cold. The patient usually feels distinctly unwell.

Severe consequences of influenza can include complications such as inflammation of the heart muscle or brain. Secondary infection by bacteria can occur too, causing sinusitis, ear infection or pneumonia *(see pages 262, 256 and 78)*.

Most patients are ill for a few days, then recover rapidly. Some have a more prolonged convalescence with mental and physical lethargy, even depression, lasting weeks or even months (post-viral syndrome).

CAUSE The influenza virus, of which there are many different strains. Infection by one strain does not result in immunity to others. The virus is spread in the same way as for the **common cold,** *page 134.*

PRESCRIPTION DRUGS

Influenza immunization may be a good idea for the elderly, and for patients with chronic diseases such as asthma, chronic bronchitis, heart disease or a generally lowered resistance to infection. Such individuals are more likely to develop the severe complications and secondary bacterial infection. People who cannot take time off work might also benefit. The vaccine is given by injection in autumn – the start of the 'flu season.

How it works: For a 'flu vaccine to be effective, it is necessary to predict which strains of virus are likely to be in circulation. Each year the World Health Organization recommends which should be included in the vaccine; it ought then to protect against about 70 per cent of infections by these strains. The effect lasts for about 12 months.

Anti-emetics, in liquid form, are useful against the vomiting, when and if it occurs. Because the side effects of these drugs are significant they should only be used in cases of persistent vomiting, and not if a patient just feels a little nauseous. This applies especially to children, in whom the side effects are commoner than in adults.

How they work: by acting on the brain, suppressing the stimulus to vomit.

Antibiotics are not usually used at the beginning of the il-

Iness; their use is discussed in **common cold,** *page 134.*

OVER-THE-COUNTER TREATMENTS
See **common cold**, *page 134.*

QUESTIONS TO ASK THE DOCTOR
See **common cold**, *page 134.*

SIDE EFFECTS
Influenza vaccine can cause a painful local reaction at the injection site. It can also cause fever and malaise, within a few hours or days of the injection, but these are usually mild. Severe, but rare, reactions can occur in patients allergic to egg protein, or to antibiotics contained in the vaccine.

Anti-emetics cause a dry mouth, skin rash and drowsiness. They should not be taken while driving or working in a potentially dangerous environment. The drowsiness is made worse by alcohol. Muscle stiffness and spasms can also occur. These are usually associated with high doses, but children, and some adults, are especially sensitive; however, an antidote is available. **Anti-emetics** should not ever be used on children under 22 lbs (10 kg) or on patients who are dehydrated – the side effects would be more likely to occur than usual.

For side effects of **antibiotics,** *see* **penumonia and pleurisy,** *page 78,* and for analgesics, *see* **common cold,** *page 134.*

SELF-MANAGEMENT
Generally the illness is more severe than the common cold: the temperature is usually higher, headache and muscle pains more severe. Nausea and vomiting are frequent in influenza, but rare in the common cold. This in mind, self-treatment as in **common cold,** *page 134,* applies equally well to influenza.

■ Remember that all medicines have side effects: if treating yourself, only take those medicines which are absolutely necessary to relieve significant symptoms and promote recovery. ■ It is impossible to isolate patients with influenza and thus there is no way to prevent them passing on the virus. The patient is most likely to pass on the virus the day before the symptoms begin. ■ The patient should start feeling better after three or four days, but an early return to full activities can delay recovery and should be avoided. If there is a delay in recovery beyond two weeks, consult a doctor.

POST-VIRAL SYNDROME
Depression, continuing weeks or even months, is in most cases mild, but occasionally requires drug therapy. If it is significantly interfering with work and social life, discuss it with your doctor. Even the most severe cases resolve over a few months, and the condition does not predispose to recurrent bouts of depression.

WHEN TO CALL THE DOCTOR
A doctor should see elderly, young and chronically ill patients. For the few cases where lethargy continues for weeks or even months afterwards, there is no specific treatment, though rest is important.

WHAT IS SHINGLES?

– An infection caused by the chicken pox virus, *herpes zoster*. The virus lies dormant in the nerves of the body for many years after the chicken pox infection, but can suddenly become activated, spreading down a nerve, causing a painful, itchy rash in the area of the skin supplied by that nerve. Often the pain, which can be severe, will precede the skin rash by a day or two. Small blisters appear, which last for some weeks. Usually several adjacent nerves on one side of the body are affected. The rash stops exactly in the mid line, which is where the nerve itself ends. Occasionally, a nerve of the face and eye is affected. Blisters developing on the cornea of the eye may lead to scarring and impaired vision if not treated promptly. General symptoms include nausea, lethargy and loss of appetite.

The rash may increase over about a week, but once improvement begins, it is unlikely to reappear in other areas, or spread further. The pain usually subsides as the rash improves, but occasionally (and especially in older people), the pain may last for many months.

The *herpes zoster* virus is not the same as *herpes simplex,* which causes cold sores and genital herpes.

CAUSE Why the virus is suddenly activated is not known, but shingles is more common in patients with impaired immunity.

PRESCRIPTION DRUGS

Antiviral agents are of limited use: viruses live within the body cells and as a result are relatively inaccessible. The antivirals listed here are available as preparations which may be applied *locally* every four hours. They must be started immediately to have any effect. Thus topical acyclovir is of limited usefulness. Taken by mouth it is more likely to reduce the duration of pain during the severe phase and decrease the incidence of prolonged pain afterwards; they may also alleviate the eye pain.

How they work: by preventing the virus from multiplying.

Analgesics: Pain is the most serious problem with shingles, and its treatment, particularly in older patients, is important. As the pain can last for months, depression, loss of appetite and general debility may occur if the pain is not adequately treated. Aspirin and paracetamol may not be sufficient.

How they work: see *pain, page 106,* and ***rheumatoid arthritis,*** *page 242.*

Compound analgesics are an option if, as is possible, the pain is really severe. Doctors do not, however, like using them because the disadvantages usually outweigh the advantages. The advantages are that each ingredient may be used in a lower dose, thus decreasing side effects. Sometimes the drugs in the preparation enhance each others' effect, giving better pain relief than that normally expected from the sum of the component parts. The disadvantages are that some ingredients need to be given more frequently than others, and are not always in the correct concentration.

How they work: see **pain,** page 106, and **rheumatoid arthritis,** page 242.

OVER-THE-COUNTER TREATMENTS
If the drugs your doctor has given are failing to control the pain, be sure to go back to discuss it. Some of the drugs already prescribed may contain aspirin or paracetamol, and if you treat yourself with these drugs in addition, overdose may result. Calamine lotion will help dry the blisters and stop the itch.

QUESTIONS TO ASK THE DOCTOR
■ How long will it last? ■ For how long is it contagious?
■ Would antiviral drugs be useful?

SIDE EFFECTS
Antiviral agents: idoxuridine solution can cause stinging on application and overuse can damage the skin. Acyclovir used locally can cause stinging on application or occasionally redness or drying of the skin. If given as a tablet it can cause nausea, headache, fatigue, impaired liver and kidney function, and also blood and nerve abnormalities. **Analgesics:** paracetamol and aspirin: see **common cold,** page 134. Ibuprofen and naproxen: see **pain,** page 106 and **rheumatoid arthritis,** page 242.

The side effects of the **compound analgesics** are those of their component parts. Codeine phosphate causes constipation. Dextropropoxyphene is a narcotic analgesic and carries the risk of abuse and addiction. It should be used with caution in patients with asthma, lung, kidney or liver disease. Side effects include nausea, constipation, retention of urine, and suppression of breathing.

SELF-MANAGEMENT
■ Relief of pain is essential: remember to take analgesics on time. Delaying reduces their effect.
■ If you are depressed, discuss this with your doctor: it is not unusual, or a sign of weakness.

PATIENT'S EXPERIENCE
"I was a fit 66-year-old when I developed shingles. I noticed an itchy sensation on my left side and a day later the skin was red and very painful. I felt generally ill, as if I had 'flu. Then blisters appeared on the skin and the pain became very severe. My doctor confirmed that it was shingles. The pain dominated my whole day and I lived for the moment that I could take the next dose of painkiller. Neither paracetamol or ibuprofen gave much relief. The one that really worked was co-codamol, but the effect wore off just before the next dose was due. The chemist also recommended calamine lotion to dry the blisters.

What worried me most of all was that the inflammation and blistering might extend inside my abdomen: the pain certainly seemed to penetrate right into me. My doctor reassured me that this was not the case.

The pain made me feel sick. I was tired all the time and did not feel like eating. My neighbour came in every day and brought me a light meal of salad and cheese or fish. I was grateful for this: left on my own, I would not have bothered to eat. Over a few weeks, the pain eased a little.

My doctor was sympathetic: however, he said that he did not feel that I needed an antidepressant unless things really got too much for me. In the end, it did improve – but even now, a year later, I can still feel the pain sometimes."

PASSING ON SHINGLES
Shingles can only be passed on as chicken pox, and to those people who have not had chicken pox.

NAMES YOU WILL HEAR

Antibiotics
Chemical name: sulphamethizole; trade names: Urolucosil, Urolex, Uroz, Thiosulfil, S-Methizole, Thiosulfil. **Chemical name:** ampicillin; **trade names:** Ampifen, Penbritin, Pentrexyl, Vidopen, Austrapen, Bristin, Amcill, Ampicin, Ampilean, Biosan, Ampil, Famicilin, Pentrex, Petercillin, Synthecillin. **Chemical name:** co-trimoxazole; **trade names:** Bactrim, Fectrim, Nodilon, Septrin. **Chemical name:** nalidixic acid; **trade names:** Mictral, Negram, Uriben. **Chemical name:** nitrofuroantoin; **trade names:** Furadantin, Macrodantin. **Chemical name:** nolidixic acid; **trade names:** Mictral, NeGram, Uriben. **Chemical name:** nitro furantoin; **trade names:** Furadantin, Macrodantin.

Potassium citrate
Chemical name: potassium citrate; trade name: Effercitrate.

RISKS WITH POTASSIUM CITRATE
Recent studies have indicated that potassium citrate may under some circumstances cause kidney damage. Raise this issue with your doctor before taking the drug.

WHAT IS CYSTITIS?
– Painful passing of urine, commonly in women. Passing urine becomes frequent, uncontrollable, and sometimes the urine contains blood. These symptoms are due to inflammation of the urethra, the tube leading from the bladder to outside the body. A pain in the lower abdomen means that the bladder is also inflamed. If the kidneys are involved, a dull backache develops, often accompanied by a fever – a condition known as pyelitis.

CAUSES The root cause is either infection or bruising. The infection may be present in the kidneys or bloodstream and descend to the bladder, but more commonly it ascends from the urethra.

PRESCRIPTION DRUGS
Antibiotics: the common remedy. Many types are available; those listed here are particularly suited to treating cystitis; typically taken as tablets.
How they work: By killing bacteria responsible for infection. However, some bacteria can become resistant to some antibiotics; the antibiotic becomes ineffective, and a different one has to be prescribed. Antibiotics also have a tendency to kill not only the 'target' bacteria, but others as well; as some bacteria are naturally helpful in fighting harmful bacteria, a course of antibiotics can leave you without natural defences.
Potassium citrate helps relieve discomfort of cystitis.
How it works: by neutralizing acid in the urine.

OVER-THE-COUNTER TREATMENTS
Potassium citrate is available under several brand names; sometimes it is referred to simply as 'pot. cit.' (pronounced ''pot sit''). A good pharmacist will recommend a dosage and trial treatment period. If this fails, see a doctor straightaway.

QUESTIONS TO ASK THE DOCTOR
■ How long should I take the antibiotics?
■ How soon will the symptoms go?
■ How will I know whether they are working?
■ What happens if I am allergic to the antibiotics?

SIDE EFFECTS
Antibiotics are usually prescribed for less than one week, but for recurrent cystitis, a course may last several weeks. Antibiotics can make you feel under-the-weather and lethargic; some people are allergic to

them, and may develop a rash. Report this to a doctor immediately.

Potassium citrate: A helpful treatment, but it tastes awful, and this may make you vomit.

SELF-MANAGEMENT

If you have had cystitis once, work against future infection – and the need to take antibiotics:

■ After using lavatory paper in the usual way, soap hands and gently cleanse anus; rinse hands, then pour a bottle of warm water over anus away from vagina.

■ Wear cotton underpants and change them daily. Avoid wearing tights. Rinse underwear well and do not use strong soap powders or bleach.

■ Always pass urine within 15 minutes of sexual intercourse and then wash the uro-genital area with cool water. Rest – if possible.

■ Drink as little alcohol as possible, and if you do, try to have long drinks, and some bland liquid afterwards.

■ Drink 3-4 pints of bland liquid or water daily.

SELF-HELP IN AN ATTACK

As soon as the attack begins:

1 Put the kettle on for two hot water bottles. **2** Drink one pint of cold water and let your stomach settle. **3** When the kettle has boiled and the hot water bottles are filled, take one teaspoon of bicarbonate of soda mixed in water or jam. **4** Take two strong painkillers. **5** Fill a jug and glass with bland liquid; keep them by you and drink often. **6** Once each hour drink strong, coffee. **7** Try to put your feet up, or go to bed. Take your jug and glass, but before resting, drink another half pint of fluid. **8** Put one hot water bottle on your back and the other high up between your legs, resting against the uretheral opening. **9** Every time you pass water, wash the surrounding area and gently dab it dry. **10** CONTINUE TO DRINK HALF A PINT OF LIQUID EVERY 20 MINUTES.

The kidneys *produce, and excrete urine. Waste materials in the blood are extracted in the kidneys and transformed into urine. This passes via the ureter tubes to the bladder where it is stored until the bladder fills up. It then passes through a valve to the urethra, down which it passes to be expelled from the body.*

SYPHILIS, GONORRHOEA, NSU

Syphilis is an infection spread by sexual intercourse. Several weeks after the disease has been contracted, a painless ulcer appears on the sex organs, and the lymph glands in the groin may become enlarged. A skin rash may follow later. Eventually the disease attacks the heart and nervous system.

Gonorrhoea causes a discharge or leakage of pus from the urethra (water passage) in men, together with a burning sensation in the penis during the passage of urine. Symptoms usually appear a few days after infection has occurred. Women with gonorrhoea usually have no symptoms.

NSU (non-specific urethritis) also causes discharge and burning in men, but the symptoms are often quite mild and occur several weeks after the infection has been acquired. Women with NSU usually have no symptoms. However, if a woman has had sexual contact with a man with NSU, she should be treated for the infection in order to prevent her from re-infecting the man, but also to prevent spread of the infection into her Fallopian tubes which can lead to infertility. *Chlamydia* is one of the organisms which can cause NSU.

Crabs (pubic lice) may be regarded as sexually transmitted disease: *see **scabies and nits,** page 286*.

PRESCRIPTION DRUGS

There is no alternative to treatment with **antibiotics** for these conditions.

Pencillin injections (typically given in the form of ampicillin) are used to treat syphilis. Approximately 14 injections may be required, depending on the stage of the infection.

Pencillin injections or tablets are used to treat gonorrhoea, usually in a single high dose. Probenecid may be given to improve the effect of the penicillin.

Nowadays, a substantial number of gonorrhoea cases fail to respond to penicillin because the organisms develop resistance to the drug. A specialist may be needed to advise on alternative therapy.

Tetracyclines are used to treat NSU, in courses of at least one week's duration. There are several different types.

Erythromycin is an alternative to tetracycline for the treatment of NSU.

QUESTIONS TO ASK THE DOCTOR

■ How did I get this infection?
■ Have you checked me for any other sexually transmitted diseases?

- How long must I avoid sexual intercourse?
- How will I know I have been cured?
- Does my partner need to be treated?

SIDE EFFECTS

Some patients are allergic to **penicillin** – it may cause a rash. Patients receiving penicillin for syphilis frequently develop a reaction early in the course of treatment: this is known as the Herxheimer reaction, which is not caused by allergy, and treatment can normally continue.

Tetracyclines and **erythromycin** may cause nausea. Most tetracyclines should be taken well before meals, and they should not be used in pregnant women because they can damage the developing bones and the teeth of the foetus.

SELF-MANAGEMENT

- Take the full course of treatment as prescribed.
- Don't have sex until you have been cleared.
- Ensure that your partner(s) have been treated.
- Restrict alcohol to minimize nausea, which could impair the treatment.
- Take this opportunity to consider the health implications of your sexual lifestyle. Remember that condoms reduce the risk of transmission of infection.

SELF-HELP IN AN ATTACK

- Remember that symptoms from these conditions will rapidly improve once the infection has been treated.
- Men with NSU may find that alcohol makes the symptoms worse.

The unacceptable face of STD: *a baby can become infected with gonorrhoea during birth; the resulting conjunctivitis may lead to blindness.*

145

Chemical name: metronidazole; trade names: Flagyl, Vaginyl, Tichozole, Neo-Tric. Chemical name: nystatin; trade names: Nystan, Mycostatin, Canstat. Chemical name: clotrimazole; trade name: Canesten. Chemical name: econazole; trade names: Ecostatin, Gyno-Pevaryl. Chemical name: ketoconazole; trade name: Nizoral.

VAGINAL DISCHARGE, HERPES, GENITAL WARTS

Vaginal discharge: A certain amount of discharge may be quite normal, but an abnormal discharge is likely to be excessive, to smell unpleasant, and to cause irritation or itching. A retained tampon is sometimes the cause.

Thrush, also known as yeast infection, can bring about a thick white discharge and irritation, commonly after a course of antibiotics, and in diabetics. Some men carry the yeast organism which causes thrush and can re-infect their partner.

Trichomonas, or TV, causes a watery and highly irritating discharge. It is almost always sexually transmitted (men carry it without symptoms) and male sexual partners should therefore be treated too.

Anaerobic vaginosis is a mixed infection causing a vaginal discharge, more noticeable after intercourse. It is not usually acquired sexually.

Herpes is caused by a virus which most of us carry in our bodies and is responsible for cold sores around the lips. Similar sores can also occur on the sex organs, and these can be acquired sexually. A first attack of herpes can be painful with multiple sores on the genitals and swelling of the lymph glands in the groin. The condition sometimes recurs, although recurrent attacks tend to be far less severe than the original one. The disease tends to burn itself out quickly.

Genital warts are caused by certain strains of wart virus (papillomavirus or HPV), and are spread sexually. It may take weeks or months before they appear. Wart infection can result in abnormality in the cancer smear and this can progress in time to cancer of the cervix. Patients with genital warts may therefore need specialist treatment. See also **viral warts,** *page 282.*

PRESCRIPTION DRUGS

Fungicides: Nystatin or imidazoles (eg econazole) are used to treat thrush, given in the form of vaginal pessaries and cream. Nystatin taken by mouth only clears the bowel. Ketoconazole by mouth can be given for severe resistant thrush, but see below.

Metronidazole is used to treat trichomonas and anaerobic vaginosis – given either as a single large dose by mouth or as a short course.

Acyclovir, the antiviral agent, can be taken by mouth as a five-day course for a severe first attack of herpes. It is far less effective as a cream. With severe recurrent herpes, it can be taken regularly to suppress attacks.

Genital warts are painted carefully with **podophyllin solution,** which inhibits the wart virus inside skin cells.

The treatment may need to be repeated two or three times a week for several weeks. Other treatments for warts include cryotherapy (freezing), cautery, laser treatment and surgery. *See also **viral warts**, page 282.*
How they work: all these preparations kill the organism responsible, or prevent it from multiplying.

QUESTIONS TO ASK THE DOCTOR
■ Have the tests confirmed a diagnosis?
■ Will I infect my sexual partner?
■ How long will the treatment last?
■ What happens if the treatment doesn't work?

SIDE EFFECTS
Some **pessaries for thrush** may suit the patient better than others, but treatment is usually safe and effective.
Ketoconazole tablets can cause liver damage and should therefore only be used for severe resistant thrush.
Metronidazole can cause nausea, and severe vomiting if taken with alcohol. It should be avoided in the first three months of pregnancy.
Acyclovir has few side effects; do not take in pregnancy.
Podophyllin may cause skin irritation, especially if spilt on healthy skin. It should be washed off four to six hours after application.

SELF-MANAGEMENT
■ Thrush: avoid unnecessary antibiotics, wear loose cotton underwear, avoid irritants (including detergents). If recurrent, has your partner been checked?
■ TV: Ensure your partner has been treated.
■ Herpes: Obtain definite diagnosis and advice from a specialist. Identify and avoid anything that could cause recurrences – and this includes stress. Look after your general health, rather than waste time on unproven remedies. Make sure you understand when you should avoid sex – it often helps if your partner also understands your condition.
■ Warts: Persist with the treatment until you are cured. Use condoms to prevent spread to your partner. Have regular cancer smears.

SELF-HELP IN AN ATTACK
■ Thrush and TV: Bathe in plain or slightly salty water; avoid irritants. Use yoghurt on the vagina if no other treatment is available: it can be a fairly effective temporary measure.
■ Herpes: Pamper yourself. Keep sores clean and dry. Avoid intercourse till completely healed.

PATIENT'S EXPERIENCE
"I was having recurrent herpes; it made me depressed and anxious. The doctor told me I had wasted time on quack remedies and sent me to a herpes counsellor. To my surprise she spoke as much about organising my life and looking after my health generally as about the condition itself. I tried to get a firmer grasp on my life, and after a while I realized that no drug treatment was necessary. I suppose I might have started taking better care of myself generally. I found I could discuss the problem with my boyfriend; we have a good relationship. Soon the herpes started to improve, and now I only get an attack once or twice a year, usually when I have a heavy cold."

MALARIA

Chloroquine, proguanil, quinine, mefloquine.

NAMES YOU WILL HEAR
Chemical name: chloroquine; **trade names:** Nivaquine, Avloclor. **Chemical name:** proguanil; **trade name:** Paludrine. **Chemical name:** pyrimethramine plus dapsone; **trade name:** Maloprim. **Chemical name:** pyrimethramine plus sulfadoxine; **trade name:** Fansidar. **Chemical name:** mefloquine hydrochloride; **trade name:** usually prescribed by chemical name. **Chemical name:** amodiaquine; **trade name:** Camoquin.

At the root of malaria *is a parasite called* Plasmodium. *Swallowed by a mosquito, it multiplies in the insect's stomach, producing hundreds of cells which migrate to the saliva glands. When the mosquito bites a human, the parasite enters the bloodstream and quickly makes its way to the liver, where it again multiplies, and can live for years. From the liver, the parasites enter the bloodstream periodically, invading the red blood cells, again developing and multiplying. When mature, they rupture the red blood cells – which causes fever.*

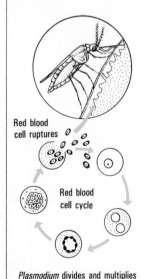

Red blood cell ruptures

Red blood cell cycle

Plasmodium divides and multiplies

WHAT IS MALARIA?
– A common tropical infection, responsible for the deaths of well over a million people worldwide every year. Fever and illness follow infection after one week or more, but sometimes illness may be delayed many months or even years. Apart from fever, symptoms may include any of the following: shivering, headaches, vomiting, cough, diarrhoea, drowsiness or confusion. The disease is impossible to diagnose conclusively without laboratory tests. Anyone with the above symptoms either during or after a trip to a malarial area should suspect they have the infection. There are four major varieties of malaria: all cause chills and fever, but one, *Plasmodium falciparum*, causes severe illness, and is commonly fatal if not treated quickly.

Two of the four species of malaria have a stage of the parasite that may remain dormant in the liver for months or years. Malaria due to these species – *P. vivax* and *P. ovale* – may recur several times over a period of years, even after treatment of the acute infection with standard drugs. This calls for further medication – see under **PRESCRIPTION DRUGS.**

CAUSES A single-celled parasite that invades red blood cells, carried from person to person by mosquitoes.

PRESCRIPTION DRUGS
Resistance to antimalarial drugs is becoming an increasing problem, especially in the case of *P. falciparum*. Consequently drug use has to be revised frequently and only broad generalizations can be presented here.

Preventive: tablets, typically **chloroquine** and **proguanil,** are taken regularly by any visitor to a malarious area, starting a week before the visit and continuing until a month after leaving the area. The actual drugs recommended depend on the place(s) to be visited, and the current patterns of drug resistance; up-to-date advice is essential.
How they work: malarial drugs interfere with the metabolism of the parasite, but exactly how is not fully understood.

To treat an attack: An acute attack must be treated quickly with a drug to which the parasite is sensitive. Chloroquine and quinine have a major role, but there are alternatives and the choice depends on the area in which the malaria was contracted. The method of giving the drug depends on the severity of the attack: tablets are usually effective for mild or moderate illness, but intravenous therapy is needed for severe cases.

How they work: see **Preventive,** above.

OVER-THE-COUNTER TREATMENTS
Chloroquine and proguanil can be bought without prescription in the UK. Aspirin or paracetamol will help the symptoms, but have no effect on the parasite.

QUESTIONS TO ASK THE DOCTOR
■ What is the latest recommendation for preventive tablets for the countries I will be visiting?
■ What variety of malaria parasite has been found in my blood test? Do I need extra treatment to eliminate parasites from the liver?

SIDE EFFECTS
Chloroquine and **paludrine** taken for prevention cause very few unwanted effects. Weekly chloroquine should not be taken for more than six years, as it may then begin to damage vision. Occasionally, **Maloprim, Fansidar** and amodiaquine have dangerous effects on the bone marrow and skin and are therefore not recommended for prevention except in unusual circumstances. **Quinine** (taken to treat an attack) commonly causes a high-pitched ringing sound in the ears, but this is not dangerous and does not affect hearing.

SELF-MANAGEMENT
The malarial parasite is extremely cunning: it develops resistance to anti-malarial drugs. Treatment is therefore varied on a local basis. So before you set out on a trip, find out the currently recommended treatment for that area. Your doctor will advise. Be sure to take preventive tablets *regularly*; continue for a month after leaving the malarious area. Avoid mosquito bites by sleeping under a mosquito net and wearing protective clothing out of doors, especially around dusk. Insect repellant is of dubious worth: it gives no guarantee against mosquito bites and possibly a false sense of security.

SELF-HELP IN AN ATTACK
It is wise to seek medical attention urgently as soon as you think you may have malaria: do not wait to see how things go. If, however, you are far from medical facilities, take a full course of treatment tablets as soon as fever develops. Take plenty of fluid.

Antibiotics
Chemical name: benzylpenicillin; trade name: Crystapen. **Chemical name:** gentamicin; **trade names:** Garamycin, Cidomycin, Genticin, Lugacin, Alcomicin, Refobacin. **Chemical name:** chloramphenicol; **trade name:** Chloromycetin. **Chemical name:** co-trimoxazole; **trade names:** Bactrim, Fectrim, Nodilon, Septrin. **Chemical name:** ampicillin; **trade names:** Ampifen, Penbritin, Pentrexyl, Vidopen, Austrapen, Bristin, Amcill, Ampicin, Ampilean, Biosan, Ampil, Famicilin, Pentrex, Petercillin, Synthecillin.

Anticonvulsants
Chemical name: phenobarbitone; trade names: Luminal, Gardenal, Maliasin, Nova-Pheno. **Chemical name:** diazepam; **trade names:** Valium, Alupram, Atensine, Evacalm, Solis, Tensium, Valrelease. **Chemical name:** phenytoin; **trade name:** Epanutin.

Analgesics
Chemical name: paracetamol; **trade names:** Panadol, Pamol, Calpol, Tylenol, Parasin, Parmol, Panado, Ceetamol, Atosol, Exctol, Tylenol, Ennagesic, Ilvamol. **Chemical name:** aspirin; **trade names:** Aspirin, Astrin, Bi-Prin. *See also* **pain,** *page 106.*

WHAT IS MENINGITIS?

– An inflammation of the membrane covering the brain. It causes fever, irritability, drowsiness, headache, vomiting, and a painful, stiff neck. Occasionally convulsions occur. It is much more common in children than in adults.

CAUSES Principally viruses and bacteria. Some types of meningitis are contagious. Viral meningitis is caused by a number of different viruses, including the one which causes mumps. This is the less severe form of the disease and recovery is usually complete. Bacterial meningitis is caused by a number of different bacteria. Brain damage may result, particularly in the young, and in severe cases.

Which type of meningitis the patient has developed may be determined by a lumbar puncture: fluid is withdrawn from the spinal canal and tested. The test may also indicate which antibiotics will be best.

Meningitis patients are almost always admitted to hospital for at least 48 hours for tests as soon as the disease is suspected. Patients with viral meningitis usually stay in hospital for a shorter period than those with bacterial meningitis.

PRESCRIPTION DRUGS

Antibiotics are used in all cases of bacterial meningitis. (They are not used in viral meningitis, where they have no effect.) However, antibiotics may be used initially, regardless of diagnosis, until it is certain that the cause of the meningitis is viral.

The type of antibiotic used will depend on the type of bacteria causing the infection. Because delay in effective treatment may cause permanent brain damage, two or sometimes even three antibiotics are used in combination. They are usually given by injection: to be effective, the dose has to be of a size which cannot be effectively administered by a tablet. Duration of treatment is also longer than for most other infections, usually about ten days. The lumbar puncture is often repeated before the antibiotics are stopped, to make sure that the infection has completely cleared. Antibiotics may also be changed during the course of treatment if they are not working.

How they work: by killing bacteria responsible for the infection. They are discussed in more detail under ***pneumonia and pleurisy,*** *page 78.*

Anticonvulsants: Convulsions occur in some seriously ill meningitis patients, and these drugs may have to be used as a preventive measure.

How they work: *see **epilepsy** page 110.*

Analgesics such as aspirin or paracetamol will help to lower the temperature and ease the headache. In young children convulsions can occur if the temperature is high, and it can be difficult to know whether the fever or the meningitis is the cause.

How they work: *see **pain**, page 106.*

Intravenous fluids are usually given as a drip into a vein to correct dehydration.

With viral meningitis the patient is not usually very ill and the treatment is symptomatic. The temperature is controlled with analgesics and cool baths. Convulsions are uncommon. Recovery is usually complete.

QUESTIONS TO ASK THE DOCTOR

■ Is hospital admission necessary?
■ Is it likely to spread to other members of the family?
■ Is it likely to cause permanent damage?

Not all of these questions can be answered immediately, but once the tests have been done, a doctor should be able to discuss these points.

SIDE EFFECTS

Antibiotics used for meningitis are stronger – because of the larger doses – than those used for most other infections. The side effects may be more marked and more varied, depending on which ones are used. They commonly include nausea, vomiting, diarrhoea and allergy *(see **pneumonia and pleurisy**, page 78).* More rarely, they can affect the kidneys, ears and the blood. Tests for these complications are done while the patient is being treated. In each case, these very real disadvantages have to be weighed against the advantages, indeed the necessity, of using antibiotics. The object is to use antibiotis only if absolutely necessary.

Anticonvulsants: *See **epilepsy**, page 110.* Phenobarbitone can cause drowsiness or irritability. Children over the age of two years are not usually given this drug as they can become very difficult and badly behaved. If treatment for convulsions has to be continued for any length of time, other drugs can be used. Valium causes drowsiness: it is not used in the long-term prevention of convulsions; *see **anxiety**, page 84.*

Analgesics/antipyretics: *see **common cold**, page 134.*

SELF-MANAGEMENT

Be aware of the symptoms of meningitis and report them to a doctor without delay.

151

Metabolic and endocrine disorders

Many complicated functions of the body such as body growth and development, sexual function, nutrient distribution and responses to stress are controlled by a series of glands that produce hormones. The pancreas gland in the abdomen produces insulin, the thyroid gland produces thyroxin and these as well as other glands are all controlled by the 'master gland' – the pituitary gland at the base of the brain.

OBESITY   **154-155**

DIABETES   **156-161**

LIPID DISORDERS   **162-163**

HYPERTHYROIDISM   **164-165**

HYPOTHYROIDISM   **166-167**

Disorders of **PITUITARY GLAND 168-169**

See also: *Infertility, page 174; drugs in pregnancy, page 184; period problems, page 190; problems of menopause, page 194.*

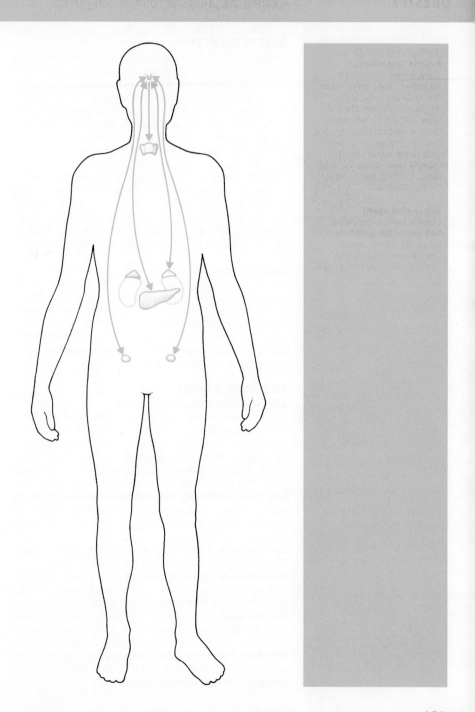

NAMES YOU WILL HEAR

Appetite suppressants
Chemical name: diethylpropion hydrochloride; **trade names:** Apisate, Tenuate Dospan, Dietec, D.I.P., Nobensine-75, Regibon. **Chemical name:** fenfluramine; **trade names:** Ponderax, Ponderax Pacaps, Ponderal, Pondimin. **Chemical name:** mazindol; **trade names:** Teronac, Sanorex. **Chemical name:** phentermine; **trade names:** Duromine, Ionamin, Fastin, Pronidin, Minobese.

Bulk-forming agents
Chemical name: methylcellulose; **trade names:** Celevac, Cellucon, Cologel, BFL, Cellulon, Nilstim. **Chemical name:** sterculia; **trade names:** Normacol, Inolaxine, Karagum, Prefil.

WHAT IS OBESITY?

The word 'obese' means excessively fat, but what you understand by excessive depends on what you regard as normal. Doctors are divided in their understanding of what constitutes obesity. Most tables of 'ideal weight' are based on old statistics from a US insurance company. Their relevance is disputed. However, there is no doubt that very fat people suffer illness and may be at risk of premature death. These people are at least 30 per cent over average weight for height.

Doctors may still advise people thinner than this to lose weight because they have conditions such as high blood pressure or arthritis, where excess weight may worsen the problem, while not actually causing it. Apart from this, there is no evidence that mild obesity, say 10 per cent over 'ideal weight', affects health.

CAUSES Simply eating more than necessary. But why? Individual needs vary, but obese people cannot recognize when they have had enough; they do not respond in the normal way to feelings of hunger or satiation. They are influenced more than other people by the taste, smell and appearance of food. They have 'learned' to overeat. Once obese, you can remain so while eating no more than anyone else.

PRESCRIPTION DRUGS

Appetite suppressants play a very minor part. Those listed are only used under careful medical supervision. Their effect is short-lived, and there is a risk of dependency developing. Most obese patients will lose about 1 lb (0.5 kg) per week while taking these drugs, but the appetite, and the weight, usually return after stopping them. The drugs help with permanent weight reduction only when combined with a programme of learning to eat less by recognizing the cues indicating one has had enough, and by ignoring those cues that lead to eating for pleasure.

How they work: probably by affecting the way the brain feels hunger, so suppressing the desire to eat.

Bulk-forming agents are available on prescription, but may also be bought without one. They are a means of supplementing the fibre content of the diet.

How they work: Everyone's diet should contain sufficient fibre, but the use of high-fibre, low-calorie supplements helps some people to feel satisfied on fewer calories. A high-fibre diet also leads to a reduction in blood cholesterol, which may lower the risk of coronary heart disease. See **lipid disorders**, page 162.

OVER-THE-COUNTER TREATMENTS

Many forms of diet foods and drinks are available. Advertisers' claims are carefully worded, but in reality these products are expensive low-calorie meals. You can create your own much more economically.

'Very low calorie diets', containing less than 800 calories per day, are being marketed, usually through non-medical 'consultants'. They are effective, but their safety and long-term effectiveness are still being assessed.

QUESTIONS TO ASK THE DOCTOR

■ Do I really need to lose weight?

SIDE EFFECTS

Appetite suppressants: Diethylpropion and most other anorectic drugs (except fenfluramine) have a mild stimulant action, which can lead to dependence. While it may seem useful to take a drug that makes you feel less tired, the risk of addiction far outweighs any apparent benefit.

Fenfluramine causes mild sedation, especially when first started; drowsiness and depression are the two most common reasons for stopping the drug. Sudden withdrawal can lead to severe depression. There is little risk of addiction.

Bulk-forming agents: Provided adequate fluid is taken, bulking agents are free from serious side effects, but people do find them unappetizing.

SELF-MANAGEMENT

Obesity is not a simple problem, nor are there easy answers. But since it has been estimated that more than a third of the population of most Western countries aged over 30 is more than 10 per cent overweight, some modification of eating habits would seem to make sense.

Fat is both the most concentrated form of calories, and the least obvious constituent of many processed ('junk') foods. It is associated with raised levels of cholesterol in the blood, and with the risk of heart disease. So reducing fat intake is worthwhile. Carbohydrates (sugar, starch) are converted by the body to fat if not needed as a source of energy. Sugar itself is also a common hidden ingredient in processed foods. A diet based on fresh vegetables, and bread, with meat, fish, eggs and cheese as sources of protein will provide fewer calories and more fibre than a diet composed mainly of processed food, sweets and biscuits.

PATIENT'S EXPERIENCE

"I began to put on weight after having my first baby. I got to 11 stone (70 kg). As I am only 5ft 4 inches tall, I felt very fat. For three years I tried all sorts of diets, but couldn't lose weight. I felt really ugly. Then my doctor suggested I join a group run by the health visitor. I carefully counted my calorie intake, and was surprised at how much I was eating. With the help of the group I found I could eat less. I started jogging, and began to feel more confident. I lost two stones (13 kg) in a year. My weight has remained around nine stones, apart from after my second pregnancy, when my GP gave me a short course of tablets, which helped get it down."

EXERCISE

■ One hour's walking, or $\frac{3}{4}$ hour's cycling or $\frac{1}{4}$ hour's swimming every day should result in an extra two to four pounds' weight loss each month.
■ A useful target is half a stone (3 kg) weight loss per month.
■ Regular exercise *combined* with a suitable diet, is the most effective way to lose weight. It can help lower serum cholesterol, too.

MORAL SUPPORT

Losing weight is difficult. Doing it alongside others with the same problem can be enormously helpful: don't dismiss joining a local weight-watchers' group.

Chart showing acceptable weight ranges: *see page 49.*

NAMES YOU WILL HEAR
Short-acting insulin
Chemical name: soluble or regular insulin; trade names: Insulin, Insulin (beef), Hyparin Insulin (beef), Insulin Injection (beef). Chemical name: neutral insulin; trade names: Neutral Insulin Injection (beef), Hypurin Neutral (beef), Neusulin (beef), Quicksol (beef), Velosulin (pork), Human Actrapid, Human Velosulin, Humulin S (human).

Intermediate and long-acting insulin
Chemical name: insulin zinc suspension (amorphous); trade names: 125 Semilente (beef), Semilard MC (pork), IZS Semilente (beef), Regular Iletin. Chemical name: insulin zinc suspension (crystalline); trade names: Ultralente (beef), Human Ultratard, Humulin Zn (human), Ultralente Iletin. Chemical name: insulin zinc suspension (mixed crystalline and amorphous); trade names: IZS Lente (beef), Hypurin Lente (beef), Neulente (beef), Tempulin (beef), Lentard MC (pork), Human Monotard, Lente Iletin. Chemical name: isophane insulin; trade names: Isophane Insulin Injection (beef), Hypurin Isophane (beef), Insulatard (pork), Monophane (beef), Neuphane (beef), Human Insulatard, Human Protaphane, Humulin I (human), NPH Iletin. Chemical name: neutral and isophane mixed insulin; trade names: Initard (50% neutral: 50% isophane, pork), Mixtard (30% neutral: 70% isophane, pork), Human Actraphane (30% neutral: 70% isophane), Human Initard (50% neutral: 50% isophane), Human Mixtard (30% neutral: 70% isophane), Humulin M1 (10% neutral: 90% isophane, human), Humulin M2 (20& neutral: 80% isophane). Chemical name: biphasic insulin injection; trade name: Rapitard MC (25% neutral pork: 75% crystalline beef insulin). Chemical name: protamine zinc insulin; trade name: Hypurin Protamine Zinc.

Continued on page 158

WHAT IS DIABETES?

A surprisingly common metabolic disorder, in most countries affecting one to two people in a hundred. Two types account for most cases:

Insulin-dependent diabetes: tends to occur in children and young adults. There is a severe deficiency or absence of the hormone known as insulin, normally produced by the pancreas gland. This causes poor metabolism of carbo-hydrates, proteins and fats. Typical symptoms are loss of weight, despite a healthy appetite; thirst and passing large volumes of urine. There is also a tendency for ketones to accumulate in the blood. (Ketones are products of fat metabolism arising in abnormally large quantities as a result of diabetes. They may be detected in the urine or smelt on the breath.) About 25 per cent of all diabetics have this form of the disease, which is fatal within a year unless treated with insulin.

Non insulin-dependent diabetes: the common form tends to occur in older people who are overweight. There is not such a severe shortage of insulin in older patients as in the insulin-dependent type, but the insulin which is produced does not work efficiently. A similar though less severe disruption of body metabolism is caused. Symptoms of thirst and passing large volumes of urine may occur, but often the disease comes on gradually and may only be recognized when the urine, which normally contains no sugar, is tested.

Diabetes can also occur during pregnancy, brought on by hormonal changes. This resolves immediately after the baby is born.

In diabetes the blood sugar (glucose) level rises because without insulin it can no longer be driven into the body's cells. When glucose in the blood reaches a certain level, it spills over into the urine. After several years of diabetes, damage to body organs may occur, particularly to the eyes, kidneys and nervous system; but if the disease has been well controlled the risk is significantly reduced.

CAUSES: In insulin-dependent diabetes, the cells which make insulin are destroyed by the body's own immune system. Why this happens is not known, but it is thought that in susceptible people a stimulus, such as a virus, triggers the process. The cause of non insulin-dependent diabetes is also not fully understood, but there are many factors which increase the risk, including obesity, increasing age, heredity. Less often, diabetes develops after attacks of pancreatitis (acute abdominal pain caused by the inflammation of the pancreas). It also occurs in association with other diseases of the endocrine glands.

PRESCRIPTION DRUGS

Insulin: obtained from the pancreas glands of cattle and pigs. It is not quite the same as human insulin which is now produced by genetic engineering (bacteria are treated to produce insulin identical to the human variety). Insulin is given by injection under the skin because it is a protein and would be digested and destroyed if taken by mouth. By combining it with retarding substances, the rate of absorption into the bloodstream can be delayed. Many insulin-dependent diabetics can control their diabetes with just two injections a day of a mixture of short- and longer-acting insulin, but the best control, allowing flexible meal times, is with three or more injections a day. Using a pump, strapped to the body or hidden in clothing, it is possible to inject slowly over 24 hours, giving boosts when food is eaten. This can give excellent control of blood glucose.

How it works: Injected insulin works in the same way as natural insulin, driving glucose into the body's cells and restoring fat and protein metabolism. The aim is to match the pattern produced by a normal pancreas, but even with a pump this can never be done exactly.

Oral hypoglycaemic agents: These sub-divide into two groups – sylphonylureas and biguanides – and are only useful in non-insulin dependent diabetes. **Sulphonylureas** are particularly useful if diabetes has not been controlled by diet alone and the patient is not obese. Long-acting types are taken once daily before breakfast. Short-acting types may be taken before meals.

How they work: by stimulating the cells which produce insulin. They are therefore ineffective in patients whose insulin-producing cells have been destroyed.

Biguanides are useful in non insulin-dependent patients who are still obese.

How they work: by reducing absorption of carbohydrates from the gut. They may also increase uptake of glucose into cells and reduce the formation of glucose from glycogen (starch) in the liver. They are dependent on the presence of insulin for their action.

Guar: a naturally-occurring plant fibre (obtained from the cluster bean) which is not absorbed from the gut. It is available as granules or mini-tablets and is taken in a drink or, most effectively, when mixed with food.

How it works: by increasing the consistency of food in the gut, slowing the rate of carbohydrate absorption. It

PATIENTS' EXPERIENCES
"I used to inject a mixture of soluble and isophane insulin before breakfast and before my evening meal, but I found that my early-morning blood sugars were high. I increased the number of units of isophane insulin before my evening meal to bring these sugars down. There was no improve-ment; some mornings my sugar was high and on others it was low; I also started sweating through the night. I decided to increase my isophane further, but was admitted to hospital in a 'hypo' that night. The doctor explained that the second injection of isophane was acting most strongly in the early hours of the morning bringing my blood sugar very low; the high sugar before breakfast was my body's over-reaction to this. I now split my evening injection, and give the soluble before my bed-time snack. My blood sugars are now much better and I wake up in the morning feeling more refreshed."

Insulin, oral hypoglycaemic agents, guar, glucagon

Oral hypoglycaemic agents

Sulphonylureas
Chemical name: acetohexamide; **trade name:** Dimelor. **Chemical name:** chlorpropamide; **trade names:** Diabinese, Glymese, Melitase, Diabinese, Promide, Chloromide, Chloronase, Novopropamide, Stabinol. **Chemical name:** glibenclamide; **trade names:** Daonil, Dabeta, Semi-Daonil, Eugluton, Libanil, Malix, Gutril, Diamicron, Euglucon. **Chemical name:** glibornuride; **trade name:** Glutril. **Chemical name:** gliclazide; **trade name:** Diamicron. **Chemical name:** glipizide; **trade names:** Glibenese, Minodiab. **Chemical name:** gliquidone; **trade name:** Glurenorm. **Chemical name:** glymidine; **trade names:** Glondafon, Lycanol. **Chemical name:** tolazamide; **trade names:** Tolanase, Tolinase. **Chemical name:** tolbutamide; **trade names:** Glyconon, Pramidex, Rastinon, Artosin, Chembutamide, Mellitol, Mobenol, NeoDibetic, Novobutamide, Oramide, Orinase, Tolbutase.

Biguanides
Chemical name: metformin; **trade name:** Glucophage, Diabex SR. **Chemical name:** buformin; **trade name:** Silubin, Retard.

Guar
Chemical name: guar gum; **trade names:** Glucotard, Guarem, Guarina, Lejguar.

Glucagon
Chemical name: glucagon; **trade name:** Glucagon Novo, Glucagon Lilly.

reduces surges in blood glucose after meals.

Glucagon: another naturally-occurring hormone produced in the pancreas gland. It is not affected by diabetes and is not used for treating diabetes itself, but it is very useful in treating patients whose blood glucose has fallen to very low levels. It must be given by injection either under the skin or into muscle.

How it works: it causes blood glucose to rise by breaking down glycogen in the liver to glucose.

OVER-THE-COUNTER TREATMENTS
None.

QUESTIONS TO ASK THE DOCTOR
■ How much weight should I aim to lose?
■ How often and at what times of day should I test my blood glucose?
■ Will I always need to take tablets/insulin?
■ What will happen if I forget to inject my insulin? What should I do in this event?
■ I am travelling by plane to another country; how should I adjust my insulin regime?
■ Why should I monitor my diabetes with blood/urine tests even if I feel well?
■ Will I be able to have children and will they inherit diabetes?
■ What can I do to reduce the risk of diabetic complications?

SIDE EFFECTS
Insulin: Injecting too much insulin, not eating enough, and unaccustomed exercise without appropriate adjustment of diet or insulin dose can cause the blood glucose to fall too far. When this happens, the patient may first feel weak and hungry, then, as the blood glucose continues to fall, there is sweating, irritability, nervousness and dizziness; if this is not corrected, unconsciousness may follow. Not all diabetics experience identical symptoms in these insulin reactions, which are called 'hypos'. Insulin-dependent patients should experience a hypo under medical supervision so they know their own symptoms. Minor allergic reactions can occur at the sites of injection but these soon settle; if they do not, a change to a purer form of insulin may help. Sometimes the fat under the skin where insulin has been given decreases (atrophy) or increases (hypertrophy), leaving a lumpy appearance. If this should happen, change the site of your injection; a more purified insulin may also help.

Sulphonylureas can also lower the blood glucose too far if a meal is missed or with unaccustomed exercise. Some of these drugs can cause flushing of the face after drinking alcohol. If you are prone to this you may be at less risk of long-term complications. There is a tendency to gain weight while taking these drugs, so it is especially important to keep to your diet. Occasionally the drugs cause skin rashes and very occasionally they reduce the production of blood cells from the bone marrow.

Biguanides do not reduce blood glucose below normal, so 'hypos' do not occur. Patients who are obese often find it easier to lose weight while taking these drugs. They can reduce appetite and may cause an upset stomach; they are better taken with food. Diarrhoea is a common side effect, but this usually settles in about ten days. Very rarely, a serious upset of the metabolism can occur, but this is almost exclusively in patients with poor kidney function.

Guar may cause flatulence and abdominal distension.

Glucagon is used to treat coma caused by low blood glucose. It may be given by a relative or friend, and works within ten minutes. If there is no response, an injection of glucose into a vein by a doctor is necessary. Occasionally, glucagon causes nausea and vomiting.

SELF-MANAGEMENT

Patients needing insulin treatment have to be their own doctor, nurse, dietician and laboratory technician. From time to time, the dose of insulin may need adjustment and it is preferable that you learn how to do this safely yourself.

■ Try not to let your diabetes interfere with work or hobbies. Discuss with your doctor/specialist.

■ Join a local or national diabetes group. You will meet others who have learnt to overcome most of your problems.

■ Dietary treatment is important in all forms of diabetes and in many cases may be the sole remedy. The main principles of diet are:

■ To maintain body weight appropriate to height.

– To avoid all forms of sugar (except during a 'hypo').

– To eat less fat.

– To eat more fibre.

– To eat regular meals.

■ Monitor your diabetic control by measuring blood or urine glucose. If you are treated with insulin, blood tests are preferred. Blood glucose can be measured on a drop of blood from a finger prick using special reagent

A chain

B chain

The structure of insulin: *Proteins, of which insulin is one, have large, complicated chemical structures built up from building blocks called amino acids, shown as numbered circles in the diagram. Different combinations of these amino acids, of which there are about 30, make up different proteins. Insulin is composed of two chains of amino acids linked by sulphur bridges (-S-S-). Beef insulin differs from human insulin in the amino acids in positions A8, A10 and B30. Pork insulin differs from human insulin only in the amino acid at B30. Insulin is not a flat structure as depicted in the diagram; the chains are coiled to produce a three-dimensional molecule.*

strips which are read in a meter or by observing a colour change. Blood tests should be done before all meals at least two days a week. If you wake through the night for any reason, use the opportunity to check your blood glucose – the result may be surprising. For ideal control, blood glucose should be between four and seven mmol/L (72 to 126 mg%). But if you have frequent 'hypos', you should not try to control your diabetes as tightly as this.

Insulin-dependent diabetes cannot be so well-controlled by testing urine for glucose because usually glucose is only spilt into the urine when the blood glucose reaches ten mmol/L (180 mg%), and is merely a reflection of what the blood glucose has been since the bladder was last emptied. Urine testing may be adequate if you are not taking insulin; the urine should ideally be free from glucose at all times.

■ Learn how to adjust your insulin according to blood glucose results, meals and exercise. If blood glucose is high at the same time on two successive days, you may increase the appropriate insulin dose by two to four units; similarly, if you have 'hypos' regularly at the same time of day, you should reduce your insulin. Eating a snack between meals can also prevent 'hypos', and is necessary for most insulin-treated patients. Exercise will lower blood glucose, so take extra carbohydrate beforehand; you may also need to reduce your insulin.

■ Always carry glucose with you in case of a 'hypo'.
■ Don't smoke. Risk of damage to blood vessels, eyes and kidneys is vastly increased in diabetic smokers.
■ The blood vessels and nerves in the feet are particularly vulnerable to damage in diabetics, so inspect your feet regularly and report any signs of damage to your doctor or chiropodist (including ulcers, black areas or blisters). Never walk barefoot. Always wear well-fitting shoes with soft uppers. Do not immerse your feet in water warmer than 110°F/43°C. Do not sit too close to fires or use hot water bottles.
■ If you wish to become pregnant it is important that your diabetes is well-controlled before you conceive.
■ Even if you feel you are managing your diabetes well it is important to see your doctor regularly. He will be able to look for and treat complications which may not show symptoms until a late stage has developed.

SELF-HELP IN ATTACKS

Hypoglycaemia ('hypo' – low blood glucose) As soon as you recognize an attack coming on, take some glucose or a glucose drink. Have a snack as soon as possible afterwards. If you are driving your car, stop, get out of the driving seat and take some glucose and a snack before continuing – preferably someone else should drive. If you are found unconscious, then a relative or friend may give an injection of glucagon, provided they have been trained in its use. When you recover you should have a glucose-containing drink to prevent another 'hypo'. If you have not recovered in ten minutes, an ambulance should be called or you should be taken direct to hospital for an injection of glucose.

Intercurrent illness: If a diabetic is taken ill with an infection or fever, and has been vomiting or eaten little, there is a temptation to reduce the insulin. This is a mistake. Because of the stress of the current illness, the patient may need more insulin. Try to take the carbohydrate allowance in a more easily digestible form – as glucose drinks if necessary. If you start to pass large volumes of urine, feel thirsty, start losing weight or show ketones in the urine, consult your doctor.

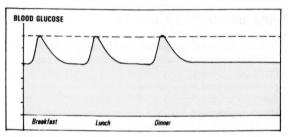

Blood glucose and insulin levels in non-diabetics taking three meals a day. *Insulin rises sharply with each meal to keep the blood glucose below six m mol/L. Insulin is present in the blood at all times, even if no food is eaten.*

Blood insulin levels in a diabetic *injecting a crystalline insulin zinc suspension in the evening and three soluble insulin injections before the main meals. Note how this approximates to the pattern of blood insulin levels in non-diabetics in the graph above.*

WHAT ARE LIPIDS?
– A collective term for fatty substances such as cholesterol and triglycerides – which are essential for making cell membranes, bile acids and some hormones; or as a source of energy. If there is too much of them in the blood there is an increased risk of heart disease. *See **angina**, page 46* and ***myocardial infarction**, page 52*.

Cholesterol and triglycerides are derived partly from diet, and partly from the body, which makes them.

CAUSES Heredity, or life-style (mainly diet); or both.

PRESCRIPTION DRUGS
Cholestyramine and **colestipol** are the first-line drug treatments for high-cholesterol, particularly in patients with a family history of hypercholesterolaemia (too much cholesterol in the blood).

How they work: by binding to bile acids in the intestine, causing them to be lost in the stools. The body uses cholesterol to replace these bile acids and thus its supply of cholesterol is depleted. Note that these drugs are not absorbed by the body, but lost in the stools together with the bile acids.

Probucol, clofibrate, bezafibrate, gemfibrozil and **nicotinic acid** plus its derivatives, are taken as tablets or capsules. Probucol lowers only cholesterol; the rest lower cholesterol and triglycerides.

How they work: complex and only partly understood.

Marine triglycerides: fish oils. Eskimos, whose diet is rich in fish, do not get much coronary heart disease; on this principle, oils have been developed to lower blood lipids. See OVER-THE-COUNTER treatments.

A new group of drugs which powerfully inhibit the manufacture of cholesterol in the body is under investigation.

OVER-THE-COUNTER TREATMENTS
Products such as Evening Primrose Oil, garlic and lecithin are variously promoted as lowering blood fats and/or reducing the tendency of the blood to clot within blood vessels. Evidence on their effectiveness is controversial and more careful research in man is required before they can be recommended as a serious remedy. The fish-oil concentrate, MaxEPA, is available (UK) on prescription and from chemists and health food shops.

QUESTIONS TO ASK THE DOCTOR
■ Why do I require drug treatment rather than a diet?

■ Is it safe to use this drug with others?

SIDE EFFECTS

The commonest side effects with **cholestyramine** and **colestipol** are constipation, nausea and bloating. Building up the dose gradually can help reduce these. A high roughage diet or a bulking agent should control constipation. **Probucol** is well tolerated but occasionally causes diarrhoea. **Clofibrate, bezafibrate** and **gemfibrozil** occasionally cause nausea, muscle pains or impotence. Clofibrate has been less widely used since it was suggested that it might be associated with an increase in unwanted side effects, such as gallstones, although it is still useful in certain patients. **Nicotinic acid** in large doses can cause nausea, flushing, itching and inflammation of the liver. Many of these will disappear spontaneously if the dose is increased gradually.

These drugs are not recommended in pregnancy or during lactation; probucol is discontinued six months before pregnancy. As with most drugs, inform your doctor if you are trying to become pregnant. If you start an unplanned pregnancy while taking one, stop the medication and get immediate medical advice.

SELF-MANAGEMENT

■ Diet, including weight reduction if necessary, is the first approach to lowering blood fats. If you can adhere to your diet, you may not need to take drugs at all. Even when taking drugs, keeping to the right diet may reduce the dose or improve the result. Take advice from a dietician.

In many, however, the high fat level is inherited, and not due to poor diet. For these patients it is often impossible to get a desirable level of blood fats without resorting to drugs.

Drugs for high lipid levels, like those for high blood pressure, only work while you are taking them. A prolonged reduction in lipid levels, and thus a reduction in risk of heart and blood vessel disease is only achieved if they are taken regularly and long-term.

■ If you think you are getting side effects from your drugs, seek medical advice.

■ Cholestyramine and colestipol are likely to work best if taken with or close to meals. They may interfere with the absorption of other drugs, which should therefore be taken at least an hour before.

■ If you are taking anticoagulants *(see page 64)*, let the clinic know of any change in your drug treatment in case it interferes with your lipid control.

Anti-thyroid drugs

WHAT IS HYPERTHYROIDISM?

The thyroid gland controls the rate at which body cells use energy. If the gland is over-active, the skin becomes hot and sweaty, the heart rate increases even during sleep; sleep is very light, and the patient may become over-active during the day. The heart muscle becomes excitable, with a rapid pulse, and an irregular rhythm known as atrial fibrillation – *see disorders of heart rhythm, page 56*. In more extreme forms the condition is described as *thyrotoxicosis* and there is often marked weight loss. Menstruating women will find that their periods become lighter and scantier. Often, but not always, there may be swelling of the thyroid gland producing the condition known as *goitre*, and some patients develop protruberant eyes, a condition called *exophthalmus*. Thyrotoxicosis occurs in women eight times more commonly than in men; it can occur at any age group but is more difficult to detect in the elderly. In young people the onset is often sudden.

Thyrotoxicosis can often be confused with an anxiety state – *see page 84* – it really can be difficult to tell them apart. Diagnosis of hyperthyroidism is made by blood tests to measure the levels of the hormone in the body, but a thyroid scan may be needed prior to commencing any treatment.

CAUSE Usually, a so-called *auto-immune* reaction in which the body inadvertently reacts against its own cells.

TREATMENT

There are three options:
1 Drug treatment: This usually stops production of most of the thyroid hormone.
2 Surgery, in which most of the gland is cut away and the remaining portion thus produces less hormone. This is often necessary in young people who have failed to respond to drugs and also in those with a goitre that is pressing against the wind-pipe.
3 Radio-active iodine: Thyroid gland tissue is destroyed by giving radioactive iodine. This diminishes the amount of hormone produced. It is often the treatment of choice in patients past child-bearing age.

Carbimazole is a widely used anti-thyroid drug. Treatment usually lasts for two years, and is then stopped. About 50 per cent will relapse and need some form of further treatment.

A beta-blocker such as propranolol is often used for temporary control of symptoms prior to surgery or other treatments. With all treatments there is a long-term risk of developing an under-active thyroid (hypo-thyroidism); *see page 166.* Low-dose replacement therapy with thyroxine is given in these circumstances.

OVER-THE-COUNTER TREATMENTS
None.

QUESTIONS TO ASK THE DOCTOR
■ Which treatment is best for me and why?
■ How long will it take to work?
■ What happens if the disease comes back after stopping treatment?
■ How often do I need a blood test?
■ How often do you need to see me?
■ Is the treatment safe if I am pregnant or breast-feeding?

SIDE EFFECTS
If an anti-thyroid drug is working properly, the symptoms of thyrotoxicosis will recede within four to eight weeks. However, the gland may become under-active *(see **hypothyroidism,** page 166),* and replacement therapy with thyroxine will be needed. The thyroid gland itself may swell as a result of treatment, and a goitre may develop; or a pre-existing goitre may enlarge, making surgery necessary. Skin rashes are relatively common and the doctor may change drugs if this occurs. Rarer side effects include headaches, nausea, hair loss, jaundice and, perhaps most important, the white cells in the blood may be reduced in number. This makes the patient susceptible to infections. Any sore throat or other infection should be reported. As with all treatments for thyrotoxicosis, there is a long-term risk of the thyroid gland eventually becoming permanently underactive, in which case replacement therapy will be needed. Beta-blockers are usually free of serious side effects but some patients may develop a tight chest if they have a tendency towards asthma. Cold fingers and feet are common and a few patients develop excessive tiredness while others complain of vivid dreams.

SELF-MANAGEMENT
Avoid stimulants such as ephedrine, found in some cough and cold treatments. Once treatment is finished, have an annual check of thyroid function. If you go to hospital or see another doctor, tell about your hyperthyroidism.

NAMES YOU WILL HEAR
Chemical name: L-thyroxine; **trade names:** Eltroxin, Oroxine, Synthroid. **Chemical name:** liothyronine (L-tri-iodothyronine); **trade names:** Tertroxin, Cytomel, Thyrolar.

WHAT IS HYPOTHYROIDISM?

The thyroid gland, one of a number of endocrine or hormonal glands, is in the front of the neck. It produces two hormones, the main one being thyroxine (T4), the other tri-iodothyronine (T3). These act on all the cells of the body to regulate the rate at which food is converted into energy. Iodine is essential for the manufacture of both the hormones. If the gland is not making the hormones, different illnesses result depending upon the age of the patient. **Cretinism** occurs in babies and young children. Body cells are starved of energy and are unable to develop; the infant is stunted and mentally handicapped. Treatment is usually undertaken in hospital. It is a very rare condition. **Myxoedema** occurs in adults and is relatively common. It nearly always comes on very slowly and may go unrecognized by patient, relatives and doctor. It is at least ten times commoner in women than in men and usually occurs after the age of 45. The body temperature falls; the heart rate slows; weight increases; the skin becomes rough and coarse, the hair thins and the face and eyelids can become puffy. Brain activity can become sluggish, especially in the elderly. Menstruating women may have heavy periods. If suspected the condition can easily be diagnosed by a blood test. It is then simply a question of starting treatment. Further blood tests will be necessary to make sure that the dose of hormone given is correct.

CAUSE Both conditions are caused by the thyroid gland not working. In the past, and even today in developing countries, iodine deficiency caused the gland to swell; the swelling is known as a goitre. In developed countries the main causes of underactivity are inflammation in the gland, or as a consequence of previous treatment for *hyperthyroidism* – see page 164 .

PRESCRIPTION DRUGS

L-thyroxine tablets are the usual treatment. Treatment is usually for life, in a once-a-day dose.
How it works: simply by replacing the substance that the body is unable to make.
L-tri-iodothyronine is rarely used except in severe cases when a rapid response to treatment is needed.
How it works: in the same way as L thyroxine.

Replacing the hormone does not mean that a child with cretinism will grow normally, or be mentally normal; but it will prevent any further deterioration. In adults with myxoedema, the majority of symptoms such as dry hair, coarse skin, cold intolerance and

Parathyroid glands — Thyroid gland

Trachea

slowness will slowly improve. However, it may be difficult to lose the weight that has been gained. A calorie-controlled diet, and considerable self-control, may be necessary.

OVER-THE-COUNTER TREATMENTS
None.

QUESTIONS TO ASK THE DOCTOR
■ How do I know that I am on the correct dose?
■ What should I do if I forget to take my tablets for a few days?
■ How often do I need to have a blood test?
■ How often will you want to see me?
■ Do I need to diet?

SIDE EFFECTS
Side effects in adults with myxoedema are usually related to either under- or over-dosage. Too little **L-thyroxine,** and the symptoms will not disappear. Too much, and the patient may develop some of the signs and symptoms of ***thyrotoxicosis,*** *page 164.* These may include a rapid pulse with palpitations, an irregular pulse, excessive weight loss, inability to sleep, hot sweaty skin and restlessness. In the elderly, the replacement of the hormone is always done gradually, building up by small increases to the full replacement dose. This may take months; suddenly giving a full dose may strain the heart and lead to angina or heart failure. If you develop any chest pain or discomfort, or breathlessness when you are starting treatment, especially if you are elderly, see your doctor soon.

SELF-MANAGEMENT
Be especially careful to maintain the directed dose; don't miss the blood tests arranged by your doctor. Maintaining stable replacement is the key to successful treatment. You will need a full check-up at least once a year. If you go into hospital or see a different doctor, don't forget to mention your thyroid condition, as it may affect treatment of other conditions.

THE PITUITARY GLAND AND ITS DISORDERS

The pituitary gland consists of two lobes, the anterior (front) and posterior (back). These are controlled by the hypothalamus – part of the under surface of the brain – to which the gland is joined by the pituitary stalk.

The most common diseases of the pituitary are benign tumours or adenomas of the anterior lobe. If these grow large, they may cause headaches and loss of visual field to one or both sides due to compression of optic nerve pathways. Large tumours may also cause decreased hormone secretion, characteristically affecting first the growth hormone (of minor consequence in adults) and also the gonadotrophins – the hormones which stimulate the testes and ovaries. Thus sexual disfunction is an early symptom of pituitary disorder, readily recognized by menstrual abnormality, or, in men, impotence and loss of libido.

Later, the production of hydrocortisone by the adrenal glands may be impaired, and this can have serious consequences: reduced ability to withstand such stresses as fevers, gastroenteritis, trauma or, surgery.

Thyroid deficiency is the other major consequence of pituitary tumour. Associated with it are lethargy, cold intolerance and modest obesity.

Some tumours of the pituitary are implicated in hormone overproduction, especially of prolactin, which interferes with function of the ovaries and testicles, and sometimes causes inappropriate milk production (galactorrhoea). Others cause growth hormone excess, leading to enlargement of soft tissue generally, and of certain bones: the condition known as acromegaly.

Pituitary overproduction of ACTH, the hormone which stimulates the production of hydrocortisone is a rare but serious condition called Cushings disease.

Pituitary tumours develop essentially only in the anterior lobe, and so do not directly affect the posterior lobe. But damage to the hypothalamus, which governs activity of both lobes, can cause not only all the features of anterior pituitary disease, but also loss of vasopressin or antidiuretic hormone (ADH). As a result, the kidney is unable to concentrate urine – the condition known as diabetes insipidus: large volumes of urine are passed by day and night and the sufferer has to heavily quench thirst and take precautions against dehydration.

PRESCRIPTION DRUGS

Hormone replacement therapy is designed to make good the deficiencies described opposite.

Adrenal insufficiency is usually treated with hydro-cortisone (cortisol) tablets – the natural hormone – or cortisone acetate.

Thyroid under-activity is simply treated with thyrox-ine, or occasionally its precursor tri-iodothyronine.

Sex hormone deficiencies in women are treated with oestrogens and progesterone-type tablets in 21-day cycles with seven days off, either as separate tablets of ethinyl oestradiol throughout the cycle, with medrox-yprogesterone acetate in the last half, or, more conve-niently, as a low-oestrogen contraceptive pill. Males are given injections of testosterone esters.

The management of growth hormone deficiency in children is usually confined to special centres.

Patients with diabetes insipidus have had their treat-ment revolutionized by the use of a synthetic near-relative of ADH, desmopressin.

Suppression of excessive hormone production: Irrespective of the cause, excessive levels of prolactin can usually be suppressed, often to normal, by the drug **bromocriptine;** it also gives control of galactorrhoea, and restoration of potency, menstruation and fertility.

OVER-THE-COUNTER TREATMENTS
None.

QUESTIONS TO ASK THE DOCTOR
■ Is it safe to continue hormone replacement therapy if I get another illness?

SIDE EFFECTS
Even with steroids such as cortisone, the doses of **hor-mones** used as replacement therapy *do not* generally cause side effects. Occasionally they may cause poten-tially serious dyspeptic symptoms: seek medical advice soon, but don't stop taking the tablets. **Bromocriptine** can cause nausea, giddiness and indigestion which, though not dangerous are often severe, even disabling. It is therefore all the more important to lessen the chances of these side effects by building up the dose slowly, starting with half a tablet last thing at night in the middle of a snack, and aiming eventually to take tablets during the three main meals.

SELF-MANAGEMENT
See **QUESTIONS TO ASK THE DOCTOR.** It is important to understand that steroid dose should be doubled under certain circumstances – for example stress from another illness. DISCUSS THIS WITH YOUR DOCTOR.

PATIENT'S EXPERIENCE
"After suffering from headaches for years, I eventually consulted my doctor, whom I had not seen for ages. I wasn't surprised to find I had high blood pressure, but I was when told this was not the cause of the headaches but probably a disease of the pituitary gland called acromegaly. He referred me to a specialist in hormone disorders who surprised me even more by revealing how long I must have had the condition, judging from old photographs. At first I was upset by his talk of a pituitary tumour and by the delving into my sex life, which had been non-existent. But I was assured that tumour in this context meant swelling, not cancer. Treatment was with tablets of bromocriptine at first, and later a remarkably minor operation which left no scar as it was done through the nose from behind the upper lip. My skin soon became less greasy, followed by quite a marked reduction in the soft tissues in my face, hands and feet – while I also experienced a return of my libido and potency, which I had presumed had gone forever."

Obstetrics, gynaecology, urinary and children

The genito-urinary system has evolved for the dual functions of reproduction and excretion. Disorders can be hormonal, infective, or structural – and many are still poorly understood.

IMPOTENCE	**172-173**
INFERTILITY	**174-177**
CONTRACEPTION	**178-183**
DRUGS IN PREGNANCY	**184-187**
URINARY INCONTINENCE	**188-189**
PERIOD PROBLEMS	**190-193**
PROBLEMS OF MENOPAUSE	**194-195**
DRUGS IN CHILDREN	**196-199**

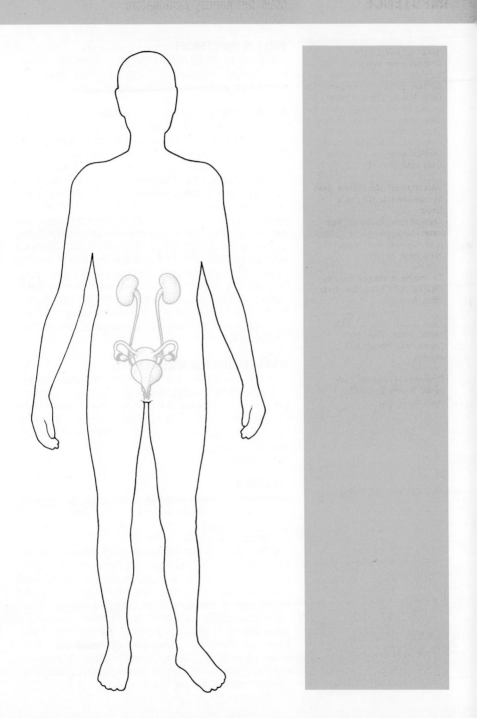

WHAT IS IMPOTENCE?

– A failure to obtain or maintain an erection for satisfactory sexual intercourse. This includes premature ejaculation and failure of pleasurable ejaculation.

CAUSES Either psychological, physical, or a combination of both. In order to have an erection, men need an adequate nerve and blood supply to the penis; male hormones are also necessary but their role in creating libido – sexual appetite – is more important. Poor blood supply is caused by: blockage of the lower aorta, as may happen with *atherosclerosis, page 52;* or by blocked small blood vessels as may may happen with *diabetes, page 156.* Poor nerve supply can have a multitude of causes: alcohol; spinal injury; antihypertensive drugs, especially beta-blockers and methyldopa; diseases such as multiple sclerosis and ageing. The underlying causes of psychological impotence are of course complex, but it is probably fair to summarize them as fear of failure; anxiety; inexperience; communication problems with sexual partner; depression; drug treatment for depression, paradoxically; and deep rooted fears related to sex.

WHAT THE DOCTOR WILL ASK YOU

How long has it been a problem? Was the onset gradual or sudden? Is it related to some work or family problem? What was intercourse like before? What is the attitude of your present partner(s)? Do you wake with erections in the morning? Can you get an erection at all? Do you ejaculate, get a sensation of orgasm? Do you masturbate?

TREATMENT

Counselling of both partners is the usual recourse for psychological impotence. This may be undertaken by a GP, a psychologist, a psychosexual clinic, or marriage guidance counsellors.

If the cause is not obviously psychological, the patient may need blood tests for hormone and blood sugar levels. If hospital investigations are considered necessary, penile tumescence (swelling) studies and penile rigidity measurements, often performed overnight, can confirm absence or presence of erections while asleep. If they are present, the problem is probably psychological. Injection of **vasodilator** drugs directly into the penile tissue will re-establish erections in most patients if the penile blood supply is adequate. This can be self-taught.

Penile implants (semi-rigid or inflatable) are an excellent option in irreversible impotence: failure rate is low – less than 5 per cent. The implant is inserted inside the penile tissue. Semi-rigid implants give a semi-permanent erection, but are not too unsightly.

Testosterone is only prescribed when the level of this hormone is low, typically as a result of removal of testes. In such cases it will restore performance.

QUESTIONS TO ASK THE DOCTOR
- Why have I become impotent?
- Am I too old to be treated?
- If my wife is no longer interested, will I be treated?
- Would marriage guidance counselling help me?

SIDE EFFECTS
Intracorporeal **vasodilators** do have drawbacks which make them unsuitable in the long term: bruising and scarring of the penile tissue can occur or a painful, prolonged erection. Penile implants have a low failure rate. The main problem is infection, but this is uncommon if antibiotics are given at the time of operation and the surgery is done carefully.

Testosterone can cause jaundice: regular liver function tests are required. If there is evidence of liver damage, the treatment is stopped. The hormone also increases the individual's level of aggression.

SELF-HELP (PSYCHOLOGICAL IMPOTENCE)
Admit to yourself that impotence is a problem and see a doctor. This creates a situation in which the problem can be discussed between the man, his partner and the doctor in a relatively rational manner. Also, frankly discuss with your partner aspects of each other's behaviour that you like or dislike, if this seems to cause problems. Try a return to petting without necessarily having sexual intercourse. Many counsellors advise a ban on intercourse at the beginning of treatment – to get rid of the large component of fear of failure.

Inflatable penile implant
Two implants, one for each of the erectile spaces of the penis.

WHAT IS INFERTILITY?

The practical definition is when the female has failed to conceive after two years of normal sexual relations. If pregnancy has occurred, but the outcome has been unsuccessful, the couple are considered to be subfertile, a condition outside the scope of this section.

If pregnancy is to occur without medical assistance, it usually does so in the first year; however, about a quarter of pregnancies do occur in the second year. Estimates of the true level of infertility vary in different societies and social groups; however, it is generally agreed that at least ten per cent of couples are infertile and recent studies indicate that the real prevalence is nearer 20 per cent.

Of those who have investigation and treatment, between 30 per cent and 60 per cent will eventually produce a live baby. Sadly, however, there remains a large group who will never be able to produce a child of their own. Modern treatments are certainly offering hope, but this too can bring problems. Having hopes raised, only to be dashed, can only prolong the agony of facing up to, and dealing with, childlessness. Couples faced with the possibility of infertility need more than average patience and realism.

CAUSES The most common factor remains disorders of ovulation. These can be detected in over 40 per cent of infertile couples. Abnormalities of the husband's semen are discovered in 30 per cent. Blocked or damaged Fallopian tubes and scarring also involving the ovary are also common, found in 20 per cent of women.

Problems with the neck of the womb and immunological factors are rare causes.

Less than four per cent of couples have unexplained infertility – that is to say all the tests are normal. Many of these couples do eventually conceive.

In about ten per cent, abnormalities in both partners are detected. This does not mean pregnancy cannot occur; treatment of both partners should take place simultaneously.

TREATMENT

The treatment depends, of course, on the cause.

Disorders of ovulation are complex and involve the use of a wide range of drugs.

Many of the problems with the Fallopian tubes, and often with the ovaries, are caused by previous infection. Usually this has been silent and symptomless, but where a diagnosis of salpingitis, (infection in the tubes), has been made, drug treatment should be intensive and active: see below. Sometimes endometriosis is the cause of infertility, or associated with it, and here drug therapy is combined with surgery *(see **period problems**, page 190).*

If the Fallopian tubes and/or ovaries are physically damaged, rather than infected, microsurgery is the first line of treatment. Success rate varies from 20 per cent to 80 per cent, depending on the nature of the problem. The next option is IVF, (*in vitro* fertilization) – a 'test tube pregnancy', which usually involves the use of drugs to produce superovulation. The overall success rate of IVF remains low, probably less than ten per cent, but as the technique is refined, success rates may well rise as high as 30 per cent.

New techniques using drugs to produce superovulation are currently being researched.

When the only problem identified is with the husband's semen, the first-line treatment is surgical; drug therapy may also be used; both tend to be unrewarding.

PRESCRIPTION DRUGS

To understand specific drug treatment of infertility, it is essential to appreciate the biochemical events of the female reproductive cycle: read what follows in association with the diagram and caption on page *193.*
Steroids have been used to treat cervical and immunological problems in the woman and also to treat the male. The treatment is not without risk or side effect and conception rates are no higher than those that occur naturally.

How they work: by suppressing antibodies that sometimes interfere with normal sperm movement.

A variety of drugs including **oestrogens, progestogens** and **clomiphene** have been used to treat those with unexplained infertility. One study showed a 50 per cent success rate using a six-month treatment programme. The first two months of treatment involved no drugs, blood tests and continual emotional support and encouragement of the female partner. The following four months involved a variety of different drug combinations to induce ovulation. One of the patients who successfully conceived had been trying to have a child for 12 months, and she conceived during the first two months of the programme.

Ovulation inducers: Choice depends on the cause of ovulatory failure. The commonest problem is oversen-

sitive feedback with suppression of the pituitary production of FSH by circulating oestrogen. Cyclofenil and
clomiphene citrate block the oestrogen receptor sites in
the brain, thus resetting the mechanism. Where this
does not work on its own, another drug may be added,
for example, chorionic gonadotrophin. This works by
adding a surge of LH when it is needed. The injections
of both FSH and LH can be used to mimic the natural
production by the pituitary. Pergonal, Profasi and
Metrodin are used for this.

More recent techniques involve suppressing or
down-regulating natural production of LH/FSH to get
better control with injected hormones.

Other sophisticated techniques act even more
radically, and involve hormones produced in the brain
which actually release LH and FSH. A special pump
may be used to inject gradually the gonadotrophin-
releasing hormone. Combinations of these drugs are
used in the IVF regime.Bromocryptine can be used to
lower the level of prolactin, thus allowing FSH and LH
to stimulate the ovaries.

OVER-THE-COUNTER TREATMENTS
None.

The moment of conception – *in a
test tube. The technique involves
removing a number of eggs from
the ovaries and culturing them with
sperm. Four days later, a few of
the successfully fertilized eggs are
returned to the womb.*

QUESTIONS TO ASK THE DOCTOR
■ At what time in the month am I most fertile?
■ What is the success rate with this/these drugs?
■ Are there any special problems I am likely to run into when taking drugs, like having twins, for example?
■ If my husband's sperm count is low, are there any simple measures that may improve it?
■ If all the tests are normal, is there anything else we can do?

SIDE EFFECTS
The milder **ovulation inducers,** cyclofenil and clomiphene citrate, produce fairly minor side effects such as flushes, sometimes breast tenderness, irritability, mid-cycle pain and feeling bloated. Occasionally, particularly with higher doses, over-stimulation of the ovaries occurs, with pain and cyst formation. Up to 10 per cent of clomiphene-induced pregnancies are twins.

More complex regimes of ovulation treatment require careful monitoring of hormone levels to reduce the risk of over-stimulation of the ovaries. Such complex treatment is not available in all hospitals. Bromocryptine commonly produces side effects and the dose has to be built up slowly. It should always be taken with meals to avoid nausea and vomiting. A general feeling of malaise, headaches and dizziness are also common. **Steroids** can produce severe side effects *(see **anaemia**, page 224)* but in short courses these are unusual.

SELF-MANAGEMENT
■ Don't let your life revolve around the presence or absence of the next menstrual cycle. Don't blame yourself, your partner or your doctor for your failure to conceive. Cultivate interests other than your desire for a child.
■ The period of maximum fertility starts 19 days before a woman's next period is due and lasts about five days.
■ If the sperm count is low, it may be improved by wearing loose fitting underpants and trousers.
■ Let neither partner get so obsessed about sexual intercourse and its frequency that the other begins to wonder whether their role has been down-graded to that of baby-producer.
■ Keep hopeful, but be realistic. If success eludes you, do not deny to yourself the fact that you may never have a child. Try to change your view so that pregnancy would become a bonus rather than the likely eventual outcome.

NAMES YOU WILL HEAR
Chemical names: combined contraceptive pills contain ethinyl oestradiol in varying doses and a progestogen. Progestogen-only pills (in italics) contain just progestogen. Trade names: Trinordiol, Logynon, Trinovum, Marvelon, Neocon, Norimin, Ovysmen, Brevinor, Microgynon 30, Ovranette, Eugynon 50, Minilyn, Norinyl-1, Anovlar, Gynovlar, Femulen, Micronor, Microval, Triphasil, Biphasil, Nordette, Eugynon, Orthonovum 1/50, Microlut, Triquilar, Marvelon, Brevinor-1, Lyndiol, Femulen, Noriday, Orthonovum 777, Ortho-novum 1/35, Brevicon, Minovral, Ovral, Norinyl-1 & 50, Trinordiol, Trinovum, Nordiol, Micronovum, Mocroval.

WHAT IS CONTRACEPTION?

– Literally, the prevention of pregnancy. This can be achieved by using hormones, barriers, or coils or, more permanently, by sterilization. The ideal contraceptive, one that is one hundred per cent effective and one hundred per cent safe does not exist, so couples must decide which method is most appropriate. Means of prevention divide into two broad types: hormonal (this page, and pages 179-180); and 'others' (pages 181-183). 'Others' comprise barriers, coils and sterilization.

PRESCRIPTION DRUGS

The combined pill: This is the most popular hormonal method. Many different brands are available, but they all contain two hormones: oestrogen and progestogen.

How it works: by stopping the woman making an egg each month. It also makes the womb less receptive to the egg, and makes it harder for sperm to swim into the womb. It should be taken regularly for 21, 22 or 28 days depending on which type you have. If it is taken for 21 or 22 days, bleeding usually occurs in the seven or six days when the pill is not taken. If a 28-day packet is taken, bleeding usually occurs in the last few days of taking the pill.

The progestogen-only pill (POP): This pill is little-used in the UK. Many brands are available, but they all contain one hormone called progestogen. It is taken every day without a break, and should be taken at the same time of day every day.

How it works: Although it may prevent the normal release of eggs, it mainly works by making it harder for sperm to swim into the womb. It also makes the womb less receptive to the egg.

The 'morning after' pill: An emergency-only measure. It is mis-named: you can take it up to 72 hours after unprotected intercourse. It consists of a strong dose of oestrogen and progestogen (usually given as two tablets) followed by another dose 12 hours later.

How it works: either by stopping the egg being released, or, if this has already occurred, it can prevent the egg settling in the womb.

Injectables: A large dose of one hormone, progestogen, by injection every three months.

How it works: prevents the egg being released; also makes it harder for the sperm to swim into the womb.

OVER-THE-COUNTER TREATMENTS

None.

QUESTIONS TO ASK THE DOCTOR

■ Why is it so important to start taking the pill at the right time of my menstrual cycle?
■ What should I do if I am sick or have diarrhoea while on the pill?
■ Can other medicines interfere with taking the pill?

SIDE EFFECTS

The combined pill is nearly one hundred per cent effective in preventing pregnancy. It has many beneficial effects such as making periods lighter and less painful. It also reduces the risk of infection in the Fallopian tubes. It reduces the chance of cancer of the womb and ovary. Annoying problems such as sickness and breast tenderness usually settle in a couple of months. However, taking the pill does carry some serious, albeit rare, risks. These include blood clots (which may cause strokes and heart attacks) and, in a few people, increased blood pressure. Studies of the risk of cancer of the neck of the womb, and of breast cancer, are conflicting and confusing. Some have found an apparent link between breast cancer and the use of this pill at a young age (less than 25), or before the birth of the first baby. Other studies have completely failed to find any such link. Until further evidence is available, the experts feel there should be no change in prescribing policy. If concerned, discuss this with your doctor.

The progestogen-only pill is not as effective as the combined pill, especially in younger women. It may be taken by many women for whom the combined pill is unsuitable – for example, breast-feeding mothers, heavy smokers and diabetics. The major problem is irregular bleeding: some women taking it have no periods, others bleed much of the time. It is not suitable for women who have previously had a pregnancy in a Fallopian tube.

The 'morning-after' pill: Many women suffer sickness after taking these pills. Their next period may be either earlier or delayed. It is not suitable for women who have previously had a blood clot. It may not work in one in 50 of those treated.

Injectables: Some women have heavy bleeding after the injection, and the injection cannot, like a pill, be stopped once given. It takes some women longer to become pregnant once they have stopped using this method, compared with the other hormonal methods.

SELF-MANAGEMENT AND SELF-HELP

■ When asking for the pill, be honest with your doctor

about any health problems, either of your own, or among close blood relatives. The pill may not be suitable for you if there is a history of cardio-vascular disease in close relatives.

■ Stop smoking. This dramatically reduces the risk of any of the serious problems associated with taking the combined pill.

■ Remember to take the pill. If you forget a combined pill (and anything longer than 12 hours is a forgotten pill) you must use additional precautions for the next seven days. If that seven days takes you beyond the end of the current packet, you must take two packets consecutively – do not have a break that month.

If you take the POP you have only three hours to remember your pill. If forgotten you must use additional precautions for 48 hours.

■ If you bleed while taking your pills, do not worry; carry on taking the pill and mention it to your doctor at your next visit.

■ If you have heavy bleeding after the injection, see your doctor, who may give you some tablets that will help with the problem.

■ If you miss a period with any of these methods, carry on taking the pill and arrange to see your doctor.

■ See your doctor immediately if you: develop pain or swelling of the legs; develop pain in the chest or stomach; develop breathlessness or cough up blood; have a bad fainting attack or collapse; develop an unusual headache, blurred vision or difficulty with speech; develop numbness or weakness of an arm or leg; notice your skin or eyes have become yellow.

BARRIERS, COILS, STERILIZATION BARRIERS

These comprise caps, diaphragms, the sheath and the 'Today' sponge; all require enthusiasm from the couple if they are to be effective.

Caps and diaphragms should be used with a spermicide to ensure maximum effectiveness. They are not as effective as the hormonal methods in preventing pregnancy. They may be inserted into the vagina several hours before intercourse; however, if intercourse does not occur within three hours, additional spermicide is required. They need initial fitting by a specially-trained nurse or doctor and require practice before they can be fitted reliably by the user.

Sheaths are male-only and can have a high failure rate, especially when used by less experienced couples. They can protect against many sexually transmitted diseases.

The 'Today' sponge is, like the sheath, available over-the-counter. It should be moistened prior to use. Insert it into the vagina several hours before intercourse, but do not remove once intercourse has occurred for at least six hours. Unfortunately it has a high failure rate – approximately one in five users become pregnant during 12 months' use.

SELF-MANAGEMENT AND SELF-HELP
■ If using a cap or diaphragm, check every time that the cervix is properly covered.
■ Ensure that the sheath covers the penis before *any* genital contact occurs.
■ Withdraw the penis before it becomes too soft. Hold the base of the condom during withdrawal so as not to spill any semen.
■ Use each condom once only.
■ If the sheath should break or come off, or if you find the cap or diaphragm was not in the correct place, see your doctor who may prescribe the 'morning after' pill.

INTERUTERINE DEVICES (COILS)
A coil is a solid object placed in the womb to prevent pregnancy. There are three varieties: inert, copper-bearing and hormone-releasing. The device is usually inserted immediately after a period. It may also be used to prevent pregnancy if unprotected intercourse has occurred and hormonal treatment cannot be given. It may be used up to five days after the egg was released.

EFFECTS AND SIDE EFFECTS
The main effect is to stop the fused egg and sperm attaching to the womb. The hormone-releasing IUDs may also prevent sperms swimming into the womb.

Most coils cause periods to become heavier and longer than normal; periods may also become more painful than usual. They also appear to increase the risk of pelvic infection. (This is infection in the Fallopian tubes – a serious matter which may prevent a future pregnancy.) Coils are not the ideal method for women who have never had children. However, they are a useful method for women who have already had at least one child as there is then little increased risk of infection.

Coils prevent pregnancy first and foremost inside the womb, so if pregnancy occurs in a woman using a coil it is more likely to be in a Fallopian tube. Coils should not be used by women who have had previous tubal pregnancies.

SELF-HELP AND SELF-MANAGEMENT
■ Since the coil may increase the risk of pelvic infection, think very carefully before using one if you have already had an infection.
■ If you have more than one partner (or at the time of changing a partner), use a sheath as well as a coil to help prevent infection.
■ Your doctor will leave the threads attached to your coil so you can feel them by the neck of your womb. Check for these threads after your period. If you cannot feel them, use additional contraception and see your doctor.
■ See your doctor immediately if you miss a period, develop bad stomach pains, get pains when you make love or develop a heavy vaginal discharge.

QUESTIONS TO ASK THE DOCTOR
■ What type of coil should I have?
■ How long can the coil remain in the womb?
  Different types of coil can be left different lengths of time.

STERILIZATION
This is the most effective form of contraception of all and very difficult to reverse. Either partner may be sterilized. Technically, the procedure is easier in the male. However it may not always be appropriate for the male to be sterilized – men are fertile for most of their lives, whereas women are only fertile for 30 to 40 years. A woman can often be sure she never wants children even if she was with a new partner, whereas a man cannot be so sure what any future, possibly younger, partner might want. The procedure is straightforward in either sex. However, counselling is most important. Both partners must be certain they want no further children, whatever may happen. Sterilization is not a solution to sexual problems, a failing marriage or contraceptive problems.

SIDE EFFECTS
In the male, the operation – a vasectomy – is usually performed under out-patient conditions under local anaesthetic. The tubes that carry the sperm from the testes to the penis are cut and tied or cauterized. This does not interfere with subsequent sexual performance. The operation takes a few weeks to become effective.
  In a woman the operation is usually performed under general anaesthetic, although local anaesthetic can be

used. The Fallopian tubes which carry the eggs to the womb are either cut, burnt or blocked with clips or rings. The stomach wall has to be opened surgically to gain access.

QUESTIONS TO ASK THE DOCTOR
■ How is the operation performed?
■ How much time off work is required?
■ How long after the operation is it effective?

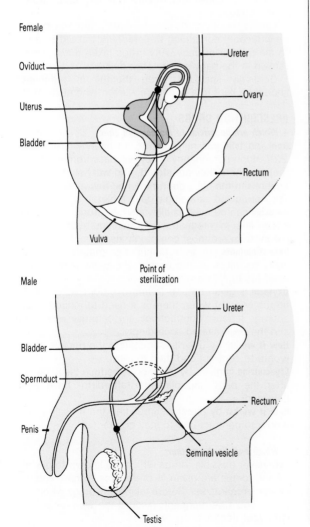

Female

Oviduct

Uterus

Bladder

Ureter

Ovary

Rectum

Vulva

Point of sterilization

Male

Bladder

Spermduct

Penis

Ureter

Rectum

Seminal vesicle

Testis

NAMES YOU WILL HEAR
Chemical name: rubella vaccine; **trade name:** Almevax. **Chemical name:** ferrous fumarate and folic acid; **trade names:** Pregaday, Bramiron, Hematon, Filabon.

Analgesics during labour
Chemical name: nitrous oxide and oxygen; **trade name:** Entonox. **Chemical name:** lignocaine hydrochloride with adrenalin injection; **trade name:** Lignocaine and Adrenalin Injection.

Oxytocics
Chemical name: oxytocin; **trade names:** Syntocinon, Pitocin. **Chemical name:** ergometrine maleate and oxytocin; **trade name:** Ergometrine and Oxytocin Injection. **Chemical name:** ritodrine; **trade name:** Yutopar.

Antacids – *see* **peptic ulcer**, *page 26.*

Beta-stimulants – *see* **asthma**, *page 74.*

Anti-emetics – *see* **dizziness**, *page 96.*

Antibiotics – *see* **pneumonia and pleurisy**, *page 78.*

Antihypertensive drugs – *see* **hypertension**, *page 48.*

Laxatives – *see* **constipation**, *page 30.*

Antihistamines – *see* **hay fever**, *page 260.*

PREGNANCY

During the first three months after conception, most of a baby's organs are being formed. This is a vulnerable time: any illness in the mother or drugs taken during this period has the potential to cause abnormalities or deformities in the baby (the foetus). After the first three months, the foetus is almost completely formed; it continues to grow, and the organs to mature. Any drugs taken during this period, or indeed illness in the mother, is unlikely to cause abnormality, but may affect growth of the foetus.

Labour usually starts spontaneously, but may have to be induced if continuing the pregnancy could be a risk to the mother or baby. Any drugs taken during labour remain in the baby's body after delivery.

Generally speaking, drug therapy in pregnancy should be kept to a minimum – even when essential.

PRESCRIPTION DRUGS

– Which are beneficial to mother and child:

Iron and **folic acid** help to prevent anaemia *(see page 224)* during pregnancy. They will pass from mother to foetus, where they are stored, and will help to prevent anaemia in the baby during the first few months of life. They are given as a single daily tablet.

Antacids can be used to alleviate heartburn, which may occur late in pregnancy. Aluminium hydroxide and magnesium are most commonly used.

Beta-stimulants are given to inhibit premature labour, initially by injection into a vein; the dose may be continued in tablet form.

Oxytocin is given by drip to improve contraction of the uterus (womb) when there is a need to induce or encourage labour. Contractions are carefully monitored and the dose altered accordingly.

How it works: by directly stimulating the muscle of the womb to contract and then to relax.

Ergometrine is given by injection to reduce bleeding just after the baby and placenta (afterbirth) have been delivered.

How it works: by directly stimulating the muscle of the womb to contract and to stay contracted.

– Which benefit the mother:

Whenever possible, drugs which are known to be safe for the foetus are given in preference to new and improved preparations. Before taking any drugs when you are or could be pregnant, discuss the possible effects with your doctor.

Anti-emetics (promethazine and meclozine) should only be used for persistent vomiting and not for nausea. See SIDE EFFECTS.

Certain **antibiotics** are safe in pregnancy, including penicillins and erythromycin. It is seldom necessary to use one which causes problems. Those to avoid include sulphonamides, tetracyclines, and cotrimoxazole.

Anti-asthmatic preparations can be safely used during pregnancy. Some, such as salbutamol, are beta-stimulants and can delay the onset of labour; treatment may have to be changed just before the baby is due.

In some women hypertension (high blood pressure) is a complication of pregnancy; it requires treatment as it can decrease the blood supply to the foetus and retard growth. Not all **antihypertensives** are safe during pregnancy, but many drugs are safe and effective.

Antidiabetic preparations: Young diabetics are usually on insulin, and the dose will probably have to be adjusted during pregnancy. Proper control of diabetes during pregnancy is vital, otherwise there is risk to the foetus.

Anti-epileptics must be continued during pregnancy if a patient is subject to fits. Unfortunately, some anti-epileptic drugs can affect the foetus, so if you are an epileptic, discuss this with your doctor *before* getting pregnant. He may be able to recommend a more suitable drug.

Many **analgesics,** including aspirin and indomethacin, are better not used during pregnancy. A few, such as ibuprofen, are relatively safe. Discuss with your doctor.

Pain relief during labour: Nitrous oxide and oxygen mixture can be used to ease the discomfort of contractions without loss of consciousness. It is usually inhaled through a mask which the mother can use herself as and when necessary. Pethidine is a strong analgesic which can be given by injection during labour.

Epidural anaesthesia is an injection of local anaesthetic (lignocaine) into the spine. It suppresses all pain stimuli from nerves in the lower half of the body, and can be used for normal deliveries, forceps-assisted deliveries and even Caesarian section operations. The mother is fully conscious, but pain-free.

X-rays may be a risk during pregnancy, depending on whether they are of the abdomen, and the dose.

OVER-THE-COUNTER TREATMENTS

Many commonly-used drugs may affect the foetus. Before taking anything, think whether it is absolutely necessary and safe. Drugs you can take include

PATIENT'S EXPERIENCE
"I was 12 weeks pregnant with my first baby when I developed a high temperature, vomiting and pain on passing urine. I had stopped smoking a few months before I became pregnant and had been quite well. I was afraid to take any medicines and went straight to my doctor. He sent a specimen of urine to the laboratory and started me on an antibiotic which he said was safe in pregnancy. He said that I could take paracetamol for the pain, but that he would not give me anything for the vomiting unless it was very severe. The symptoms improved quite quickly and I was well for the rest of my pregnancy."

paracetamol and laxatives which work by increasing the bulk of the stool. Drugs to avoid include: aspirin, laxatives which stimulate the bowel, antihistamines, cough mixtures containing iodine, cigarettes, alcohol and drugs of addiction. See SIDE EFFECTS.

QUESTIONS TO ASK THE DOCTOR
■ Are you sure this drug is safe during pregnancy?
■ What kind of sedation can I have during labour?

SIDE EFFECTS
Iron and **folic acid:** *See anaemia, page 224.*
Oxytocin can cause excessive uterine contractions which in turn may affect blood supply to the foetus. It can also cause hypertension and fluid retention in the mother: the latter tend to be dose-related, and are thus usually controlled. **Ergometrine** cannot be used until after delivery as it causes marked and sustained uterine contraction.
Beta stimulants: *See asthma, page 74.* Some **anti-emetics** have been used for many years with no adverse effects, but they have also been associated with foetal abnormalities. **Tetracyclines** can discolour the teeth of the child, **sulphonamides** can damage the red blood cells and cause anaemia; **co-trimoxazole** can, in theory, cause foetal abnormalities.
Methyldopa has no specific side effects in pregnancy, likewise insulin in the correct dose. **Anti-epileptic drugs** which may cause foetal abnormalities include sodium valproate, phenytoin and phenobarbitone. Substitutes can sometimes be found, but if one of the above drugs is the only one which adequately controls the fits, its benefit will outweigh the risk to the foetus. *See epilepsy, page 110.* **Aspirin** causes abnormalities of blood clotting in the foetus and may lead to haemorrhage. Many of the **anti-inflammatory analgesics** can cause heart problems in the foetus and prolonged labour. Ibuprofen can however be used: for side effects *see rheumatoid arthritis, page 242.*
Nitrous oxide and **oxygen mixture,** and **pethidine,** may suppress uterine contractions (prolonging labour) but this is not usually significant. Epidural anaesthetic may cause headache and a fall in blood pressure. Sometimes the anaesthetic fails to reach all nerve fibres, and pain is not suppressed.
Laxatives like senna which work by increasing the contractions of the bowel may also stimulate uterine contraction and precipitate labour; in large doses, they may also cause diarrhoea. **Antihistamines** may cause abnor-

malities in the foetus. Cough mixtures containing iodine may produce a goitre in the foetus. **Nicotine** inhaled with cigarette smoke constricts the blood vessels and can thus reduce blood supply to the foetus, resulting in a small baby and an increased risk of mental retardation and other abnormalities. **Alcohol** taken even in moderate amounts is implicated in higher incidence of foetal abnormality, including mental retardation. **Drugs of addiction** can cause foetal abnormalities, and if present in the mother at the time of birth, can cause irritability and withdrawal symptoms in the foetus.

SELF-MANAGEMENT

Before pregnancy, ensure that you are fit by:
■ Maintaining a healthy diet; try not to be overweight at the start of the pregnancy.
■ Giving up smoking.

During pregnancy:
■ Keep up with your antenatal examinations; they really are important for enabling doctors to detect early signs of complications such as hypertension. ■ Report any unusual symptoms to your doctor. ■ Avoid taking any drug unless it is absolutely necessary – even before you are pregnant. ■ Guard against excessive weight gain. Beside the obvious discomfort, it can exacerbate hypertension. Don't attempt to 'eat for two': small, frequent meals tend to be best, avoiding foods high in carbohydrate. Keep active: boredom can be a cause of weight gain. ■ Don't curtail normal activities unless advised by a doctor: if working, you can usually continue quite late into pregnancy. ■ Minimize constipation by using a high-fibre diet. *See* **constipation**, *page 30.* ■ Lessen the nausea of early pregnancy by eating small meals, frequently. The same applies to heartburn. ■ Minimize backache with a firm bed, sound posture and a regular daily rest. ■ Go to antenatal classes: the exercises they teach you really will help deal with the pain of labour.

Labour:
■ Air your feelings about how much pain relief you want. Preferably discuss it with your doctor before confinement; certainly raise it with the midwife as soon as you have started labour.
■ If you have a Caesarian section, consider the possibility of an epidural, and so remain conscious during the whole procedure. Many mothers prefer this, and most doctors feel that it improves bonding.

PATIENT'S EXPERIENCE
"My doctor told me that because I am quite short, I would probably need a Caesarian section instead of normal delivery. I asked him if I could have it under epidural anaesthetic and he said that it would probably be possible and explained the procedure. I was given the epidural quite soon after contractions started: I could feel my abdomen and legs going numb. They wheeled me into the operating theatre and draped sterile sheets over me ready to do the Caesarian. I couldn't see where the doctors were cutting because I was lying flat, and I couldn't feel a thing. The doctor told me that he was taking the baby out and then I heard her cry. The nurse wrapped her in a towel and gave her to me immediately. My husband and I were thrilled – he had been with me the whole time. I was able to get up and about much quicker than other mothers who had had general anaesthetics."

URINARY INCONTINENCE

Imipramine. propantheline, emepronium, terodiline

IN THE ELDERLY
The cause of the incontinence should be sought and treated appropriately. Loss of bladder control in old people should not be regarded as 'normal'.

General measures to assist old people include: enabling them to be as mobile as possible; advising against restrictive clothing; moving the bedroom closer to the lavatory, and/or providing the old-fashioned expedient of a commode; minimizing use of tranquillizers and sleeping tablets – they can make incontinence worse; reminders to go to the lavatory may be helpful, particularly in mildly confused patients. ■ Diuretic therapy, see page 52, can cause incontinence. It may be possible to adjust the timing of tablets to fit in with the patient's daily activity. If possible, diuretics should not be taken after 4 pm. Discuss with the doctor. ■ Poor motivation makes incontinence more likely: give plenty of encouragement. ■ Any acute illness or move to unfamiliar surroundings can precipitate incontinence, which may then clear up of its own accord when conditions have stabilized.

WHAT IS URINARY INCONTINENCE?
– The involuntary passing of urine. There may be no sensation that the bladder is full or that urine is being passed. It may be impossible to prevent the flow of urine, even with effort – it "comes away" regardless. "Double incontinence" refers to loss of control over both bowel and bladder emptying.

CAUSES ■ Infants normally acquire bladder control at about two years. Incontinence at night can last until five or six years. Some children will have the occasional "accident" much later than this. ■ Stress/urgency incontinence which usually occurs in middle-aged women is due to laxity of the pelvic muscles (especially after childbirth). The pelvic muscles support the bladder and when they are stretched some degree of bladder control is lost. ■ Following damage to the nerves of the bladder (for example in paraplegia and certain nerve diseases), there is no sensation that the bladder is full and no control over the passage of urine. ■ In the elderly, incontinence is the commonest consequence of nerve damage (as in *stroke, page 60,* or *senile dementia, page 124);* poor pelvic muscle tone in women; prostatic enlargement in men.

PRESCRIPTION DRUGS
Drugs are not particularly effective and they have a high incidence of side effects.
Imipramine and **amitriptyline** are used to treat urinary incontinence at night in the young and the old, if drugs are considered necessary. In children, the first line of treatment is usually behavioural, with bell alarms and star charts.
How they work: by causing retention of urine. It depresses nervous impulses to the bladder, and allows it to dilate. Also, children sleep less deeply and thus recognize the sensation of an enlarging bladder.
Propantheline, emepronium bromide and **terodiline** can help the patient urinate less frequently.
How they work: by decreasing contraction of the bladder muscles, so increasing bladder capacity.

Physiotherapy can improve pelvic muscle tone – or just practising the exercises for the pelvic floor which are taught in antenatal classes.

OVER-THE-COUNTER TREATMENTS
None with any proven value. However, barrier creams are useful in dealing with the redness, and the damage of the skin of the buttocks which is a secondary result

of incontinence. Disposable sheets backed with plastic help to save laundry, as do absorbent pads worn inside underwear.

QUESTIONS TO ASK THE DOCTOR
■ Is my child's bed-wetting severe enough to justify drug treatment, or would a buzzer system be better?
■ Is the incontinence reversible?
■ Is it necessary to test the urine for infection?

SIDE EFFECTS
Imipramine can cause a dry mouth, blurring of vision and constipation. It can also reduce blood pressure, and cause dizziness or fainting, convulsions and irregularities in heartbeat. It should be used with caution in patients with heart disease, epilepsy, liver or thyroid disease and glaucoma. It is sedative, and should not be taken when driving or working in a potentially dangerous environment. The adverse effects are aggravated by alcohol. **Propantheline** can cause a dry mouth, blurring of vision, constipation and a rapid heartbeat. It can precipitate glaucoma and heart failure. Urinary retention may occur.
Emepronium and **terodiline** may cause similar problems.

SELF-MANAGEMENT
Children:
■ Tensions associated with potty training can have long-lasting effects, and the same applies to being dry at night. ■ Don't take a toddler out of nappies if he or she is likely to wet the bed. ■ Routine measures including limiting fluid intake after 4 pm; getting the child up to urinate after three or four hours' sleep (this need not involve waking the child completely); and using a star or reward system for dry nights. ■ Don't put undue stress on being dry and don't show anger over wet sheets. A child is not in control of the bladder when asleep. ■ Family tension may be a cause. If bed-wetting continues beyond five, consult your doctor.

After nerve damage:
This can cause total loss of bladder control. ■ If a man has sufficient penile length, a sheath designed to empty into a bag may be helpful. Otherwise absorbent pads and plastic-backed sheets are the only other relatively simple options. ■ The skin must be kept clean and dry to reduce the risk of bed sores. Apply barrier cream after cleaning. ■ Catheters are only used in selected cases: they can cause bladder infection.

PATIENT'S EXPERIENCE
"My mother, aged 83, was becoming more and more senile. When the doctor put her on some pills for her heart, she suddenly became incontinent. I phoned the doctor and he explained that the pills were diuretics to make her pass more urine. He said I should remind her to go to the lavatory every half-hour after taking a tablet. He also said that the second tablet of the day could be taken at 4 pm, to give it a chance to work before bedtime.

Things went well enough until she had a bout of arthritis in her knees. She just could not reach the lavatory in time. I persuaded her to wear an absorbent pad which made her less apprehensive of accidents.

The arthritis improved, and so did the incontinence, but then a few months later it recurred for no apparent reason. I thought the cause might be worsening senility, and that nothing more could be done. My mother also appeared to accept the situation. However, I mentioned it to the doctor when he next checked her heart. He sent off a urine specimen to be checked for infection. The test was positive, and, after a course of antibiotics, the incontinence disappeared completely."

SUDDEN ONSET
Sudden urinary incontinence in any age group should be investigated by a doctor for the possibility of bladder infection. This will mean sending a specimen of urine to a laboratory. It is very important to provide a clean "mid-stream" specimen – the urine should go straight into a sterile container which a doctor or nurse can provide.

WHAT ARE PERIOD PROBLEMS?

– Several different and distressingly common conditions including: **heavy periods; frequent periods; infrequent** or **absent periods** (amenorrhoea); **painful periods** (dysmenorrhoea); **bleeding between periods** (intermenstrual bleeding) and **pre-menstrual tension/syndrome** (PMT/PMS). The last is a complex of symptoms including fluid retention, bloating and irritability prior to periods. These are the commonest complaints; a less common problem is endometriosis, an abnormality in the growth and location of the lining of the womb which gives rise to painful periods.

CAUSES Generally, it is thought that the most usual cause of period problems is an imbalance in the levels of hormones – oestrogen and progesterone. Very rarely there may be a more serious underlying cause. In particular:

Heavy periods (menorrhagia) are often 'normal' periods which simply become heavier as a woman grows older. Other (rarer) causes include having a coil (IUCD) in place; fibroids; an underactive thyroid gland, *see **hypothyroidism**, page 166;* and blood clotting disorders.

Painful periods (dysmenorrhoea) can start soon after puberty (primary dysmenorrhoea) and are caused by hormone imbalances which cause high levels of prostaglandins to be present in the uterus. These are believed to cause uterine contractions/cramps. Period pain which starts later on in life (secondary dysmenorrhoea) can be due to endometriosis or to chronic pelvic infection (pelvic inflammatory disease or salpingitis).

Bleeding between periods can be due to miscarriage (abortion), tubal (ectopic) pregnancies, the progesterone-only pill (POP) *see **contraception**, page 178;* the coil, cervical erosion, polyps and very rarely cancer (of the cervix, ovary or uterus).

Lack of periods (amenorrhoea) can be due to pregnancy, severe weight loss (***anorexia**, page 220*), ***stress**, page 88,* and, very rarely, ***tumours of the pituitary gland**, page 168* or an underactive thyroid gland – *see **hypothyroidism**, page 166.*

The cause of PMT/PMS is not fully understood, but again hormone imbalances are probably implicated.

PRESCRIPTION DRUGS

Hormones help relieve the symptoms of period disorders. They don't usually 'cure' the condition and their effects tend to wear off soon after stopping them. Progesterone is often used on a cyclical basis (for example one to three weeks in a month) to help reduce imbalances in the levels of oestrogen and progesterone. The treatment can stop or reduce the amount of bleeding. Oestrogen can be used on its own to induce an artificial period, but is more often used in combination with progesterone in the combined oral contraceptive pill. This is usually taken for three weeks in every month and as well as acting as a contraceptive (by inhibiting ovulation) it helps regularize periods and reduces pain and bleeding.

Danazol is a hormone which inhibits the production of hormones from the pituitary gland, the master gland in the brain which controls all hormones. It is useful in the treatment of endometriosis and is also used to reduce heavy bleeding. It is a particularly expensive drug.

Antispasmodic drugs can relieve painful periods.

How they work: by relaxing the muscle in the wall of the uterus. See *irritable bowel syndrome, page 32.*

Prostaglandin inhibitors such as mefenamic acid are used for reducing heavy and painful periods.

How they work: by blocking prostaglandin production. See *pain, page 106.*

Antifibrinolytic drugs also reduce bleeding and are quite useful in treating heavy periods.

How they work: by acting on the blood clotting system. Vitamin B6 (pyridoxine) is very helpful in the treatment of PMT. Its action is not understood.

Mild diuretics are also useful in PMT as a remedy for water retention. They are often taken on a cyclical basis, for example one or two weeks prior to a period.

How they work: *see page 54.*

A dilation and curettage (D & C) is a relatively simple procedure in which most of the lining of the womb is scraped away. It then re-grows, with new, healthier tissue, possibly less likely to give rise to period problems.

OVER-THE-COUNTER TREATMENTS

Simple painkillers such as paracetamol and aspirin will help relieve mild period pains. Self-treatment is perfectly appropriate. Many over-the-counter preparations contain combinations of simple painkillers, antispasmodics and caffeine (which acts as a stimulant). These are more expensive than simple painkillers, and probably no more effective. If period pain does not respond to aspirin or paracetamol, a visit to the doctor is required. Hormone treatments, including the pill, are not available over-the-counter.

PATIENT'S EXPERIENCE

"I started having period pains on the very first day of my first period aged 12 years. For many years while I was at school I was told period pains were normal and to carry on as usual. I rarely took tablets for the pain and occasionally had to be sent home from school because I felt so awful. When I first went on the pill I was pleasantly surprised to find my periods were less heavy and painful. After coming off the pill I found it took almost a year for the pain to recur. I then asked my doctor if I could try something else. He suggested mefenamic acid tablets three times a day from the moment my period started, continuing for two days. I still have some pain, but I find that by taking the tablets I can at least manage to carry on with work. Some people say period pains lessen as you get into your early 20s, but I'm 28 now and they are just the same as when I was 12 years old. Others say that they improve after having a baby – I suppose that is something to look forward to."

QUESTIONS TO ASK THE DOCTOR
■ How many days in each month should I take tablets?
■ How long should I continue the treatment?
■ What will happen to my periods?
■ Do the tablets have a contraceptive effect?
■ Is the treatment curative, or for symptoms relief only?
■ Would a D & C be helpful?

SIDE EFFECTS
Oestrogen: nausea, vomiting, weight gain and fluid retention. Rare, and adverse, side effects include liver problems, rashes, depression, headache, blood thrombosis and cancer of the uterus. Withdrawal bleeding occurs two to four days after stopping oestrogen treatment.

Progesterone: the main side effect is a withdrawal bleed on reducing the dose or stopping the drug. Others include headache, depression and, rarely, liver problems.

Antifibrinolytic drugs: principally nausea.

Antispasmodics: dry mouth, blurred vision, palpitations, difficulty passing urine and constipation. *See **irritable bowel syndrome**, page 30.*

Prostaglandin inhibitors: drowsiness, dizziness, nausea, diarrhoea and stomach ulceration.

SELF-MANAGEMENT
Because of the close relationship of the brain to the pituitary gland, any illness which has an effect on the brain can affect the menstrual cycle. This applies to many physical illnesses as well as psychological problems such as stress. It follows that avoidance of stress can be of help in avoiding period problems. Maintaining a normal body weight is also important for regular periods.

SELF-HELP
■ If the problem is really severe, rest in bed with a hot water bottle over the lower abdomen. A hot bath may also help. Take regular analgesics. Change sanitary towels or tampons regularly. With persistently heavy/painful periods, try and organize your life so that you have a lighter than normal day or two when your period first starts. Take regular aspirin or mefenamic acid as soon as the period starts, before the pain comes on. Consider going on the pill if you are in need of contraception. For inexplicable bleeding between periods or bleeding after the menopause, always consult a doctor.

The Menstrual Cycle
Numerals refer to days from start of menstrual cycle

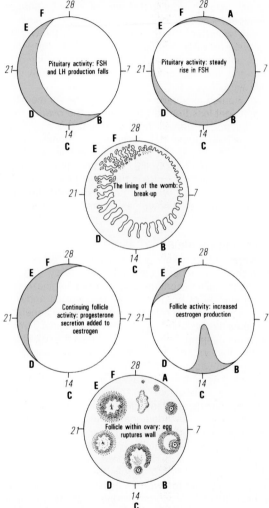

The ovaries are controlled by a small gland in the brain called the pituitary. It secretes several hormones, three of which affect the ovaries. Two of them, follicle stimulating hormone (FSH) and luteinizing hormone (LH) are actually responsible for ovulation.

A In the first half of the menstrual cycle, there is a steady rise of FSH: it stimulates the ovarian follicles which contain the eggs.

B As the follicles approach the moment for releasing the eggs, they produce increasing amounts of the hormone oestrogen. It is discharged into the bloodstream and carried through the body, in particular to the lining of the womb which it stimulates and enriches in preparation for the fertilized egg.

C But the rising levels of oestrogen have another effect: they trigger the pituitary gland to produce a massive surge of luteinizing hormone. This is vital: it allows the egg to rupture through the wall of the follicle and pass into the abdominal cavity so that it can be 'harvested' by the Fallopian tube down which it can travel to the womb.

D With the release of the egg, the follicle's job continues. In addition to producing oestrogen, it now secretes a second hormone, progesterone, which further develops and enriches the lining of the womb, to make it as attractive as possible to the fertilized egg which will arrive and burrow in to the lining of the womb four days later.

E The oestrogen and progesterone circulating in the bloodstream in increasing quantities, now exert a negative feedback effect on the pituitary gland's production of FSH and LH. The higher the levels rise, the less FSH and LH the pituitary is able to produce. Without these two hormones to maintain and stimulate the empty but active follicle, its cells wither away and die. Only if replicas of FSH and LH are produced from the womb from an implanted pregnancy will the follicle continue to produce oestrogen and progesterone.

Without a pregnancy in the womb, oestrogen and progesterone levels fall dramatically at the end of the menstrual cycle. Denied continuous stimulus of oestrogen and progesterone, the enriched and enlarged womb lining breaks up and menstruation ensues.

F The third hormone produced by the pituitary is counter-productive to pregnancy. Prolactin is usually produced in increasing amounts during pregnancy and, with stimulation of the nipples after delivery, levels continue to rise to maintain lactation.

However, prolactin suppresses the ovaries' ability to produce follicles. For a number of reasons, the levels of prolactin can rise dramatically when it is unwanted, and these reduce the prospects of pregnancy.

193

WHAT IS THE MENOPAUSE?

– Strictly speaking, the date of the last menstrual period, usually around the age of 50. A 'surgical' menopause occurs in younger women who have the uterus (womb) or ovaries removed; if only the womb is removed and the ovaries are left behind, the periods stop, but the changes in hormone balance which occur with the menopause do not take place until years afterwards.

All women experience these changes. As menstrual periods get less frequent and cease, the ovaries make less oestrogen (female hormone) and this may cause hot flushes. Some get dryness or soreness in the vagina. The bones get thinner, and this increases the risk of fractures later in life. For some, these changes can be lived with; for others they are unendurable. The worst affected will want to consider oestrogen treatment, otherwise known as hormone replacement therapy or HRT.

PRESCRIPTION DRUGS

Oestrogen can be given in several different ways.

1 Women who have had a hysterectomy can take oestrogen tablets continuously, or use a vaginal cream, or an implant of hormones can be inserted under the skin. The treatment offers some interesting benefits: it prevents flushes and sweats; prevents vaginal dryness; prevents thinning of the bones and thus the risk of fractures later in life; prevents premature ageing and changes in vagina and urethra.

2 Women who have a uterus run a slight risk that its lining will be stimulated to form cancer if they take oestrogen on its own. In order to take oestrogen safely, they must take an additional hormone, progestogen, for at least ten days every month. When the progestogen is stopped, the lining of the womb may be shed, as in a normal period. These monthly withdrawal bleeds are necessary to remove the risk of cancer and do not mean that the woman has become fertile again. If these drawbacks can be tolerated, HRT will, for these women: prevent flushes and sweats; prevent vaginal dryness; prevent ageing changes in vagina and urethra and the 'urethral syndrome'.

3 Oestrogen cream can be used to prevent dryness and soreness in the vulva and vagina. This may be a problem during intercourse and the treatment is simple and effective. It should be used for about a fortnight initially, then every few days as often as necessary. A lubricant jelly applied before intercourse can also help.

4 New methods such as skin patches and vaginal rings are being developed in order to deliver oestrogen in small doses. It is worth consulting your doctor about availability.

OVER-THE-COUNTER TREATMENTS

Calcium tablets are widely available, and are used to prevent osteoporosis – thinning of the bones. They are nothing like as effective as oestrogen for this purpose, but they may be useful to women on diets low in calcium. Hormone treatments such as oestrogen are not available without a prescription.

QUESTIONS TO ASK THE DOCTOR

■ Are you sure that hormone therapy really will help my menopause problem?
■ What are the side effects?
■ How long should I take HRT? Should I have oestrogen alone, or oestrogen with progestogen?

SIDE EFFECTS

Because of the risks of taking **oestrogen,** a doctor should ask the menopausal patient about major past illnesses such as breast cancer. Make sure the doctor takes your blood pressure, does a breast examination and a smear test. Hormone replacement therapy can then be started unless something needs further investigation. Before taking the final decision to start HRT, doctor and patient have to weigh, against the advantages listed under **PRESCRIPTION DRUGS,** the following disadvantages:

If a woman has a uterus: possible monthly bleeding; supervision by doctor; unknown long-term risk of breast cancer and coronary heart disease; also of dependency on oestrogen.

If a woman has had a hysterectomy: medical supervision is required, but only for heart and blood pressure; unknown long-term risk of breast cancer. Oestrogen alone probably lessens risk of heart disease unless the patient has had a thrombosis; possible dependency on oestrogen. All these risks are very slight and long-term results with patients on HRT are reassuring.

As long as side effects do not develop, HRT can continue for many years after the menopause if necessary. Even a few years' treatment can mean significantly less risk of bone fractures in old age. If you think you want to stop taking the tablets, discuss with your doctor taking a few months off HRT – you can always start again if your menopausal symptoms return.

DURATION OF HRT
As long as side effects do not develop, HRT can continue for many years after the menopause if necessary. Even a few years' treatment can mean significantly lesser risk of bone fractures in old age. If you think you want to stop taking the tablets, discuss with your doctor taking a few months off HRT – you can always start again if your menopausal symptoms return.

COMMONSENSE MEASURES TO MAINTAIN HEALTH AFTER THE MENOPAUSE
■ **Exercise:** Energetic walking or aerobics improve the bones, heart and lungs. ■ **Sunshine:** Even a few minutes out of doors every day will increase the Vitamin D content of the body. This helps with the absorption of calcium. ■ **Diet:** Calcium in the form of low-fat dairy products, and also in tinned fish and green vegetables, helps the bones to stay healthy. ■ **Don't smoke,** and don't drink heavily. These poisons harm your bones, liver and heart.
■ **Regular sex** (with a lubricant if necessary) keeps the vagina healthy.

NAMES YOU WILL HEAR

Antibiotics
Chemical name: amoxycillin sodium; trade names: Amoxil, Moxacin, Moxilean, Novamoxin, Penamox, Polymox. Chemical name: co-trimoxazole; trade names: Bactrim, Fectrim, Nodilon, Septrim. Chemical name: erythromycin; trade names: Erythrocin, Erythromid, Ilotycin, EpMycin, Erostin, Emu-V, Ethryn, Eromel, Ilocap, Ilosone, Rythrocaps.

Anti-worm preparations
Chemical name: mebendazole; trade name: Vermox. Chemical name: piperazine salts; trade names: Antepar, Pripsen.

Analgesics/antipyretics
Chemical name: paracetamol; trade names: Panadol, Pamol, Calpol, Tylenon, Paracin, Parmol, Panado, Ceetamol, Atosol, Exctol, Tylenol, Ennagesic, Ilvamol. Chemical name: aspirin; trade names: Aspirin, Astrin, Bi-Prin. *See also* **pain**, *page 106.*

Fluoride preparations
Chemical name: sodium fluoride; trade names: En-De-Kay, Fluor-a-day Lac, Zymafluor, Floran, Zymafluor.

Many illnesses covered in this book occur in children; their drug therapy is discussed under the relevant section. There are, however, some illnesses, and specialized applications of drugs, which occur almost exclusively in childhood. Some of the most important genereal issues are covered here, but see particularly comments on children's problems under diarrhoea, *page 28;* asthma, *page 74;* insomnia, *page 92;* pain, *page 106;* common cold, *page 134;* eczema, *page 278.*

PRESCRIPTION DRUGS

Antibiotics are frequently prescribed for children. The most common illnesses in childhood are due to viral infections and include the common cold, many of the ear infections and diarrhoea. Antibiotics have no effect against viruses, but bacteria may cause a secondary infection and it is often difficult to tell whether the illness is viral or bacterial. Parents are naturally eager for their child to recover as quickly as possible and some are reluctant to 'wait and see' – which is all that is needed for viral infections. So the pressure is on the doctor to prescribe an antibiotic early in the course of the illness.

At the same time, parents have reason to be anxious about the excessive use of antibiotics. Side effects may occur; they are usually mild, but they can be severe. Diarrhoea is a particularly common one; thrush is another. Bacteria can become resistant to the commonly used antibiotics *(see* **pneumonia and pleurisy,** *page 78),* and then they will not work when they are really needed. A second course of the same antibiotic should not be used within three months, as the bacteria are more likely to be resistant.

If needed, however, repeated courses of antibiotics will not weaken or damage your child's body. If you are concerned about repeated courses of antibiotics, raise the issue with your doctor. Most doctors are only too happy to withold an antibiotic until it is really necessary.

If a child has a recurrent runny nose and cough, and seems to go from one course of antibiotics to the next, and if in addition there is a family history of hay fever, eczema or asthma, discuss the possibility of allergy with your doctor. Many children whose problems are really due to allergies like hay fever are treated with antibiotics on the assumption that they have an infection. The presence of fever helps to discriminate: allergies rarely cause fever, but infections often do.

How they work: *see* **pneumonia and pleurisy,** *page 78.*

Anti-worm preparations: Children get worms from accidentally swallowing the eggs of worms, which are present in, for example, sandpits or parks and gardens. Several different types of worm are involved, the most common being thread worms and whip worms. These, and most others, can be treated with a single dose of mebendazole. Another common anti-worm drug is piperazine.

How they work: by inhibiting the metabolism of the worm. The worm is paralyzed, allowing it to be excreted from the bowel.

OVER-THE-COUNTER TREATMENTS

No drug should be used in children without specific reason. Some, including paracetamol, aspirin and iron tonics can cause severe illness in overdose. Analgesics/antipyretics are commonly used to treat pain and fever. Paracetamol is safe in the correct dose for age, and may be used even in babies as early as three to six months for the treatment of colic, fever and teething. Dose should be four to six hourly. Aspirin should not be given to children under 12 because of the risk of Reye's syndrome *(see **common cold**, page 134)*.

*(see **common cold**, page 134)*.

PATIENT'S EXPERIENCE
"My little boy had been at nursery school for a few months when I noticed that he was frequently scratching his bottom. I took him to the doctor who thought that it was worms. I asked him where he thought that my little boy had picked it up, and he said it was most likely he had swallowed some sand with worm eggs in it, either at nursery school or in the park. He gave me a prescription for some medicine which lasted a few days and told me to go back within a few weeks if the symptoms had not disappeared."

Sound brushing is as essential to teeth care in the young as any artificial assistance from fluoride preparations
Use the size of brush recommended by your dentist. Begin brushing the inside surfaces. Keep the bristles at 45° to the teeth and use an up-and-down movement.

After brushing the inside surfaces, *brush the chewing surfaces; then the outside surfaces. Encourage a child to adopt this sequence as a routine.*

Fluoride preparations, taken regularly, can significantly reduce the amount of decay in developing teeth, and is recommended where there is not sufficient fluoride in the drinking water (ask your local dentist). It can be started at a few months old and should be continued until at least ten years. It is given as a single daily dose. The value of giving fluoride during pregnancy has not been established.

How they work: by making the dentine and enamel of teeth more resistant to acid.

A fever strip: *easy to use for a quick indication; get an accurate reading with a thermometer*

TAKING TEMPERATURE

Lift arm and tuck the thermometer under, holding it in place for two to three minutes

QUESTIONS TO ASK THE DOCTOR
■ Is an antibiotic absolutely necessary, or could we wait and see if she gets better without it?
■ Is it ever necessary to repeat worm treatment?
■ What can I give my baby for teething?

SIDE EFFECTS
Antibiotics: *see pneumonia and pleurisy, page 78.* Mebendazole rarely causes side effects, though headache, abdominal pain and diarrhoea have been reported. It should not be used during pregnancy.
Analgesics/antipyretics: *see common cold, page 134.*
Fluoride can, in chronic overdose, cause discolouration of the teeth. If a large number of tablets are taken, nausea, vomiting, abdominal pain, diarrhoea and paralysis can occur.

SELF-MANAGEMENT
■ Use only drugs which are absolutely necessary.
■ If a child has a drug reaction, contact doctor at once.
■ Some drugs pass to the baby in breast milk. Many prescription and non-prescription drugs can adversely affect a baby, so always check with your doctor first. The common ones to avoid while breast-feeding include aspirin, indomethacin, tetracyclines, some anti-migraine preparations and antidepressants. Many other

GIVING MEDICINE

A dropper *makes a useful tool for giving a baby medicine; whatever the method used, wrapping a child in a towel will help to prevent struggling and resulting spillage*

drugs are not known to be safe, so don't take any drug unless it is absolutely necessary.

■ Dosage: Drug dose in children is most accurately calculated by the child's weight, whereas the recommended dose on the bottle is often given by age group. If your child is underweight or overweight for his or her age, this must be taken into account.

■ Worms: Treatment for worms must be accompanied by washing of hands and nails regularly. The worm lays eggs around the anus. This causes itching and eggs deposited under the nails while scratching are transferred to the mouth, perpetuating the infection.

■ Children under a year old are particularly sensitive to drugs. Always check that the drug is recommended for that age or weight range. In children under three months, the liver and kidneys may be immature, and drugs that are broken down in the liver or excreted by the kidneys will need to be used in reduced doses.

■ Many liquid medicines contain sugar, which causes tooth decay. If medicines have to be taken for a long period, sugar-free preparations or tablets may be available; or give the child a drink of water afterwards.

■ Teething is often difficult to diagnose with certainty, and can be distressing. If a baby really appears to be in pain, a dose of paracetamol can be used safely; if it appears to ease the pain, use it every four hours.

Malignant disease and the immune system

For many people, the words cancer or leukaemia carry an automatic death sentence, but this is certainly not true today. In several types of malignant disease treatments have progressed a long way: cures are not uncommon, and the majority can hope for effective long-term control of their disease.

LUNG CANCER	**202-205**
BREAST CANCER	**206-207**
ADULT LEUKAEMIAS	**208-209**
CHILDHOOD LEUKAEMIAS	**210-211**
LYMPHOMAS	**212-213**
AIDS	**214-215**
ORGAN TRANSPLANTS	**216-217**

NAMES YOU WILL HEAR

Cytotoxic drugs
Chemical name: cyclophosphamide;
trade names: Endoxana, Endoxan-
Asta, Cytoxan, Procytox, Endoxan.
Chemical name: ifosfamide; trade
name: Mitoxana. Chemical name:
doxorubicin; trade names: Adriamycin,
Adriablastina. Chemical name:
vincristine; trade names: Oncovin,
Pericristine. Chemical name: vindesine
sulphate; trade name: Eldisine.
Chemical name: cis-diammino-
dichloro-platinum; trade names:
Cisplatin, Platinol, Platinol. Chemical
name: carboplatin; trade names:
Paraplatin, Paraplatin. Chemical
name: mitomycin; trade name:
Mitomycin-C. Chemical name:
etoposide; trade name: Vepesid.

Steroids
Chemical name: dexamethasone;
trade names: Decadron, Dexacortisyl,
Oradexon, Oradexon. Chemical name:
prednisolone; trade names: Codelsol,
Delta Phoricol, Deltacortril, Deltalone,
Deltastab, Precortisyl, Prednesol,
Sintisone, Nisolone, Delta-Cortef,
Deltasolone, Prelone, Lenisolone,
Meticortilone, Predeltilone.

Antiemetics
Chemical name: prochlorperazine
mesylate; trade names: Stemetil,
Compazine, Anti-Naus, Mitil, Vertigon.
Chemical name: metoclopramide;
trade names: Maxolon, Primperan.
Chemical name: domperidone; trade
names: Motilium.

WHAT IS LUNG CANCER?

– Abnormal cell development in the lungs. There are four main types, classified by part of the lung or bronchi from which the cancer cells originate. The abnormal cells can grow either in the lung itself, giving rise to shortness of breath, wheezing, pain and coughing up of blood; or they can spread to other areas of the body such as the bones, liver or the brain, in which case a variety of symptoms may arise from these sites.

The cancers known collectively as non-small cell may remain localized for many years, and are frequently amenable to local treatment by surgical resection or radiation therapy. About 20 per cent are of quite a different type termed small cell lung cancer. These can spread rapidly, but they are often remarkably sensitive to the anti-cancer drugs.

A particular problem of lung cancer can occur when the tumour presses on the large blood vessels just above the heart. The face and arms become swollen, a condition known as superior mediastinal obstruction (SMO). The central nervous system can also be involved if a tumour presses on the brain or spinal cord.

The outlook with this disease is better than commonly supposed. Some patients – including those with widespread disease – survive several years. Control of symptoms such as pain and nausea are much improved.

CAUSES The two proven causes of lung cancer are cigarette smoking, particularly those brands with a high tar content; and exposure to asbestos, for example in building workers or dock labourers. Specialists suspect that up to 80 per cent of cases are attributable to smoking; otherwise (leaving aside asbestos involvement) the cause is unknown.

PRESCRIPTION DRUGS

Cytotoxic drugs: These can be given either alone or in combination, and while usually given by injection, some are available in tablet form.

How they work: By killing the cancer cells giving rise to the tumour. However, some normal cells are often damaged in the process, and this causes side effects. At some point the cancer cells may become resistant to the drug or drugs used. A change may have to be made, either to different drugs or by introducing a different type of treatment such as radiotherapy (radioactive rays are beamed at the cancer to kill the cells). *See also breast cancer, page 206.*

Corticosteroids: If SMO is present, or there is tumour spread to the brain or other parts of the central nervous system, corticosteroids can improve the symptoms dramatically.

How they work: by reducing the swelling around the tumour and relieving the pressure on the nerve cells.

Antiemetics: Most of the cytotoxic drugs cause some degree of nausea, and this can usually be controlled by oral or rectal administration of antiemetics. Occasionally an intravenous infusion of a higher dose of antiemetic may be required.

How they work: by acting on the centre in the brain responsible for the stimulus to vomit.

For **analgesics** and **antibiotics,** *see pages 106 and 78.*

OVER-THE-COUNTER TREATMENTS
None.

QUESTIONS TO ASK THE DOCTOR
- How long will the course last?
- What side effects will I get?
- What if any of these become particularly severe?
- How do I get further supplies of the tablets?
- Which tablets are part of the treatment and which are to control side effects?
- How often do I need to have a blood test?
- How long will it be before you know if the treatment is working?
- What should I eat and drink?

SIDE EFFECTS
Cytotoxic drugs are usually given by injection every three to four weeks or in tablet form daily for seven to 14 days, in which case the side effects may be less marked, but more prolonged. The principal side effects are nausea, with or without associated vomiting, loss of hair, and damage to the normal cells produced by the bone marrow. The normal cells of the lung, kidney or heart can be affected, but this is rare.

Nausea may be due to either a local effect on the stomach, or directly on a 'trigger zone' in the brain.

Hair loss is due to damage to the follicles by the cytotoxic drugs and is nearly always temporary. Cooling of the scalp at the time of drug administration can occasionally prevent this occurring.

The effects on the bone marrow are more complicated and potentially serious: if the red cells are affected, anaemia may occur and blood transfusion may be required. If a cytotoxic drug affects the platelets, which are important for blood clotting, bleeding can occur from the nose, intestine or into the skin and appear as a rash. However, the white blood cells are most commonly affected; when their number falls below a critical level, there is a high risk of infection which may urgently require antibiotics. Often there is no obvious site for this infection, and a sore throat, fever, rigors or general malaise are the only signs.

Other less common side effects are mouth ulcers, diarrhoea, a skin rash and nerve damage. *See also breast cancer, page 206.*

Steroids can cause a range of side effects, including some serious ones, but as the drugs are usually given only short-term for lung cancer, increased appetite, retention of fluid with weight gain and change of mood are the only side effects commonly seen. Patients with high blood pressure associated with diabetes have to be monitored carefully when on steroids.

Antiemetics are unfortunately not without side effects themselves: they may cause drowsiness, skin rash and in some cases where high doses are used, muscle weakness, tremor or twitching of the limbs: these may be disconcerting, but are usually temporary.

SELF-MANAGEMENT
When taking anti-cancer drugs, moderation in one's habits without withdrawing from normal social activity is the best approach.

■ Try to continue to eat a balanced diet, avoiding spicy or fatty food which may upset you. If you do not feel like eating, at least keep drinking to keep your fluid intake and output high. Small quantities of alcohol, perhaps avoiding neat spirits, is unlikely to be harmful.

■ Continue moderate activity along the lines you are used to, whether that is swimming, walking, housekeeping or golf, but do stop when you are tired, and take plenty of rest.

■ Do get a wig, do go out, do meet your friends or have them round to see you. Try and maintain your self-esteem as much as possible and confide in your close family and friends – they can prove understanding and helpful.

■ Organize your house to minimize the amount of routine work or movement you have to do: for example, move the bedroom downstairs, or instal a downstairs lavatory.

■ While infection is a risk, most of the organisms involved come from within your own body; however, it is best to avoid children with chickenpox.

■ Take advantage of any counselling services available through your general practitioner as well as the cancer nurse specialists.

SELF-HELP
■ Keep your clinic appointments and have blood tests on time – the results can help to give advance warning of complications.
■ Take the tablets only for the prescribed time. You may have a mixture of cytotoxic drug tablets and painkillers. If in doubt, write the names and frequency down, and check it over with your doctor.
■ Infection: If you have a fever, sweating, shivering or rigors, contact your doctor or hospital immediately for advice.
■ Bleeding: For a nose bleed, sit quietly with a cold compress over the bridge of your nose and your head slightly forwards. If bleeding does not stop in 15-20 minutes, contact your doctor. Coughing up blood may be disconcerting, but is rarely serious.
■ Breathing difficulties: Sitting up and leaning forward often helps; use several pillows. Remain calm. If your breathing suddenly becomes worse, seek medical advice.

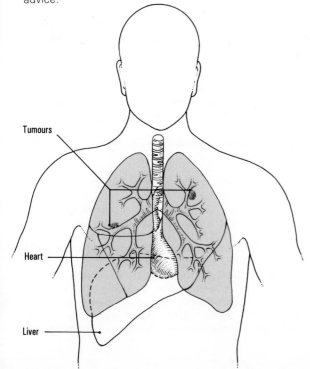

Tumours

Heart

Liver

Lung cancer *often begins in the bronchi or breathing tubes which join together in the centre to form the trachea. Symptoms arise when the cancer cells grow inwards blocking the tube, often collapsing part of the lung. If there is a raw edge or ulcer, bleeding may occur and specks of blood will appear in the sputum. The cancer can spread locally to the rest of the lung, by the lymph glands and channels to the centre of the chest, and by the bloodstream to the bones, liver or brain.*

NAMES YOU WILL HEAR

Hormonal treatments
Chemical name: tamoxifen; **trade names:** Nolvadex, Tamofen, Kessar, Noltam. **Chemical name:** aminoglutethimide; **trade name:** Orimeten. **Chemical name:** medroxyprogesterone acetate; **trade names:** Depoprovera, Provera, Farlutal. **Chemical name:** megestrol acetate; **trade name:** Megace. **Chemical name:** stilboestrol; **trade name:** Tampovagan. **Chemical name:** ethinyloestradiol; **trade names:** Lynoral, Edrol, Estigyn, Estinyl, Primogyn. **Chemical name:** drostanolone propionate; **trade name:** Masteril. **Chemical name:** nandrolone; **trade names:** Durabolin, Deca Durabolin.

Cytotoxic drugs
Chemical name: doxorubicin; **trade names:** Adriamycin, Adriablastina. **Chemical name:** epirubicin; **trade name:** Pharmorubicin. **Chemical name:** mitozantrone; **trade name:** Novantrone. **Chemical name:** vincristine sulphate; **trade names:** Oncovin, Pericristine. **Chemical name:** cyclophosphamide; **trade names:** Endoxana, Endoxan-Asta, Cytoxan, Procytox, Endoxan. **Chemical name:** fluorouracil; **trade names:** Fluorouracil, Fluoroplex, Adrucil. **Chemical name:** methotrexate; **trade names:** Emtexate, Maxtrex.

WHAT IS BREAST CANCER?

– Abnormal growth of cells originating in the breast. Most lumps in the breast are minor abnormalities of fatty tissue and are benign. They do, however, need medical assessment in order that the minority of lumps due to breast cancer can be detected.

Early breast cancer is treated by surgery often combined with radiotherapy. The intention is to remove every malignant cell and thus to effect a complete cure. Surgeons used to remove the whole breast (radical mastectomy), but nowadays this is only done in advanced cases. Whenever possible, only the lump is removed, with the object of restoring body shape to near-normal. But since the disease may be present in microscopic form, surgery cannot be a guarantee against recurrence in another site.

When breast cancers do give rise to tumours in other sites, they are known as secondary cancers or metastases. Drugs have an important role in the treatment of overt symptomatic metastases; they can also be used to eliminate undetectable ones. This is known as adjuvant treatment and is given to patients when there is a possibility of 'secondaries' being present and developing later. Radiotherapy may be used instead of, or in addition to drugs.

Improvements in treatment mean that the outlook for breast cancer gets better and better. This is a form of cancer which can be cured, provided treatment is started early enough.

PRESCRIPTION DRUGS

Hormonal (endocrine) treatments: usually given as tablets, although some are administered as injections one to three times a week.
How they work: A substantial proportion (50 to 60 per cent) of breast cancers are known to depend on hormones (in particular oestrogen) for their growth. The drugs interfere with the action of the hormone on the cancer cells.
Cytotoxic drugs ('chemotherapy') is often administered by injection into a vein. This can be done on an outpatient basis, but may require hospital admission for one or two days. Chemotherapy is given in cycles of one to five days every three to four weeks.
How they work: Cytotoxic drugs are all poisons: they affect normal as well as abnormal cells. The recovery powers of normal cells are greater than those of the cancer cells and provided that the drug is given intermittently, the normal cells will recover between doses

while the abnormal ones will not. The dose of cytotoxics which can be given is limited by the amount of damage which the normal tissues can stand.

Anti-emetics may be used to treat the side effects of cytotoxic drugs: *see **lung cancer**, page 202.*

QUESTIONS TO ASK THE DOCTOR
- Is the treatment chemotherapy or hormone therapy?
- What side effects can I expect?
- What can I do to lessen the side effects?
- How will I know the treatment is working?

SIDE EFFECTS
Hormonal treatments are associated with mild side effects. The commonest is probably nausea, but this is usually transitory and does not require stopping the drug. Tamoxifen given to pre-menopausal women may produce disturbances of menstruation and hot flushes. In post-menopausal women it causes almost no side effect. Fleeting skin rashes are common with aminoglutethimide. Androgens are associated with the growth of unwanted hair and deepening of the voice. Oestrogens give rise to vaginal bleeding. The latter two groups of drugs are rarely used.

Chemotherapy side effects range from the unpleasant to the seriously adverse. The latter may not give rise to any symptoms until very advanced and need to be detected by monitoring the patient.

The common side effects are nausea, vomiting and alopecia (hair loss). Hair always grows again. Some drugs may give rise to unpleasant tingling sensations. Prolonged tiredness may also occur, and a feeling of weakness. The serious side effects are changes to the bone marrow resulting in increased susceptibility to infection and likelihood of abnormal bruising and bleeding. These will usually be found by the doctor before they become a problem, but sore throat, mouth ulcers or bruising may be the first signs and should be reported immediately. *See also **lung cancer**, page 202.*

SELF-MANAGEMENT
- Prevention: regular, monthly self-examination of the breasts is the best way to ensure early detection. Ask your doctor to teach you the technique.
- Many forms of self-help for breast cancer patients are available, including diet and visualization techniques. They should only be undertaken with the advice of an expert and the approval of a hospital specialist.
- Self-help groups can give invaluable moral support.

PATIENT'S EXPERIENCE
"When I first went to my doctor with a blotchy rash which had suddenly appeared I had no idea that I was suffering from breast cancer. I was referred to a skin specialist who biopsied the rash and discovered that it was due to secondaries from breast cancer. She referred me to the breast clinic who found a lump in my breast and removed it. They confirmed that it was breast cancer. Because of the widespread rash, I was told that mastectomy or other local treatments were not suitable and I was told I would need chemotherapy.

For the first course of treatment I went into hospital for three days, but since then I have attended as an outpatient. Whenever I arrive at the hospital, my blood is taken for tests and I have to wait for the results. So far the results have always been satisfactory. They put a drip in my arm and then give the injections. There have been no unpleasant sensations during the injections, but afterwards I feel sick until the following day. Three weeks later I go back for another course. After two treatments the rash started to disappear and nine months after I started chemotherapy there is no rash and I feel well. I have continued my office job throughout this time."

Cytotoxic drugs

NAMES YOU WILL HEAR
Cytoxic drugs
Chemical name: busulphan; **trade name:** Myleran. **Chemical name:** chlorambucil; **trade name:** Leukeran. **Chemical name:** cytarabine; **trade names:** Cytosar, Cytosar U, Alexan. **Chemical name:** daunorubicin hydrochloride; **trade names:** Cernbidin, Ceonbidine. **Chemical name:** doxorubicin; **trade names:** Adriamycin, Adriblastina. **Chemical name:** etoposide; **trade name:** Vepesid. **Chemical name:** mitoxantrone; **trade name:** Novantrone. **Chemical name:** thioguanine; **trade name:** Lanvis. **Chemical name:** vincristine; **trade names:** Oncovin, Pericristine.

WHAT IS ADULT LEUKAEMIA?

– A malignant blood disorder which, in adults, is divided into acute and chronic forms. There is further division into myeloid and lymphoid sub-types, depending on the type of white blood cell involved. Diagnosis is by examination of the blood and bone marrow.

Acute leukaemia in adults, in contrast to that in children, is usually of the myeloid type, although acute lymphoblastic leukaemia may occur in adults of any age. The first symptoms reported to a doctor are usually related to anaemia (tiredness and breathlessness) or bleeding (particularly from the gums, nose and into the skin), or infection (again particularly in the mouth, skin and chest). These problems arise due to a lack of normal red cells, platelets and white cells.

Chronic leukaemias in adults are again of two types. Chronic myeloid leukaemia, also known as chronic granulocytic leukaemia, is most common in middle age. Symptoms include fever, tiredness and malaise. Enlargement of the spleen and liver may cause swelling of the abdomen. Chronic lymphatic leukaemia is a more indolent condition often occurring in older age groups. This may be discovered during a routine blood count, or may present with anaemia, bleeding or infection. Enlargement of the lymph glands, particularly in the neck, under the arms and in the groins, is another common feature. Enlargement of the spleen may produce swelling and a feeling of fullness in the abdomen.

CAUSES In most cases unknown, but exposure to certain drugs, and to radiation, may be responsible for a small percentage of cases.

PRESCRIPTION DRUGS

Cytotoxic drugs are given by tablet or injection to control the growth of the abnormal white blood cells. The chronic leukaemias usually respond well to less intensive treatment with tablets, while the acute leukaemias are treated with intensive combinations of drugs given both orally and directly into the blood stream.

Acute myeloid leukaemia in adults is treated using intermittent intensive combinations of drugs with 'rest' periods to allow the normal bone marrow to recover. Acute lymphoblastic leukaemia in adults is treated with similar regimes to those used in children.

Chronic myeloid leukaemia is, in the early stages, usually readily controlled using tablet treatment. Control may become more difficult after one or two years, and in some cases the disease changes its character and acute leukaemia develops. Bone marrow transplantation may be the preferred treatment, once the disease is under control, for some cases of acute leukaemia and also for some cases of chronic myeloid leukaemia. Chronic lymphatic leukaemia is usually only treated, particularly in older people, if it is causing problems, and indeed no treatment may be required for long periods. Swelling of the lymph glands or anaemia are usually treated with a course of tablets.

Drug treatment forms only a part of the total care of a person with leukaemia, and transfusions of blood (to correct anaemia) and platelets (to correct bleeding) are commonly required. Antibiotics are given to control and treat infections.

How the drugs work: *see* ***lung cancer,*** *page 202.*

QUESTIONS TO ASK THE DOCTOR
■ What sort of leukaemia do I have?
■ How long will treatment last?

OVER-THE-COUNTER TREATMENTS
None.

SIDE EFFECTS
Cytotoxic drugs are all poisons. They may thus damage healthy cells as well as leukaemic cells. Damage to healthy tissues may produce loss of hair, soreness of the mouth and diarrhoea. Damage to normal bone marrow cells may produce anaemia, bleeding problems and a temporary increase in susceptibility to infection. Some cytotoxic drugs may cause nausea and vomiting and anti-emetic drugs are often given routinely to prevent this. Some of the drugs used to treat the diarrhoea may damage heart, lungs and liver. All these potential side effects are closely monitored during treatment and doses are modified to minimize the problems.

SELF HELP
■ Pay close attention to personal hygiene, especially in the mouth.
■ Report to your doctor immediately should you feel ill, especially with fevers or other signs of infection, particularly when your white blood cell count is low.
■ Avoid exposure to people with obvious infections, again when your white blood cell count is low.
■ Treatment of leukaemia, especially acute leukaemia, may be physically and emotionally very demanding, and you can help yourself through the programme by being aware of what is happening, and why.

WHAT IS LEUKAEMIA?
– A malignant condition involving the white blood cells: normal blood production is affected leading to anaemia, infection and bleeding. There may be enlarged lymph nodes in the neck, armpits and groins and an increase in the size of the liver and spleen. Bone pain, especially in the back and knees, may occur. Leukaemia afflicts one in 2,000 children. Eighty per cent have acute lymphoblastic leukaemia (ALL); these days, 60 per cent are cured. A small number have myeloid leukaemia, which responds less well to treatment. This disease is similar to that in adults. Both are diagnosed by examination of the blood count and of the bone marrow.

CAUSES No cause can be found in most children. But it can be caused by excessive radiation, and it does occur in association with some other rare childhood diseases. Certain animal leukaemias are transmitted by viruses, for example in cats, but no such virus has been identified in man.

PRESCRIPTION DRUGS
Cytotoxic drugs ('chemotherapy'): the mainstay of treatment. Some of the drugs can be taken as tablets or medicines, others have to be given by injection, usually directly into a vein. Treatment for ALL is administered as a programme usually lasting two years or more. Initial intensive drug treatment is given to obtain a remission, when the disease is no longer detectable in blood or bone marrow. Local X-ray treatment to the head is then applied to reduce the risk of nervous system involvement. Further treatment, mainly oral, is continued to maintain remission until treatment is completed. Acute myeloid leukaemia is treated more intensively and for a shorter period with a different combination of cytotoxic drugs. Certain cases may best be treated after initial therapy by a bone marrow transplant.
How they work: cytotoxic drugs are cell poisons, and act by killing leukaemia cells. Once the bone marrow is cleared of these cells, normal blood production will resume.
Antibiotics: Co-trimoxazole is given three days a week throughout treatment to reduce the risk of serious lung infection. Other antibiotics may be given to treat specific infections.
How they work: by killing the bacteria responsible.
Acyclovir: an anti-viral agent given as a course to prevent or treat chicken pox, shingles or cold sores, which can

occur more readily in a leukaemia patient, or while on treatment for the disease.

OVER-THE-COUNTER TREATMENTS
None.

QUESTIONS TO ASK THE DOCTOR
■ What time of day should my child take the drugs?
■ What should I do if my child vomits back the drug?
■ What will happen if I forget my child's treatment for a day or two?

SIDE EFFECTS
Cytotoxic drugs: Besides killing leukaemic cells, cytotoxics also damage healthy body tissues. Injury to the hair follicles is likely, and leads to hair loss; it always regrows. Damage to the lining of the mouth is also common, and causes local pain and ulceration. Normal blood cell production is affected. Effective treatment always leads to some periods of reduction in the white blood cell count, with a depression of immunity and a risk of infection. Some infections, especially measles and chicken pox, may prove very serious to children being treated for leukaemia. The administration of some intravenous drugs causes vomiting. Leakage from the vein during an injection may cause a local painful chemical burn.

Antibiotics: Co-trimoxazole's side effects are rare, but skin rashes may occur.

Acyclovir's side effects are very rare in children, but doctors will monitor patients' kidney function.

HOW PARENTS CAN HELP
Treatment requires continuous expert supervision, including regular blood counts, but you can help:

■ Hygiene, particularly the care of teeth and gums.
■ Ask school teachers and friends to warn you if your child is likely to come into contact with chicken pox or measles. Inform your doctor promptly: preventive treatment is available.
■ Avoid unnecessary crowds at times when the blood count is very low, but encourage the child to attend school and other normal activities whenever possible.
■ Don't have a child immunised while on treatment.
■ Do not over-indulge your child, despite the serious nature of the illness.
■ Keep yourself well informed about the frequent developments in treatment.

WHAT ARE LYMPHOMAS?

– Tumours affecting the body's immune system. They usually develop first in the lymph glands, but can also start in, and spread to, spleen, liver, bone marrow, bowel and sometimes other organs. Several types exist, including Hodgkin's lymphoma and non-Hodgkin's lymphomas. Common symptoms are enlarged neck glands, weight loss, fever and sweats. Diagnosis is confirmed by biopsy – removing a lymph gland or other tissue and examining it under a microscope. The extent or stage of the disease is found by X-ray tests, body-scan or sometimes by an abdominal operation. The disease is lethal without treatment; however life expectancy can be as high as 20 years given diagnosis at an early stage, and good response to treatment. Indeed some cases are cured.

CAUSE Unknown. The disease is not infectious.

TREATMENT

Lymphomas tend to respond well to drugs and radiotherapy. Radiotherapy alone may be used if only neck glands are involved and it cures some cases.
Combinations: The disease will respond to treatment with a single drug, but it does tend to recur. For this reason a combination of drugs is used as the chances of the tumour developing resistance to all the drugs are extremely small. A typical combination is **nitrogen mustard, vincristine** (Oncovin), **prednisolone** and **procarbazine** – MOPP for short – widely used in treating Hodgkin's disease. A two-week course including injections might be given to start treatment, followed by a break, then the next course. At least six courses are given.

New combinations are frequently being tested, and often these lead to improvements in treatment.
How they work: by killing tumour cells. Normal body cells can also be damaged in the process, but this can be minimized by using the appropriate dose and by having rest periods between courses of treatment.

OVER-THE-COUNTER TREATMENTS
None.

QUESTIONS TO ASK THE DOCTOR
■ What sort of lymphoma have I got?
■ How far has it spread?
■ Will it respond to treatment?
■ What will be the side effects of the treatment?
■ Can I continue at work?

SIDE EFFECTS

Patients receiving **combination** treatment have to allow for: reduction in the blood cell count – needs to be detected early by regular blood tests; mouth ulcers, nausea and diarrhoea – may be prevented or treated; scalp hair loss, and sometimes body hair loss – the hair always regrows; cessation of menstrual periods; sterility in men; proneness to infection. **Vincristine** additionally causes tingling or burning in the hands and feet; **bleomycin** and **doxorubicin** cause breathlessness. Most of the side effects are distressing but manageable; fever, rash, bleeding, persistent headache and breathlessness should be reported to a doctor without delay.

SELF-MANAGEMENT

Get treated at a specialized centre: these have the necessary experience to give the best results. Try to accept that you may have a massive emotional reaction as well as lymphoma. Doctors can help you with both: try to accept help. Keep up your interest in your work, family and friends. Do something that you really enjoy every day. Live within your capabilities; think of ways of doing things easily. If hair loss bothers you, get a wig matched and fitted, sooner rather than later. If you are male and might want children, consider storing sperm before chemotherapy. You may find a self-help support group useful.

The lymphatic system *consists of a series of tiny vessels which drain fluid from all tissues of the body. Along these channels are sited lymph glands which act as filters before the fluid is returned to the blood stream.*

Lymph vessels

Lymph glands

AIDS (Acquired Immune Deficiency Syndrome)

– The disease develops when the body's defence against infection – the immune system – is badly damaged by the human immunodeficiency virus (HIV). A variety of serious infections may develop affecting the lungs, brain, digestive system and skin. Unusual tumours may also develop.

Most AIDS sufferers are infected without being initially aware of symptoms. After a highly variable period of time, swollen glands may develop, particularly in the neck and armpits. Later, other symptoms may develop, including fever and night sweats, loss of appetite, weight loss, profound fatigue, prolonged diarrhoea and skin rashes. Full-blown AIDS may eventually develop in perhaps 35 per cent of infected people: but the final percentage is not known, because the disease has only recently spread to developed countries.

AIDS patients often first go to their doctor with a form of pneumonia, (caused by the organism *Pneumocystis carinii*), complaining of shortness of breath, dry cough and fever. Kaposi's sarcoma may also develop: pinkish-purple blotches – firm to the touch – on any part of the skin. These symptoms *may* be associated with other illnesses and don't necessarily mean AIDS, or an AIDS-related condition.

If you are worried, see your doctor soon, or attend a clinic which specializes in AIDS.

CAUSE HIV infects white blood cells (lymphocytes), which have a key role in defence against infection. Their numbers are severely reduced, leaving the body open to attack by various micro-organisms to produce opportunistic infections.

There is no cure for AIDS as yet; nor is there a protective vaccine, although attempts to develop one are underway.

PRESCRIPTION DRUGS

Antiviral drugs have a role: they can prevent the virus from multiplying and infecting other cells in the blood.
Zyclovucline may be prescribed in patients who have AIDS or related conditions but has to be taken six times daily to be effective. Treatment must be continued indefinitely to hold the virus in check.
How it works: by selectively blocking the metabolism of the virus, and preventing it from multiplying.
Antibiotics – many different types – may be used, both to treat acute infections and to prevent recurrences.
Cotrimoxazole is often used to treat pneumonia, and is

usually injected into a vein in hospital.

How they work: by killing the bacteria responsible for infection.

Cytotoxic drugs such as etoposide or vincristine are sometimes used in the treatment of severe Kaposi's sarcoma.

How they work: cytotoxics are all poisons: they rely on healthy cells' ability to recover from their effect, while malignant or abnormal cells are completely destroyed.

QUESTIONS TO ASK THE DOCTOR

■ How can I be certain I am infected?
■ What are the advantages and disadvantages of getting tested for HIV infection?
■ Whom should I tell?
■ Could I infect others?
■ What is "safe sex"?
■ Is it safe to have vaccinations?

SIDE EFFECTS

Zyclovucline sometimes affects cells in the bone marrow, causing anaemia: patients have to be regularly monitored. The antibiotic **cotrimoxazole** commonly produces skin rashes in AIDS patients: inform your doctor at once if this occurs.

Cytotoxic drugs: *see lung cancer, page 202.* Etoposide may produce hair loss, but the hair usually regrows when the drug is stopped.

SELF-MANAGEMENT

■ Take care of yourself: see your doctor for regular checks: take plenty of rest when you need it and aim for at least eight hours' sleep at night.
■ Regular exercise is beneficial, but don't overdo it. A local AIDS support group can advise you on this and other issues.
■ Meals should be well-balanced and include plenty of fresh fruit and vegetables.
■ Stop or considerably cut down on smoking: it makes you especially prone to chest infection.
■ Don't get pregnant: there may be a 50 per cent chance of infecting your baby, and pregnancy may accelerate the development of AIDS.
■ Never share items likely to be contaminated by blood. These include tooth brushes, razors and scrubbing brushes. It follows that acupuncture, tattooing, ear-piercing and electroysis should be avoided because of blood- contaminated equipment. Don't allow a barber to shave you.

FURTHER SAFETY MEASURES

■ Don't donate blood, milk or semen or any body organ. Don't carry a kidney donor card.
■ Cover cuts with water-proof plasters until healed.
■ Be honest about your present and past sexual activities with your partner and practise safe sex: a local support group or doctor will advise you.
■ Drug misusers must stop taking drugs, or if this is impossible, don't inject.
■ Spills of blood or body fluid: cover with paper tissues and carefully apply diluted bleach – one part of strong bleach to nine parts water. If possible, leave in contact for 30 minutes before wiping up and flushing down the WC. Wear rubber gloves for this.

ORGAN TRANSPLANTS

Immunosuppressives

THE NEW TRANSPANT

A transplanted organ, whether kidney, heart, lung or any other, is bound to be regarded by the body as foreign. Rejecting it is the body's natural response; from the day of the operation this tendency has to be countered by use of sophisticated modern drugs, some developed specially for the purpose. Although this section is relevant mainly to kidney transplants, much of the information also applies to heart and lung transplants.

PRESCRIPTION DRUGS

The typical first choice of immunosuppressive is actually to give two together: azathioprine and the steroid prednisolone.

How they work: Azathioprine stops blood cells dividing: when given in the right dose, it has a selective effect on lymphocytes, thus inhibiting rejection. Prednisolone, as a steroid, suppresses inflammation and therefore rejection. Cyclosporin is a more efficient immunosuppressive than azathioprine-with-prednisolone, and it carries less risk of infection; however it has the major drawback of causing kidney damage and the dose has to be adjusted to exactly the right level.

Other drugs given to correct biochemical changes in the blood and bones, which commonly arise from kidney failure, include **antihypertensives,** *see page 28.* Because patients on immunosuppressive drugs are unusually vulnerable to infection, antibiotics are also likely to be given: among those commonly used are gentamicin, flucloxicillin, cotrimoxazole and cefitaxime.

SIDE EFFECTS

Immunosuppressives not only damp down the body's defences against a foreign organ; they also undermine its natural immunity to bacteria, viruses and funguses. The special-ist's main concern is therefore to adjust the dose so that it is just enough to prevent rejection and no more. The other major problem is kidney damage with cyclosporin: if the drug is given, patients have to be very carefully monitored. Cyclosporin also has the minor side effects of hirsutism and gum overgrowth. Azathioprine has none. For side effects of antihypertensives, beta-blockers and antibiotics, *see pages 28, 26 and 78.*

OVER-THE-COUNTER TREATMENTS

None.

QUESTIONS TO ASK THE DOCTOR
■ For how long do I have to take each drug?
■ Can you help me fix in my mind the correct dose for each drug? How many tablets are equivalent to how many mg?
■ What are the symptoms of deterioration in graft function?
■ Are there any drugs or immunizations which are unsafe in combination with immunosuppressives?
■ What happens if I forget a dose of immunosuppressive?
■ Are there any foreign countries where I run particular risk of infection?

SELF-MANAGEMENT
■ Never stop taking immunosuppressives unless specifically told by the specialist: if you do, the transplant may be acutely rejected.
■ Have an adequate supply of the drugs at all times.
■ Be vigilant for signs of infection: fever, boils, pain in the chest, cough, pain on passing urine.
■ Assist your doctor by accurately reporting side effects; co-operate with all routines to check the level of immunosuppressives in the blood. This will include self-monitoring of blood pressure (twice a day with a sphygmomanometer); taking the temperature once a day; collecting a urine sample at least 24 hours before each clinic appointment.
■ Keep a list of telephone numbers of your specialist and hospital by you at all times.
■ Keep to the recommended diet.
■ Remember, keeping a transplant going well is team work.

What happens in a kidney transplant

Old (non-functioning) kidneys *may or may not be removed depending on their condition.*

Pelvic girdle

Bladder

New kidney, *with its artery and vein joined to the iliac artery and vein.*

Colon and blood vessels *serving colon fill the avilable space this side, so the transplant is always installed on the other side.*

Blood and nutritional

Nutrition involves everything from eating a diet containing suitable foods to the way the individual cells are reached by the bloodstream. Psychological, dietary and hormonal factors are all relevant to nutritional disorders.

Disorders of EATING	**220-223**
ANAEMIA	**224-227**
VITAMIN DEFICIENCY	**228-229**
FOOD INTOLERANCE	**230-231**

See also: *Malabsorption, page 36; alcoholism, page 94; fatigue, page 90; lipid disorders, page 162; obesity, page 154; diabetes, page 156; hyper- and hypothyroidism, pages 164-167; adult leukaemias, page 208; childhood leukaemias, page 210.*

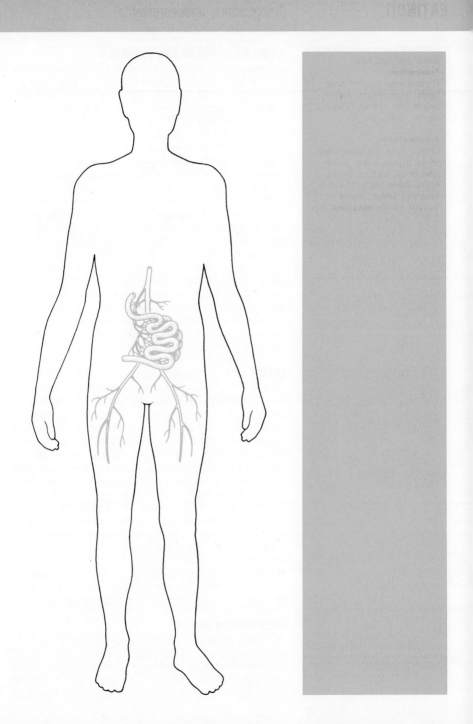

NAMES YOU WILL HEAR
Tranquillizers
Chemical name: diazepam; **trade names:** Valium, Alupram, Atensine, Evacalm, Solis, Tensium, Valrelease; see also anxiety, page 84.

Antidepressants
Chemical name: amitriptyline; **trade names:** Tryptizol, Lentizol, Domical, Elavil, Laroxyl, Tryptanol, Saroten, Amiline, Deprex, Levate, Meravil, Novotriptyn, Amilent, Trepiline, Tryptanol; see also **depression**, page 116.

ANOREXIA NERVOSA AND BULIMIA

– These are the technical terms for the two commonest disorders of eating. Anorexia is voluntary starvation accompanied by substantial weight loss and malnutrition. Bulimia is overindulgence in food followed by self-induced vomiting or use of large doses of laxatives, causing diarrhoea. Bulimia develops into anorexia, or alternates with it. Some patients with bulimia have a history of obesity. The problems are most common in adolescent girls, although they may occur at any age. Men are rarely affected.

The anorectic is obsessed with food, weight and diets. There is excessive fear of becoming fat, and a loss of judgement regarding food requirements and body image: the anorectic often believes she is overweight when in fact she is extremely thin.

Other common symptoms of both conditions include amenorrhea (interruption of normal menstrual bleeding); loss of scalp hair; increase in the fine hair on the face and arms; obsessional commitment to physical exercise and a general restless activity. In patients who regularly vomit after meals, acid from the stomach can cause rapid tooth decay.

CAUSES Ultimately unknown, though it appears that a number of complex factors come together to cause both conditions: ■ There is often conflict within the family, including a poor mother-daughter relationship, sibling rivalry and alcoholism in parents. Families (and especially mothers) must not be thought of as the sole cause, but they are involved in the problem. ■ The typical anorectic is often an 'easy' child, insecure and eager to please her parents. Until adolescence she does not challenge their expectations; then, she finds she has her own ideas of how she wants to develop. Anorexia seems – almost literally – to be the embodiment of this conflict. ■ Social pressure: slimness as a mark of female attractiveness is of course a goal for many adolescent girls.
■ Hormonal changes do occur, but they are thought to be a result of the malnutrition, rather than a cause of it.
■ Brain mechanisms: poorly understood as yet.

PRESCRIPTION DRUGS

The basic aims of treatment are **1** to restore a safe weight on a balanced diet: this is not the solution to the problem but may be necessary for survival – and it can be impossible for a therapist to work with a patient whose thinking is impaired by gross malnutrition; **2** to help the patient to readjust psychologically. Severe cases of anorexia are treated in psychiatric units; many specialists would argue that drugs play a minor role in the treatment of eating disorders. However, **tranquillizers** can help decrease the anxiety which the patient feels when she does eat. The most commonly used are the benzodiazepine group.

How they work: *See **anxiety**, page 84.*

Antidepressants may be used, too, but they are relatively ineffective. The most commonly used group are the tricyclic antidepressants.

How they work: *see **depression**, page 116.*

It is essential for doctors, patients and anyone else concerned to understand that giving drugs and enforcing weight gain without tackling the root cause are ineffective, even dangerous.

OVER-THE-COUNTER TREATMENT

Appetite stimulants and food supplements may seem appropriate to friends and family, but the anorectic herself has no use for them and they don't work.

SIDE EFFECTS

Tranquillizers should be used for the shortest time and in the lowest possible dose because of the risk of dependence. *See **anxiety**, page 84.*

Tricyclic antidepressants: *see **depression**, page 116.*

QUESTIONS TO ASK THE DOCTOR

■ Are the drugs really necessary?
■ What can the family do to help?
■ Can the family obtain outside support if necessary?

SELF-MANAGEMENT

First of all, understand that:

■ Doctors are anxious not to over-diagnose anorexia. Many teenagers have food fads; doctors tend not to act unless weight is ten per cent below the average for age and height. At this level, the danger to health is significant.

■ It is natural for parents to react with anger, guilt and despair; it is difficult for them to cope with the way the anorectic appears to reject their love and care.

■ The patient's behaviour is driven by fear of lack of control over life. A constructive approach, of understanding, support and working together often requires the help of a psychologist working in a hospital setting to bring about step-by-step changes in behaviour. Doctors and therapists will attempt to explore family problems, many of which parents may feel they have handled successfully. This is a threatening experience, but airing the problems *can* help.

IF YOU SUSPECT ANOREXIA OR BULIMIA:
■ Don't delay in seeking help. The family cannot usually undertake the cure alone: they are too closely involved.
■ The best starting point is the family doctor, especially if he or she has known the family for some time and has their trust. The doctor may wish to refer to a specialist (usually a psychiatrist or psychologist) if weight loss is extreme.
■ Parents often find it difficult to hand over control to the doctors: the psychiatrist, for example, has respon-1F-sibilities to the patient and may not be prepared to discuss confidences with parents. Try to understand, and work with the doctors.
■ Parents often feel a need for more positive action than is first offered in terms of investigations and physical treatment. But the best result is for her to *want* to start eating again, not to be drugged and force-fed.

THE PATIENT'S PROBLEMS
■ She may have a distorted perception of her own size, and feel that she is large when she is thin. She may also be unable to assess what a normal plateful of food should be.
■ She may be deceitful about food and her weight. This is part of the illness.
■ There appears to be a deep-rooted fear that she will lose self-control if she gives in to the desire to eat.
■ She often feels insecure and incompetent.
■ She finds it difficult to ask for help because of her desire to retain control of her life.
■ Bulimia can be time-consuming: hours are devoted to secretly buying, eating and then vomiting up food.
■ Without treatment, the condition can progress to a point at which the patient is unable to help herself because of real malnutrition.

STRATEGY
Anorexia is a behavioural 'solution' to a state of internal conflict. The anorectic cannot be forced to give up anorexia before the process of recovery begins. Everyone needs defence mechanisms occasionally.
■ Counselling and psychotherapy: Find someone the anorectic can trust, and talk with, as soon as possible. The therapist must be someone who allows her to re-

tain control of her treatment; if she does not, feelings of incompetence and insecurity will be compounded.

Drug therapy: The disadvantages usually outweigh the advantages. Because the drugs' action is essentially to lower resistance, they impair self-control, the very quality on which the therapist needs to work. Any decision to use drugs must be made with the anorectic's consent.

■ Hospital admission may be necessary if malnutrition is endangering the anorectic's life. A balanced diet of proteins, carbohydrates, fats, vitamins and minerals can be given by means of sedation, feeding via a tube into the stomach, or a drip into a vein.

Going into hospital can also be useful in removing the anorectic from a tense family situation. However, the emphasis in hospital tends to be on weight gain, rather than addressing the underlying problems. It is therefore essential for the anorectic and the family to consider what the hospital's approach will be before agreeing to admission. It ought to appreciate the importance of the patient retaining control where possible; treatment must not degenerate into a struggle of wills between her and the hospital staff.

One aspect of hospital treatment is behaviour modification based on a reward system for co-operation. Privileges such as family visits, being allowed out of bed and participation in activities are made to depend on weight gain. This can involve loss of control by the patient: there may be a rapid weight gain, but after discharge there may well be an equally rapid weight loss, and possibly suicidal depression. Enforced bed rest until weight gain has been achieved can also be a torment for an already anxious, restless person. If there is to be a weight goal, it ought to be negotiated with, not dictated to, the patient.

Individual and group psychotherapy with family involvement ought to be the major part of any hospital treatment, but resources for psychotherapy are limited in some countries. Hospital treatment should, in addition, include occupational therapy.

Both in hospital and at home there must be total honesty over contents of food prepared for the anorectic. Secretly adding high calorie products will result in loss of trust and resistance to all food.

■ Chances of a happy outcome are significantly improved if the problem is presented to a doctor early, and if the onset is in the early teens, within three years of puberty. There is no correlation between disturbed behaviour and the number of episodes.

SIGNS OF RECOVERY
A change in attitude towards eating; loss of obsession with food. Weight gain is not a reliable sign of recovery and menstrual periods take many months to return to normal. Recovery also involves a sense of the patient being in charge of her own life, with an ability to make her own decisions about what she wants, and an accurate sense of her worth.

NAMES YOU WILL HEAR
Iron
Chemical name: ferrous sulphate;
trade names: Feospan, Ferrograd C,
Ferro-Gradumet, Feritard, Fespan, Fer-
in-Sol, Fesofor, Ferrosan. **Chemical
name:** ferrous fumarate; **trade
names:** Fersaday, Fersamal, Galfer,
Bramiron, Fumiron, Feroton,
Ferrofume. **Chemical name:** ferrous
gluconate; **trade names:** Fergon,
Ferro-G, Fersin, Glucohaem, Fertinic,
Novoferrogluc. **Chemical name:**
ferrous glycine sulphate; **trade names:**
Fe-cap, Ferrocontin Continus, Kelferon,
Plesmet, Ferro-Chel. **Chemical name:**
ferrous succinate; **trade names:**
Ferromyn, Cerevon, Kepler.

Injectable Iron Preparations
Chemical names: iron dextran
injection, iron sorbitol injection; **trade
names:** Imferon, Jectofer.

Folic Acid
Chemical name: folic acid; **trade
names:** Lexpec, Folettes, Folvite,
Novofolacid.

Vitamin B12
Chemical names: hydroxocobalamin,
cyanocobalamin; **trade names:**
Cobalin-H, Neo-Cytamen, Cytacon,
Cytamen, Hepacon-B12, Panalamine,
Anacobin, Bedoz, Bio-12, Cyanabin,
Neo-Rubex, Redisol, Rubion.

WHAT IS ANAEMIA?

A disorder of the red blood cells. These cells take oxygen from the lungs to the tissues of the body; the oxygen is transported on an iron-containing substance called haemoglobin which is stored in the red cells.

Anaemia may result in fatigue, breathlessness on exertion, soreness of the tongue and mouth, palpitations, dizziness and headache. Sufferers may have an unusually pale skin, with loss of normal colour in the lips, tongue and linings of the eyes. The pulse may be noticeably more rapid than usual, especially on exercise; people with heart disease or narrowing of the arteries may have worse symptoms if they become anaemic.

The effects of anaemia on the individual depend on its severity and on how quickly it has developed. Slowly-developing anaemias allow time for the body to adapt and are thus better tolerated.

CAUSES Generally, anaemias arise in the two main ways. In order to make blood properly, the bone marrow needs a supply of protein and essential vitamins and minerals such as folic acid, vitamin B12 and iron. Anaemia resulting from failure to produce sufficient haemoglobin can arise, therefore, from lack of these essential ingredients (see below); or from a disease of the bone marrow such as acute leukaemia. Secondly, anaemia can result from loss or breakdown of red cells at a rate which exceeds their production. This may occur in severe bleeding

CAUSES OF IRON DEFICIENCY A diet low in fresh fruit and vegetables can result in folic acid deficiency. The bowel may fail to absorb folic acid from the diet, for example in chronic diarrhoea. Or there may be a high demand for extra folic acid, as in pregnancy, or in some bone marrow disorders; if folic acid supply does not keep up with the demand, anaemia will follow.

CAUSES OF VITAMIN B12 DEFICIENCY Absorption of vitamin B12 from the stomach may be lowered if there has been surgery to the stomach, for example to treat ulcers. Another cause is pernicious anaemia, which results from an immune response. Less commonly, vitamin B12 deficiency can result from disease of the small bowel.

PRESCRIPTION DRUGS

Iron deficiency will usually respond to taking iron by

mouth. However, some people are truly unable to tolerate iron by mouth, or may have bowel problems preventing this remedy. These may require iron by injection. Treatment with iron corrects the anaemia of iron deficiency in six to eight weeks. A further two to three months' treatment is often given to replace the body's iron stores.

Folic acid and vitamin B12 deficiencies are treated by tablet; vitamin B12 deficiency is treated by injection. Response to folic acid and vitamin B12 is rapid, with clear evidence of improvement within a few days. The anaemia is usually completely corrected in four to six weeks. In folic acid deficiency, treatment is often continued for three to four months to replace body stores. Maintenance injections of vitamin B12 may be necessary and in this case are given every two or three months for life.

QUESTIONS TO ASK YOUR DOCTOR
■ Am I anaemic or is there some other cause for my symptoms?
■ What sort of anaemia do I have?
■ Why have I become deficient in iron/folic acid/ vitamin B12?
■ Should I modify my diet?
■ Is there an underlying cause for the anaemia that needs investigation?
■ How long will the treatment take to work?

OVER-THE-COUNTER TREATMENTS
Although the preparations containing iron and vitamin B12 are available at chemists and health food shops, don't attempt to treat yourself. This is a complex condition, and dosage has to be correct: many preparations contain too little iron or B12 to be effective.

SIDE EFFECTS
Iron: nausea, discomfort in the stomach, constipation and diarrhoea. These effects are due to iron itself and an alternative iron preparation may produce fewer side effects only because it contains less iron. All iron tablets produce darkening of the faeces. Iron given intramuscularly or intravenously may produce nausea, vomiting and flushing. Staining of the skin may also occur. Major reactions with collapse, low blood pressure and acute breathlessness are rare, but iron should not be given in this way to people with a history of allergy and asthma.
Folic acid and vitamin B12 are essentially free of significant

PATIENT'S EXPERIENCE
"I am now 26 years old and I have suffered problems with sickle cell anaemia since early childhood. My main problem at present is a tendency towards recurrent crises which produce severe pain particularly in my back and legs. I have found that over-exertion and rapid changes in temperature increase the likelihood of a crisis developing and I am careful to avoid them. If I feel a mild crisis starting, I keep warm, drink plenty of fluids and take simple pain killers. This is often all I need to do; however, sometimes the crisis worsens and I then need intensive treatment in hospital. Fortunately this is infrequent."

side effects. Neither should be given, however, until a deficiency state has been properly diagnosed.

SELF-HELP

If you have iron, folic acid or vitamin B12 deficiency, eat a well balanced diet containing a full range of vitamins and minerals. Some diets do carry a risk of developing vitamin deficiencies, for example very strict vegetarian diets may contain insufficient vitamin B12.

Look for and report immediately to your doctor any bleeding in the urine or faeces. Similarly, unusually heavy or abnormally-timed menstrual bleeding, and particularly bleeding from the vagina occurring after the menopause.

OTHER ANAEMIAS

Aplastic anaemia is a severe anaemia caused by reduced production of normal blood cells in the bone marrow. This may be due to a severe general illness, or to invasion of the bone marrow by abnormal cells, as in cancer.

Thalassaemia occurs as a result of failure of the mechanism for producing normal haemoglobin. The red cells are broken down more easily than usual. It runs in families.

Sickle cell anaemia is a similar haemolytic anaemia occurring particularly in people of west African or West Indian extraction.

PRESCRIPTION DRUGS AND OTHER TREATMENTS

Aplastic anaemia: Less severe cases may need no drugs; mildly or moderately affected people may benefit from attempts to boost bone marrow function. The agent most commonly used in this situation is **oxymethalone,** a drug similar to the male hormone testosterone. Severe (life-threatening) cases may be treated by bone marrow transplant. If this is not possible, drug treatment with the **anti-white cell agents** (immunosuppressive drugs) and the steroid **methyl prednisolone** may be tried.

Thalassaemias: Most people with thalassaemia need no treatment. However, a severe thalassaemia (thalassaemia major) causes a serious anaemia in early childhood. This is not amenable to drug treatment but needs regular blood transfusions. This causes problems: transfused blood contains large amounts of iron which accumulate in the body and can damage vital organs such as the heart and liver. To rid the body of this excess iron, **desferrioxamine** may be used – it binds the iron, enabling it to be excreted in the urine. Some children with severe thalassaemia have been effectively treated by bone marrow *transplantation,* although such treatment is not yet widely available.

Sickle cell anaemia: People with sickle cell disease are unusually anaemic but tolerate the condition well and often require no specific drug treatment other than regular folic acid. Children with sickle cell anaemia should receive prompt treatment for bacterial infections – their resistance to infection may be diminished.

Sickle crises (severe pain in the legs, back or chest due to blockage of small blood vessels by the abnormal 'sickled' red cells) may respond to simple measures at home (see SELF-HELP).

SIDE EFFECTS
Steroids: oxymetholone can cause the following: acne, fluid retention leading to ankle swelling; in women development of facial hair, deepening of the voice and irregular periods. A serious side effect can be jaundice, a yellow discolouration of the skin and eyes indicating disturbance of liver function. Report immediately to your doctor.

Methyl prednisolone can cause acute rise in blood pressure, fluid retention, muscle weakness, and, rarely, drug-induced diabetes *(see page 156);* insomnia and depression; indigestion and heartburn and generally decreased resistance to infection; weakening and thinning of the bones, especially in the spine. Long-term prednisolone's side effects are undeniably grave, but the drug's use is justified by the fact that it can be life-saving; that not all patients suffer the side effects; that careful monitoring can anticipate problems before they develop. Stopping the drug can itself be problematic, and must be done gradually under supervision.

Desferrioxamine must be given by injection. It can, very occasionally, cause pain at the infusion site and collapse with a sudden fall in blood pressure. This usually occurs at the start of the infusion; the first few doses must be carefully monitored.

SELF-HELP IN SICKLE CELL ANAEMIA
1 The frequency of sickle crises can be reduced by avoiding sudden changes in temperature, dehydration and over-exertion. If a mild crisis does start, warmth, rest, a high fluid intake, and simple painkillers may be sufficient. In a severe crisis, or if a mild crisis worsens, inform your doctor as soon as possible.
2 Seek advice from your doctor about any infection, however apparently mild it seems.

227

WHAT IS VITAMIN DEFICIENCY?

Vitamins are constituents of the diet necessary for the normal function of various organs in the body. Minimum requirements are recognized for each one.

CAUSES Restricted or deficient diet: typically a problem of vegans (those on ultra-restricted vegetarian diet); alcoholics who may not eat properly; old people living alone who find it too bothersome to cook; non-absorption of vitamins because of bowel disease; temporarily increased need for certain vitamins, for example in pregnancy or growth spurts. Certain drugs also interfere with vitamin absorption.

Vitamin A deficiency is rare in developed countries. It results in poor night vision, dry eyes, damage to the cornea and eventually blindness. The vitamin is found in animal fats, fruit and vegetables.

Vitamin B group – thiamine (B1), riboflavin (B2), pyridoxine (B6), cyanocobalamin (B12) and folic acid – are rarely deficient because they are found in a wide variety of foods. Deficiency occurs in chronic alcoholism or as the result of an extremely restricted diet. Folic acid and B12 deficiencies result in anaemia, *see page 224.*

Vitamin C deficiency causes scurvy. Mild symptoms are quite common, especially in the elderly, and include bleeding gums, bruising and delayed healing of wounds. The vitamin is found in citrus fruit, green vegetables and potatoes, but is destroyed by cooking.

Vitamin D deficiency causes rickets and is most commonly found in the elderly and in Asians who eat unleavened bread. It may also be seen in babies (especially those born prematurely) who are not given vitamin D supplements. The vitamin is necessary for hardening of bone and for normal strength in muscles. In young children the deficiency results in bending of the long bones; in the elderly the bones become soft. Vitamin D can be produced in the skin in the presence of sunlight; it is also found in fish oils and animal fat.

Vitamin K is important for chemicals necessary for blood clotting. Produced by bacteria in the bowel, and absorbed with fat, it may be deficient in the newborn because just after birth the bowel is sterile. It may also be lacking in people who cannot absorb fats from the bowel. The vitamin occurs in milk and green plants. Deficiency causes prolonged bleeding.

REPLACEMENTS

Vitamin A can be given as a single daily dose, alone or in combination with Vitamin D or a multivitamin preparation. The recommended daily dose is 1,300 to 5,000 units. Higher doses can be given less frequently.

Vitamin B group can be given by tablet or injection.

Vitamin C is given as a single daily dose of 200 mg to prevent or treat scurvy, particularly in the elderly or those on a poor diet.

Vitamin D can be given as drops for the very young, or as a tablet or injection. The usual daily dose is 400 units.

Vitamin K is given routinely by injection to newborn babies for reasons given above, and because a baby's liver tends to be immature at birth and, with reduced vitamin K, fails to produce enough clotting factors.

OVER-THE-COUNTER TREATMENTS
All the vitamins listed are available without prescription. Multivitamin preparations have no advantages over single preparations, and many are expensive.

QUESTIONS TO ASK THE DOCTOR
■ If I am a vegetarian, do I need extra vitamins?
■ Do old people need extra vitamins?
■ Does my baby need vitamin supplements?
■ Do I need to let you know if I am taking vitamins?
■ Can I take extra vitamins during pregnancy?

SIDE EFFECTS
Vitamin A in excess can cause rough skin, dry, sparse hair and increased calcium in the blood. Very large doses can cause irritability and increased pressure within the brain. Large doses should be carefully avoided during pregnancy as the high blood level of calcium can affect the baby.

Vitamin B group and **vitamin C** don't have significant side effects. There is no evidence that massive doses of vitamin C increases resistance to the common cold.

Vitamin D is potentially dangerous as high doses can increase the level of calcium in the blood. This can cause vomiting, dehydration, constipation and kidney stones. Do not use during pregnancy or while breast-feeding because of risk to the baby.

Vitamin K can cause excessive clotting in patients on anticoagulants, but has no other side effects.

SELF-MANAGEMENT
■ A commonsense, balanced diet is all that is necessary to prevent vitamin deficiency.
■ Restricted diets must be critically examined for vitamin content.

PATIENT'S EXPERIENCE
"I was feeling run-down in the middle of the winter and I went to see my doctor because I felt that I needed a vitamin tonic. She asked me questions about my diet, and said that although I was a vegetarian, it diet did contain sufficient vitamins. She took a blood test for anaemia and when I returned for the results, it was normal. I was not convinced because I was still so tired and irritable. We spoke for a while about my job which hadn't been going very well. She said she felt that my job was affecting me and suggested that I take a holiday. This has helped a bit, and I am actively trying to cut down stress at work: maybe I do feel better."

VEGETARIANS
– Do not generally need extra vitamins if their diet is varied. If it is very restricted, as with vegans (no dairy produce), vitamin supplements may well be necessary.

VITAMIN PREPARATIONS
■ The body's requirements for vitamins is generally much less than is contained in most of the vitamin preparations. There is no advantage to taking excessive doses of vitamins and in some cases, overdose can cause illness.
■ Avoid multivitamin preparations: if there really is a deficiency of a vitamin, replace it with the correct dose.
■ Vitamin D is usually added to baby milk mixes.

WHAT IS FOOD INTOLERANCE?

The expression "One man's meat is another man's poison" is of Roman origin: it has long been acknowledged that foods can produce adverse reactions in sensitive individuals. This phenomenon is now known by the general term of food intolerance and includes several recognized conditions:

Food aversion is a psychologically based inability totolerate certain foods; an extreme, but typical example is **anorexia** – see page 220.

True food allergy is a sensitivity to a particular food mediated through the immune system. Fish allergy, associated with severe swelling of the lips, is a classic form. The allergy is readily demonstrated by a skin reaction when testing solution is applied. Many foods cause allergy, including nuts, egg and mushrooms.

Chemical or pharmacological reactions produced in the body by some foods or drinks are normally minor, if noticeable at all, but if the subject is particularly sensitive or takes the food in large quantities, symptoms may appear. The commonest substance which acts in this way is the caffeine in coffee, tea and Coca-Cola. Large quantities of coffee in sensitive subjects can produce headache, palpitations, anxiety and insomnia.

Enzyme deficiency: the body is unable to break down specific foods. Lactase, for example, is a bowel enzyme which breaks down dairy products. Individuals lacking it develop chronic abdominal pain and diarrhoea.

Certain substances can, in addition, cause reactions in sensitive individuals by mechanisms which are not yet understood. These include additives, which are added to food as preservatives, colouring agents, tasting agents and substances which affect texture and moisture. Monosodium glutamate, the flavour-enhancing agent in Chinese food, can cause pain and tingling in the chest which can be mistaken for a heart attack. Tartrazine, a yellow colouring used in many foods, can cause swelling of the lips, urticaria (large, itchy red lumps in the skin) and it can exacerbate asthma. Certain dyes, such as eosin, can produce hyperactivity in sensitive children.

PRESCRIPTION DRUGS

Drug therapy is of little value in food intolerance, as the main approach is to identify and then avoid any food which causes a major problem. However, an acute allergic reaction with swelling of the face and urticaria can be treated with an **antihistamine:** one of the newer types such as Triludan is best, since it does not cause drowsiness. **Sodium cromoglycate,** a cell stabilizer, will sometimes prevent an allergic reaction and is prescribed for food-allergic patients who are going out for a meal which may contain a food to which they are sensitive. It is not helpful on a regular basis.

OVER-THE-COUNTER TREATMENTS
None.

QUESTIONS TO ASK THE DOCTOR
■ Do you think I have a true food allergy?
■ Can you recommend a diet?
■ Is it worth seeing a specialist dietician?

SIDE EFFECTS
The main problem with food intolerance is that it can produce a wide range of symptoms which can mimic many other diseases. It is, therefore, important that the patient should be assessed by a physician to exclude any serious disease prior to investigating food intolerance. The following symptoms can be caused by food intolerance: headache, catarrh, sneezing, depression, anxiety, sore throat; palpitations, asthma; chronic pain, bloating and diarrhoea; rheumatism, eczema, urticaria.

For side effects of **antihistamines** see **sinusitis,** page 262, of **sodium cromoglycate,** see **asthma,** page 74.

SELF-MANAGEMENT
1 Check with your doctor that your symptoms do not have another cause.
2 Avoid, for one week, any food which you suspect might be related to your problem.
3 If you do not suspect a particular food, try a general elimination diet for seven days. A simple one limits you to meat, fish, vegetables, salads, fruits and water. It excludes bread and all grains, dairy products, additives, tea and coffee. For the first few days you may feel unwell due to withdrawal symptoms, but an improvement should be evident within seven days.
4 If the symptoms resolve within seven days, foods should then be added back into the diet at 24-hour intervals to identify which was causing the problems.
5 If there is no improvement after seven days, food intolerance is unlikely; return to a normal diet.
BUT:
6 If you still feel that food intolerance could be the cause of your problems, seek expert advice. It is dangerous to attempt more rigid elimination diets.

PATIENT'S EXPERIENCE
"I suffered severe migraine attacks every weekend. They occurred on a Saturday afternoon: agonizing – I was sick too, and I felt weak all over. My wife thought they were psychological: an excuse to avoid shopping with her on Saturday afternoons. Numerous drugs failed to help. Finally I went to see an allergist interested in food intolerance who noted that I regularly drank about ten cups of coffee each day when at work, but not at the weekend. He suggested that my weekend headache was similar to a drug withdrawal: the level of caffeine in my blood dropped at the weekend. I stopped drinking coffee at work during the week and, to my surprise, the headaches ceased."

Skeletal, joint and muscular disorders

The body has a complicated system of bones and joints which allow a great variety of movements. The joints are supported and strengthened by ligaments (fibrous strengthening around or inside the joints), muscles and tendons. Tendons connect the body of the muscle with fixed points on the bony skeleton. The joints are lubricated by synovial fluid produced by the membrane surrounding the joints. The upright posture of the human being has produced a range of adaptations from the basic four-legged animal skeleton, but our 'locomotor system' is still prone to wear and tear and disease.

STRAINS AND SPRAINS,   234-235
including fibrositis, tennis elbow, house-maids knee

BACK PAIN   236-237

OSTEOARTHRITIS   238-241

RHEUMATOID ARTHRITIS   242-245

GOUT   246-247

ANKYLOSING SPONDYLITIS   248-249

CRAMP   250-251

See also: *Fatigue, page 90.*

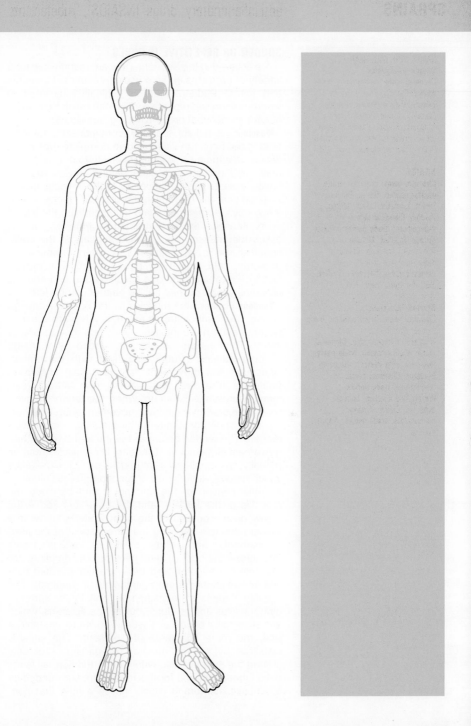

STRAINS AND SPRAINS

Simple analgesics, steroid injections, non-steroid anti-inflammatory drugs (NSAIDS), rubefacients

NAMES YOU WILL HEAR
Simple analgesics
Chemical name: paracetamol; **trade names:** Panadol, Pamol, Calpol, Tylenon, Paracin, Parmol, Panado, Ceetamol, Atosol, Exctol, Tylenol, Ennagesic, Ilvamol. **Chemical name:** aspirin; **trade names:** Aspirin, Astrin, Bi-Prin. *See also **pain,** page 106.*

NSAIDs
Chemical name: ibuprofen; **trade names:** Apsifen, Ebufac, Brufen, Fenbid, Ibumetin, Lidifen, Motrin, Paxofen. **Chemical name:** indomethacin; **trade names:** Indocid, Artracin, Indoflex, Mobilan, Rheumacin, Arthrexin. **Chemical name:** naproxen sodium; **trade names:** Laraflex, Naprosyn, Synflex. *See also **pain,** page 106.*

Steroid injections
Chemical name: hydrocortisone; **trade names:** Hydrocortisone Injection, Efcortesol, Hydrocortistab. **Chemical name:** dexamethasone; **trade names:** Dexamethasone Injection, Decadron, Oradexon. **Chemical name:** prednisolone; **trade names:** Prednisolone Injection, Codelsol, Deltastab. **Chemical name:** triamcinolone; **trade names:** Adcortyl, Kenalog.

SUDDEN OR REPETITIVE INJURIES

– Are covered in this section. They are responsible for a variety of problems in the muscles, tendons, ligaments and joints. Sudden injury is typically sustained in vigorous exercise; repetitive injury can result from as innocent an occupation as wringing out clothes.

Muscle injury results, typically, from a direct blow or by tearing the fibres; this can involve complete rupture, in which case the muscle loses its ability to contract; or it may be a partial tear – the painful 'pulled muscle' typically sustained by athletes. If the muscle tear is situated near the skin, a large bruise can appear within a few days, sometimes some distance from the site of injury. Muscles are also affected by fibrositis, or soft tissue rheumatism. This usually appears in the neck, shoulder, or lower back and is often attributed to draughts, cold, anxiety or poor posture. The muscle fibres go into spasm in one specific area, and nodules or lumps which or may not be painful can be felt.

Tendons connect the muscles to the bones. Although strong, they cannot stretch much; indeed with age they become even more inelastic, and thus more prone to injury. Tendons are usually surrounded by a sheath which produces a lubricating fluid with movement. Unaccustomed movement cancause pain known as tendonitis; it resolves within a few days without treatment. Tenosynovitis occurs when the tendon is overused or injured by repetitive movement such as a heel tab on a shoe constantly rubbing against the Achilles tendon. The tendon becomes painful and swollen, and movement is restricted. Tendons, like muscles, can be partially or completely ruptured: a painful experience which causes varying loss of function. Tennis elbow is an inflammation of the tendinous joint between the muscles of the forearm and the bone just above the elbow on the outside of the arm. Golfer's elbow is a similar condition affecting the inner aspect of the arm.

Ligaments and joints exist in various forms throughout the body. There are simple hinge joints (for example the fingers); and there are complicated ball-and-socket joints (for example the hip or shoulder). The stability of joints is maintained not only by the surrounding muscles and tendons, but by the **ligaments,** which are essentially bands of tissue. The more unstable a **joint,** the more ligaments are present. The knee is stabilized by a large number of ligaments not only around the joint but also within it. In addition, all joints need lubrication, and for this reason are surrounded by a synovial membrane which makes a fluid that continually bathes the joint. If the joint is injured, this reacts by making extra fluid and the joint, or part of it, may swell. If the front of the knee is subjected to repeated injury such as kneeling, a sac of fluid may appear over the knee (otherwise known as housemaid's knee).

PRESCRIPTION DRUGS

Simple analgesics or painkillers like paracetamol or aspirin will relieve the pain and, to a lesser extent, reduce inflammation. The catch is that once the pain is relieved, there is a temptation to return to full activity at once, and thus to worsen the injury. Combinations with codeine increases the pain relief. See **pain,** page 106.

NSAIDS will reduce swelling, redness and tenderness around an injury, and quicken healing. As they also reduce pain, there is a similar temptation to return to full activity too soon. See **osteoarthritis,** page 238.

Steroid injections, given directly in the injured area, can have great effect in reducing local inflammation. They are particularly helpful in treating tennis elbow and joint swellings. See **rheumatoid arthritis,** page 242.

Rubefacients – agents which are rubbed in or sprayed on – act by counter-irritation of the skin: the feeling of warmth detracts from pain elsewhere. There is no evidence that they help with deep pain.

OVER-THE-COUNTER TREATMENTS

Apart from steroid injections, all the other treatments listed are available from chemists. The range of NSAIDS is, however, limited; use them with caution.

QUESTIONS TO ASK THE DOCTOR

■ How long should I rest after the injury?
■ Would physiotherapy be helpful?
■ What can I do to stop it happening again?

SIDE EFFECTS

Simple analgesics are relatively free of side effects: however, if combined with codeine, they are more likely to produce nausea, vomiting and constipation (see **pain,** page 106 and **common cold,** page 134). Aspirin should not be used in children under 12 years of age. Allergic reactions can occur, often an itchy skin rash.

NSAIDs are related to aspirin and allergic reactions do occur. See **pain,** page 106.

Steroid injections, if repeated too frequently, can lead to joint and tendon damage.

Rubefacients should not be used on broken skin. Local allergic reactions are common.

PATIENT'S EXPERIENCE

"It was around Christmas, in the frost, that I slipped while running and went over on my left ankle. It was extremely painful, but I managed to walk the three miles home. Afterwards, my ankle was like a balloon: I was sure that it was broken, but the doctor said that it was just a bad sprain. I insisted on an X-ray, but he was right. It was strapped up and I had daily ultrasonic treatment from a physiotherapist at the hospital. I needed crutches to get about. The swelling slowly went down, but even at Easter I could still feel the pain if I put it under pressure. If I hadn't had to walk home, I don't think it would have swelled up so much."

NON-DRUG OPTIONS

Rest is usually necessary to allow the healing process to get under way. Strapping and resting an injured part are common measures. Physiotherapy, if available, is often helpful, especially ultrasonic sound therapy if given soon after a sprain. Surgery may be a last resort in certain conditions such as tennis elbow which have not responded to steroid injections. It is the only treatment for a complete tendon tear.

THE RICE PRINCIPLE

Apply the RICE principle for the first few days after the injury. R is for rest. This helps to stop bleeding, external and internal, and to minimize damage to the tissues. I is for ice, or a cold application: cold water, or a bag of ice cubes, or even frozen peas. Take care: excessive cold can burn skin. C is for compression: firm bandaging will stop bleeding into the tissues. Don't apply too tightly. E is for elevation: raising the affected part allows fluid to drain away and reduces swelling.

A couple of days after most sudden or repetitive injuries, it is usually possible to start gentle exercise, massage, or local heat treatment oneself, but if in any doubt consult a doctor or physiotherapist.

NAMES YOU WILL HEAR
Simple analgesics
Chemical name: aspirin; **trade names:** Aspirin, Astrin, Bi-Prin.
Chemical name: paracetamol; **trade names:** Panadol, Pamol, Calpol, Tylenon, Paracin, Parmol, Panado, Ceetamol, Atosol, Exctol, Tylenol, Ennagesic, Ilvamol. *See also **pain,** page 106.*

Narcotic analgesics
Chemical name: dihydrocodeine; **trade names:** DF 118, Onadex 118, Paramol 118, Rikodeine, Tuscodin, Paracodin, Fortuss. **Chemical name:** buprenorphine; **trade names:** Temgesic, Buprex. *See also **pain, page 106.***

NSAIDS
Chemical name: ibuprofen; **trade name:** Apsifen, Ebufac, Brufen, Fenbid, Ibumetin, Lidifen, Motrin, Paxofen. **Chemical name:** indomethacin; **trade names:** Indocid, Artracin, Indoflex, Mobilan, Rheumacin, Arthrexin. *See also **pain,** page 106.*

Muscle relaxants
Chemical name: diazepam; **trade names:** Valium, Alupram, Atensine, Evacalm, Solis, Tensium, Valrelease. **Chemical name:** orphenadrin citrate; **trade names:** Norflex, Norgesic, Disipal, Biorphen. **Chemical name:** methocarbamol; **trade names:** Robaxin, Robaxisal. **Chemical name:** chlormezanone; **trade names:** Trancoprin, Trancopal, Lobak.

THE BACK AND ITS PROBLEMS
The back bone, or spine, is divided into three main sections: neck (cervical spine), upper back (dorsal or thoracic spine), and lower back (lumbo-sacral spine).

The spine is actually a column of bones called vertebrae, separated from each other by discs, which are rings of tough fibrous tissue with an inner core made of a jelly-like substance. Their principal function is to absorb stress on impact, like a shock-absorber. With age they slowly stiffen, becoming brittle.

The vertebrae are secured by a system of ligaments and muscles which support the whole structure and allow a limited amount of movement. Each vertebra also has joints linking it with adjacent bones thus making a whole series of complex joints allowing co-ordinated movement The spine also provides protection to the spinal cord, from which, between the vertebrae, fine pairs of nerves branch off and lead to the skin, muscles and joints of the body.

Similar causes give pain in any part of the back.

CAUSES OF BACK PAIN Movements which place abnormal stress or load on the spine will cause injury and pain. This can happen suddenly, as when lifting a heavy weight, or it can come on slowly, as when performing a repetitive task. The vertebrae can be compressed in a severe injury; indeed the arch bones at the back of the vertebrae can be broken in a severe twisting injury. Ligaments of the spine may be stretched, partially torn or may rupture completely. The small joints may be strained, or, even more serious, the discs may rupture and the jelly inside can protrude and compress nerves or the spinal cord itself.

''Referred pain'' occurs when injury to the spine irritates a nerve supplying a specific part of the body. Perhaps the commonest example is sciatica, in which pain is felt in the legs, although the spine is the site of damage or inflammation. Fibrositis is a common back problem arising from muscle spasm, in turn caused by over-use of a muscle or muscles.

Arthritis in the spine is usually a 'wear and tear' process; it may reflect previous injury, or be a gradual change associated with ageing. X-rays will reveal changes caused by early 'wear and tear' arthritis in most people in their 20s or 30s.

PRESCRIPTION DRUGS
Simple analgesics – aspirin and paracetamol – are often effective, relieving pain and reducing inflammation.

See *pain, page 106,* as also for **narcotic analgesics.**
NSAIDS reduce the swelling and inflammation around an injured area, thus giving pain relief.
How they work: *see osteoarthritis, page 238.*
Muscle relaxants are of some value, especially when most of the pain is due to muscle spasm. Diazepam, a sedative can reduce associated tension and anxiety. See *anxiety, page 84.*

OVER-THE-COUNTER TREATMENTS

Aspirin and paracetamol, available without prescription, should be tried before consulting a doctor. If you report that they are ineffective, this can be a useful basis on which to plan the next step in treatment.

Ibuprofen is available from chemists in many countries and can be tried if simple analgesics have failed.

Rubefacient creams are widely available. They are a way of applying local heat to the affected part, and act by counter-irritation.

QUESTIONS TO ASK THE DOCTOR

■ What do you think has caused the pain?
■ Would physiotherapy or an osteopath be helpful?
■ Can I go to work/take exercise?
■ Should I learn back-strengthening exercises?

SIDE EFFECTS

Simple analgesics, especially paracetamol, are more or less free of side effects. However, aspirin should be used with caution and not at all in the under-12 age group. See *pain, page 106.*
Narcotic analgesics can produce drowsiness, unsteadiness and an inability to concentrate. Vomiting is sometimes a problem and most people become constipated if they take these drugs for an extended period. There is a danger of addiction. See *pain, page 106.*
NSAIDS are related to aspirin and have the same side effects but usually less so. Indigestion, a common side effect, can often be prevented by taking them with a meal, or with milk. See *osteoarthritis, page 238.*
Muscle relaxants are often sedative, but they can also cause dry mouth and blurring of vision, especially if taken in higher dosage. See *anxiety, page 84.*

SELF-HELP

■ Take simple painkillers as soon as the pain starts. Heat treatment can be started immediately: if you don't have a purpose-designed lamp, a hot bath and/or rubefacient are worth trying.

PATIENT'S EXPERIENCE

"I was working as a nurse on a geriatric ward when I got my first attack of low back pain. It was while we were lifting this old man: I had to twist and lift at the same time. The pain came on like a knife: I could hardly move. I had to go home, rest and take some painkillers. The pain went within ten days; I went back to work. However, the pain kept coming back, and I kept having to take time off.

This went on for more than a year: I was seriously thinking of changing my job when a physiotherapist at the hospital saw me in pain. She suggested some exercises, and advised me on how to lift patients the right way. It took some months for the benefit to come through; but now my back feels much stronger and I'm taking much less time off work."

REST

Once the pain has started, rest is the most important healing factor: anything that leads to further back strain should be avoided. Sitting will aggravate the pain unless the back is well supported with a cushion. A cervical collar or lumbar support may be of temporary benefit, but should not be used for too long.

PREVENTION

1 always lift weights with the knees bent and the back straight; **2** maintain strong back and stomach muscles by means of suitable exercises (ask a physiotherapist to show you the exercises); **3** sleep on a firm bed.

CAUTION

If there is much referred pain and numbness in the arms or legs, seek medical advice. If you are unable to pass urine, seek medical help urgently.

Simple analgesics, compound analgesics, non-steroidal anti-inflammatory drugs (NSAIDs)

NAMES YOU WILL HEAR
Simple analgesics
Chemical names: aspirin, acetylsalicylic acid; **trade names:** Aspirin, Astrin, Bi-Prin. **Chemical name:** paracetamol; **trade names:** Panadol, Pamol, Calpol, Tylenon, Paracin, Parmol, Panado, Ceetamol, Atosol, Exctol, Tylenol, Ennagesic, Ilvamol. **Chemical name:** dextropropoxyphene; **trade names:** Doloxene, Algaphan, Algodex, Depronal SA. *See also pain, page 106.*

Compound analgesics
Chemical name: co-proxamol (dextropropoxyphene plus paracetamol); **trade names:** Co-proxamol, Distalgesic; *see also pain, page 106.*

Non-steriod anti-inflammatory drugs
Chemical name: aspirin; **trade names:** Aspirin, Astrin, Bi-Prin. **Chemical name:** indomethacin; **trade names:** Indocid, Artracin, Indoflex, Mobilan, Rheumacin, Arthrexin. **Chemical name:** ibuprofen; **trade names:** Apsifen, Ebufac, Brufen, Fenbid, Ibumetin, Lidifen, Motrin, Paxofen. **Chemical name:** ketoprofen; **trade name:** Orudis. **Chemical name:** naproxen sodium; **trade names:** Laraflex, Naprosyn, Synflex. **Chemical name:** phenylbutazone; **trade name:** Butazolidin. *See also pain, page 106.*

WHAT IS OSTEOARTHRITIS?

A condition of the joints. It may affect any joint, and it comes with age. It is particularly likely to develop in joints subjected to undue wear and tear. Thus in overweight people the joints in the lower back, hips and knees tend to be most severely affected. Minor degrees of arthritis are extremely common, but do not necessarily cause trouble.

Nature has designed most joints so that a smooth range of movement can occur. In a normal synovial joint (see diagram) the opposing bone ends are covered by areas of smooth and glistening hyaline cartilage. These are separated by a very thin layer of a lubricating substance called synovial fluid. In osteoarthritis (OA), there is thinning or complete loss of the normally smooth joint cartilage, as well as changes in the surrounding bone.

The severity of OA varies considerably: in mild forms there may be just slight loss of joint cartilage with no symptoms at all; in severe forms the cartilage may be completely worn away so that bone grates on bone and there may be considerable damage, disability and pain. Mild forms of OA are extremely common: in certain joints, such as the one at the base of the big toe, everyone develops some of these joint changes from as early as their 20s or 30s.

CAUSES The root causes of OA are not fully understood; certainly the ageing process, and general wear and tear, are implicated. A better understanding of the causes is perhaps gained by an awareness of the different types of OA:

Primary generalized OA affects many joints. It may begin in women in their 40s and 50s, but can affect men. You may notice bony swellings around the joints at the ends and middle of the fingers, and sometimes swelling at the wrist or the base of the thumb. Often these joints ache and may be a little stiff, particularly in the morning. These symptoms are usually much milder than the pain and stiffness of say, rheumatoid arthritis *(page 242)*. Symptoms of pain and stiffness tend to vary. The joints commonly involved include the base of the big toe, the knees, the neck and the low back. Primary generalized OA tends to run in families.

Localized OA is confined to one or two weight-bearing joints such as the hip or the knee, and becomes increasingly common with age. Patients with primary generalized OA may also develop localized OA in weight-bearing joints.

NORMAL SYNOVIAL JOINT

- Bone
- Synovial membrane
- Cartilage
- Joint space containing snyovial fluid

Above, *the appearance of a normal synovial joint, with cartilage intact and synovial fluid to lubricate movement; below, the effects of osteoarthritis on the same joint – cartilage lost, and bony swelling round the joint.*

OSTEOARTHRITIC JOINT

- Bone
- Osteophyte (new bone formation)
- Swelling round joint
- Cartilage lost

Secondary OA may occur as the result of pre-existing joint disorders. These include rheumatoid arthritis and previous injury to the joint. Childhood joint problems may well be involved; the knees, typically of professional footballers, are especially vulnerable.

TREATMENT

Drugs form a major element of treatment. For details on how analgesics and compound analgesics work, *see especially pain, page 106* and *rheumatoid arthritis, page 242*

Primary generalized OA: In most patients, **simple analgesics** such as paracetamol and aspirin will provide adequate pain relief. Where there is more severe stiffness, a more powerful non-steroidal anti-inflammatory drug (NSAID) may be prescribed. But because this form of arthritis is typically very mild, a major part of the treatment will be reassurance from the doctor that no other, potentially more serious, form of arthritis is present. Your doctor may ask a physiotherapist to advise a simple hand exercise programme, or exercises to strengthen muscles around other joints involved.

Associated problems such as neck stiffness may be helped by the use of a special foam collar, and low back pain by a simple physiotherapy programme.

Localized OA in hip or knee: Again, simple analgesics are tried first with **NSAIDs** being reserved for more severe pain and stiffness. As with primary generalized OA, physiotherapy may be helpful. Weight reduction through dieting may also be advised in an attempt to reduce joint load. Splints and supports may be prescribed for unstable joints. Lastly, in severely affected joints, the patient may be referred to an orthopaedic surgeon for surgical joint replacement.

OVER-THE-COUNTER TREATMENTS

OA is best treated by prescription of the appropriate pain relief from a doctor; but in the event of a sudden painful flare-up, or a first bad spell, it is perfectly sensible to treat yourself with paracetamol bought from a chemist. Dose: a maximum of two 500 mg tablets four times daily.

None of the currently available drugs will restore an osteoarthritic joint to normal and their only function is to relieve pain and stiffness.

QUESTIONS TO ASK THE DOCTOR

■ Should I lose weight?

■ How much exercise should I take?
■ Do I need surgery? Would I have to wait long for a hip replacement?
■ Would relaxation exercises help?
■ What are the side effects of my tablets?

SIDE EFFECTS

Paracetamol in normal dosage is much safer than, and does not have the gastric side effects of, **aspirin** and the **NSAIDs.** However, in overdose, paracetamol may cause liver damage and **dextropropoxyphene** can cause respiratory depression and heart failure. *See pain, page 106.*

NSAIDs: the main side effects of these drugs include gastro-intestinal discomfort, nausea and sometimes bleeding. People with previous histories of chronic indigestion or gastric or duodenal ulcers are particularly susceptible. Other side effects include rashes, headaches, ankle swelling and a range of uncommon effects on other internal organs including the kidneys and liver.

SELF-MANAGEMENT

■ If you are overweight, lose weight by cutting down on sweets, sugar and alcohol. Ask your doctor for a diet sheet.
■ If you have OA in a weight-bearing joint, avoid over-stressing it with excessive exercise. On the other hand, a certain amount of exercise helps to maintain muscle tone. Obtain advice from your doctor on the amount and type of exercise you need. Swimming is generally a useful form of exercise for OA as it allows muscular activity in an environment where the joints are relatively protected.
■ Local warmth is often reassuring if the pain is restricted to one accessible joint. A hot water bottle well wrapped up to prevent damage to the skin can produce short-term relief of pain and discomfort.
■ *See also strains and sprains, page 234, and back pain, page 236.*

FLARE-UPS

OA sufferers may have intermittent flare-ups which may be related to the release of crystals into the joint space. These attacks may be recognized by increasing pain, warmth and tenderness in the affected joint and they do require medical attention. This will often involve rest, sometimes local injections and prescription of regular analgesics or NSAIDs.

NAMES YOU WILL HEAR

Non-steroid anti-inflammatory drugs
Chemical name: aspirin; trade names: Aspirin, Astrin, Bi-Prin. Chemical name: indomethacin; trade names: Indocid, Artracin, Imbrilon, Indoflex, Indolar SR, Indomod, Mobilan, Rheumanin, Arthpexin. Chemical name: ibuprofen; trade names: Brufen, Apsifen, Ebufac, Fenbid, Ibumetin, Lidifen, Motrin, Amersol. Chemical name: ketoprofen; trade names: Orudis, Alrheumat, Oruvail. Chemical name: naproxen sodium; trade names: Naprosyn, Laraflex, Synflex. See also **pain**, page 106.

Slow-acting antirheumatic drugs
Chemical name: chloroquine; trade names: Arlochlor, Nivaquine. Chemical name: penicillamine; trade names: Distamine, Pendramine, Cuprimine, Metalcaptase. Chemical name: sodium aurothiomalate; trade names: Myocrisin, Myochrysine.

Steroids
Chemical name: prednisolone; trade names: Codelsol, Delta Phorical, Deltacortril, Deltalone, Deltastab, Precortisyl, Prednesol, Sintisone, Nisolone, Delta-Cortef, Deltasolone, Prelone, Lenisolone, Meticortilone, Predeltilone.

Analgesics
Chemical name: paracetamol; trade names: Panadol, Pamol, Calpol, Tylenon, Paracin, Parmol, Panado, Ceetamol, Atosol, Exctol, Tylenol, Ennagesic, Ilvamol; see also **pain**, page 106.

WHAT IS RHEUMATOID ARTHRITIS?

– A chronic inflammation of the joints, which results in deformity and disability. There is joint pain, swelling and stiffness, especially in the mornings. The hands and toes are often affected early in the course of the disease. Later the inflammation spreads to other joints; almost any joint may be involved. It is an episodic disease, with periods of severity and improvement. There is no cure, but the intervals between bad episodes can last for years.

Although the joints are often the worst problem, other organs can be affected too: fatigue, loss of appetite, weight loss, fever, skin nodules, muscle pain, dry eyes, anaemia, and damage to nerves are all symptoms. Occasionally the lungs and heart are involved.

Rheumatoid arthritis can afflict children, in which case it is called juvenile rheumatoid arthritis (previously known as Still's disease). The condition usually disappears before adulthood, but damage to joints may occasionally be permanent.

CAUSES Unknown, but both inherited and environmental factors are involved.

PRESCRIPTION DRUGS

The aims of treatment are: to relieve the pain; to maintain function of joints; to prevent or minimize permanent deformity. The great variety of drugs available indicates that none is totally successful.

NSAIDS: Aspirin is still the first choice, but many suffer side effects (see below) from the high doses necessary. Aspirin needs to be taken every four hours if it is to work its best, and this is often inconvenient.

Indomethacin is also very effective, but again side-effects can be problematic. Ibuprofen, ketoprofen, and naproxen are less likely to cause side effects than aspirin or indomethacin, BUT they may also be less effective.

There are numerous other preparations available, all with similar side effects. Their only advantage is that they have to be taken less frequently. It is often important, however, for the doctor to try various preparations: some respond better to one than another.

How they work: by inhibiting the body's production of prostaglandins, which play an important part in creating inflammation.

Slow-acting antirheumatic drugs: One of these may be included in the treatment as an extra if anti-inflammatory drugs are not adequately controlling the pain and inflammation. About 80 per cent of patients will respond to one or other of these preparations, but it takes a few months for this type of drug to work properly.

How they work: unknown. Gold (sodium anrothiomalate) is thought to have some effect on the inflamed membranes of joints.

Steroids work well on joint inflammation but the benefit wears off as soon as they are stopped. Steroids have severe side effects if used continuously (see below) and should only be used when all other measures have failed to arrest severe progressive disease. They reduce the inflammation but do not restore the damaged joints. Steroids may also be given by injection directly into inflamed joints, satisfactory if only a few large joints, for example the knee or shoulder, are involved. The side effects of steroids by mouth are avoided in this way.

How they work: by blocking the chemical process which causes inflammation.

Surgery can improve the function of damaged joints, but the patient must be clear about the likely result.

OVER-THE-COUNTER TREATMENTS

Simple analgesics can of course be bought without a prescription, but this disease requires close co-operation between the patient and doctor. If the drugs your doctor has prescribed are failing to control the pain, it is best to discuss this with him and together plan a more effective form of treatment. Aspirin should not be used in combination with prescription drugs without the approval of a doctor: it can worsen the side effects of other drugs.

Paracetamol, however, does not interfere with other drugs and can be used for severe pain until you can see a doctor.

QUESTIONS TO ASK THE DOCTOR

■ Will deformity result?
■ Will physiotherapy help? What about swimming?
■ Should I rest painful joints?
■ How long should I take the drugs?
■ Will local heat treatment help?
■ Am I anaemic? Should I have a blood test?
■ Is joint replacement likely to help me? How long might I have to wait?

SIDE EFFECTS

NSAIDS: see **osteoarthritis**, page 238. **Aspirin:** see pain, page 106. **Slow-acting antirheumatic drugs** can cause skin

PATIENT'S EXPERIENCE

"I developed rheumatoid arthritis when I was 35. My first symptom was tiredness; I found it difficult to get up in the morning. Soon I realized that this was because the muscles in my arms, legs and hands were stiff and painful. The stiffness improved during the morning, but after a week the symptoms were becoming so severe that I was unable to get up in time to take the children to school. I also had some swelling of my wrists, and my fingers were constantly painful. I went to see my doctor who did some blood tests and also X-rays of my hands.

The results showed rheumatoid arthritis, and he referred me to a specialist. When I attended the specialist's clinic I was horrified to see other patients with severely deformed joints, many of them confined to wheel chairs. By the time that I saw the specialist I was in tears, as I imagined that this was what I would be like in a few years' time. The specialist explained that most patients were not severely affected and that with good treatment and some effort on my part, things wouldn't be too bad.

My GP had started me on large doses of aspirin, but I stopped taking it as it made me dizzy and gave me continuous ringing in the ears. The specialist prescribed Indocid suppositories at night to help the morning stiffness, and an Indocid tablet in the morning to help for the rest of the day. The Indocid had to be taken with food.

I also had to have physiotherapy three times a week. Here I learned the importance of exercising the muscles and not letting the joints become stiff and immobile. I also met another lady who had had several severe episodes of RA. She now had very little pain, but still continued her exercises regularly.

The pain has responded well to the treatment and I am feeling a lot more optimistic."

rashes, mouth ulcers, nausea and vomiting. Occasionally abnormalities of the blood may occur. Chloroquine may cause eye damage and penicillamine and gold injections can affect the kidneys. Patients must have regular blood and urine checks to detect these complications, and patients on chloroquine need to have regular eye examinations. Serious side effects are rare if patients have these checks. Patients on gold injections should carry a card to this effect in case of sudden reactions.

Steroids causé few problems if given only over a week or so. The serious side effects come from more prolonged use and are dose-related: *see **anaemia**, page 224*.

Steroids are, in addition, very difficult to stop. Not all of the side effects occur in every patient, but most occur in patients on steroids for more than a couple of months. The side effects are minimized if the lowest possible dose is given; it may be that taking steroids on alternate days only may decrease side effects. Against this list of grave drawbacks must be weighed the fact that steroids usually give marked relief to rheumatoid arthritis patients.

While on any of the prescription drugs described above: Let your doctor know immediately if you may be pregnant or are considering breast-feeding. Check with your doctor before taking any other drugs. This includes cold remedies, oral contraceptives, vaccines and many other prescription drugs. Avoid alcohol, while taking any of the drugs, until you have checked with your doctor.

All of the drugs used have significant side effects, but these must be balanced against the risk to the patient of letting the disease continue unchecked. Discuss the side effects of each new drug with your doctor.

SELF-MANAGEMENT
The disease has active and quiet periods. Joints become damaged during periods of active inflammation.

■ Prevention of or minimizing of permanent deformity depends to some extent on how much the patient can keep the joints mobile, even during an acute attack.

■ Take drugs regularly and on time, with food, as instructed.

■ Physiotherapy started during an acute attack should be continued to maintain mobility of the joints.

■ Exercises should be done regularly at home – indefinitely.

■ Aids and appliances are available to help patients

who have problems in the home because of weakness or deformity of joints.

■ A firm mattress and one firm pillow prevent strain on the muscles and joints of the back.

■ Contact with rheumatoid arthritis groups and social services are very useful in solving individual problems.

■ There are many useful publications about this disease in public libraries.

■ Obesity puts extra strain on joints and weight should be reduced to normal wherever possible.

■ Exercising in water is particularly beneficial.

■ Don't assume that the drugs can be stopped as soon as you feel better – check with your doctor.

■ Relaxation of body and mind help to control pain, anxiety and tension.

■ Remember, only a small proportion of patients with rheumatoid arthritis go on to develop severe disability.

■ 'Miracle cures' are usually the result of a spontaneous improvement – as far as doctors know. Climate and diet have no specific effect, but a healthy diet is always advisable. Don't be fooled into paying money for 'cures'. Discuss them with your doctor.

SELF-HELP IN AN ATTACK

■ Find out from your doctor what extra medication you can take if the pain suddenly becomes more severe. If in doubt, take two paracetamol tablets every four hours.

■ Make an appointment to see your doctor early in an attack, so that your treatment can be stepped up to meet the attack.

■ Warmth can ease the pain and a hot water bottle on an affected joint is helpful.

■ Take sufficient medication to reduce inflammation and relieve pain. This may mean regular tablet-taking, even when you are not actually in pain.

■ Don't just retire to bed without consulting your doctor: stiff, deformed joints may result. A balance must be achieved between adequate rest of inflamed joints, and maintaining muscle power and preventing deformity. Physiotherapy plays an essential part in achieving this.

■ Splints can be useful, especially at night, to rest joints and prevent deformity. These may be ready-made, or made especially for you to rest the joint in the best possible position.

■ Remember, the more pain-free you are, the more you will be able to move your joints and keep them mobile. Don't delay seeing your doctor, and don't be afraid to take regular treatment to reduce inflammation.

NAMES YOU WILL HEAR
NSAIDS
Chemical name: indomethacin; **trade names:** Indocid, Artracin, Indoflex, Mobilan, Rheumacin, Arthrexin. **Chemical name:** ibuprofen; **trade names:** Apsifen, Ebufac, Brufen, Fenbid, Ibumetin, Lidifen, Motrin, Paxofen. **Chemical name:** ketoprofen; **trade names:** Orudis, Alrheumat, Oruvail. **Chemical name:** naproxen sodium; **trade names:** Laraflex, Naprosyn, Synflex. *See also **pain,** page 106.*

Others (acute gout)
Chemical name: colchicine; **trade name:** Clochicine Tablets. **Chemical name:** hydrocortisone acetate; **trade name:** Hydrocortisone Acetate Injection.

Drugs which lower uric acid
Chemical name: allopurinol; **trade names:** Allopurinol Tablets, Zyloric, Zyloprim. **Chemical name:** probenicid; **trade name:** Benemid.

WHAT IS GOUT?

A metabolic disorder which results in an excess of uric acid in the blood (hyperuricaemia). This may be completely asymptomatic, or the uric acid may be deposited in joints causing acute or chronic arthritis, or occasionally, kidney stones. Uric acid may also be deposited in the skin, causing lumps (tophi).

The most common symptom is joint pain, often affecting the big toe, hands, knees and ankles. Almost any joint may be involved later in the course of the disease; early on, usually one joint is involved.

In acute arthritis, the onset is sudden, with the pain developing over a few hours. The joint is extremely tender: even the pressure of a sheet is painful. In the chronic forms, the pain is usually milder, although acute attacks can occur. The frequency of these attacks varies from every few weeks to every few years. Without treatment, the joints gradually deteriorate, leading to deformity. Gout is commonest in men, and in women after the menopause.

CAUSES The high uric acid levels in the blood may be due to an over-production of uric acid by the body, or a failure to excrete uric acid in adequate amounts. These abnormalities can be inherited.

PRESCRIPTION DRUGS

It is important to differentiate between the drugs used for the treatment of an acute attack and those used in the long-term control of the disease, which lower uric acid levels.

NSAIDS: Indomethacin is the drug of choice for acute pain, given either as a tablet or a suppository. It usually gives relief within two to five days. Other anti-inflammatory drugs such as ibuprofen, ketoprofen and naproxen are also useful. They are slightly less effective than indomethacin, but tend to have a lower incidence of side effects. Aspirin should not be used in the treatment of gout, as it can raise the uric acid level and aggravates the symptoms.

How they work: *see **rheumatoid arthritis,** page 242.*
Colchicine is as effective as indomethacin, but it often causes side effects.

How it works: it is thought to act against the inflammatory process caused by uric acid.

Steroid injections into an acutely inflamed joint will relieve symptoms, but the treatment is only suitable for certain large joints.

How it works: *see **rheumatoid arthritis,** page 242.*

Long-term control: Drugs to lower the uric acid tend to be used only if the level is very high, or when there are recurrent attacks of acute arthritis. These drugs should never be started during an acute attack: they can make it worse; they are given with large amounts of fluid. Allopurinol lowers the uric acid level. It can however precipitate an attack of gout, and to prevent this, anti-inflammatory drugs are usually given with it initially.

How it works: by preventing the formation of uric acid from other chemicals within the body.

Probenicid can be used instead of allopurinol or in conjunction with it.

How it works: by increasing uric acid excretion from the kidneys. It cannot be used if the patient has kidney stones or kidney disease.

OVER THE COUNTER TREATMENTS

There are no effective non-prescription treatments for gout. Paracetamol can be used for the pain, but it is not strong enough to be effective.

QUESTIONS TO ASK THE DOCTOR

- For how long should I take the drugs?
- Will deformity result?
- Would a change of diet help?

SIDE EFFECTS

NSAIDS: see *rheumatoid arthritis, page 242.*
Colchicine commonly casuses nausea, vomiting, and abdominal pain. It can also cause severe diarrhoea, rashes and kidney damage. Nerve damage and blood disorders are rare side effects.

Steroids: see *rheumatoid arthritis, page 242.*

Allopurinol is usually well tolerated, but it can cause rashes and mild gastro-intestinal disorders. Headache, hypertension, baldness and liver disorders are rare side effects.

Probenicid has few side effects, though occasionally nausea, vomiting or headache result. Very rarely, liver, kidney or blood disorders arise.

SELF-MANAGEMENT

- The disease has active and quiet periods; joint pain can become severe over a few hours, so always have an anti-inflammatory drug available.
- Resting the affected joint is essential.
- Drugs such as diuretics can make gout worse, so always remind your doctor that you have had gout if he wants to give you any new tablets.

ALCOHOL AND GOUT
Alcohol (of any type) can increase the frequency of attacks and should be restricted. Drinking heavily can precipitate an attack.

ANKYLOSING SPONDYLITIS

Non-steroid anti-inflammatory drugs (NSAIDS), steroids, analgesics

NAMES YOU WILL HEAR
Non-steroid anti-inflammatory drugs (NSAIDS)
Chemical name: aspirin; trade names: Aspirin, Astrin, Bi-Prin. Chemical name: indomethacin; trade names: Indocid, Artracin, Indoflex, Mobilan, Rheumacin, Arthrexin. Chemical name: ibuprofen; trade names: Brufen, Apsifen, Ebufac, Fenbid, Ibumetin, Lidifen, Motrin, Paxofen. Chemical name: ketoprofen; trade names: Orudis, Alrheumat, Oruvail. Chemical name: naproxen sodium; trade names: Laraflex, Naprosyn, Synflex. For more comprehensive lists of trade names of the foregoing drugs, see **pain**, page 106.
Chemical name: phenylbutazone; trade name: Butazolidin. Chemical name: piroxicam; trade name: Feldene; Chemical name: diflunisal; trade name: Dolobid; Chemical name: diclofenac; trade name: Voltarol.

Steroids
Chemical name: prednisolone; trade names: Codelsol, Delta Phorical, Deltacortril, Deltalone, Deltastab, Precortisyl, Prednesol, Sintisone, Nisolone, Delta-Cortef, Deltasolone, Prelone, Lenisolone, Meticortilone, Predeltilone.

Analgesics
Chemical name: paracetamol; trade names: Panadol, Pamol, Calpol, Tylenon, Paracin, Parmol, Panado, Ceetamol, Atosol, Exctol, Tylenol, Ennagesic, Ilvamol; see also **pain**, page 106.

WHAT IS ANKYLOSING SPONDYLITIS?
– A chronic inflammation of the joints of the back, occurring most commonly in young men.

The inflammation affects the joints between the vertebrae (the bones which make up the spine), and also the joint between the sacrum of the spine and the iliac bones of the pelvis (see diagram). This inflammation causes fusion of the vertebrae: the back loses its flexibility and becomes rigid. There may be arthritis of other joints in the body, for example the hips and shoulders.

Onset is gradual, with pain and stiffness in the lower back. Symptoms are worse in the morning and following inactivity. The pain occurs in bouts; at times there is no pain at all. As the disease progresses, the normal curvature of the lower (lumbar) spine is lost and the movements of the back are limited. This may lead to a characteristic posture: head and neck forward, upper back rounded, chest flattened. Limitation of movement can also affect deep breathing.

Ankylosing spondylitis can also produce inflammation of the eye, the main blood vessel from the heart (the aorta) and the aortic valve of the heart itself. The last is a rare cause of heart failure (see page 54).

CAUSES Unknown at present, but there is a strong familial pattern. The inherited antigen HLA B27 is linked with ankylosing spondylitis, and with some other inherited disorders.

PRESCRIPTION DRUGS
The principles of treatment are the same as for **rheumatoid arthritis** – see page 242. In ankylosing spondylitis the problem of rigidity is more severe, and every effort must be made to maintain the flexibility of the spine. This is done by using drugs to reduce pain and inflammation, by active physiotherapy and exercises to maintain mobility.

NSAIDS: See **rheumatoid arthritis**, page 242. The only difference is that in ankylosing spondylitis, phenylbutazone, not used in rheumatoid arthritis, is often the most effective drug.

Steroids: These are sometimes used to treat the eye inflammation as well as the joints: see **rheumatoid arthritis**, page 242. Local injections of steroids into the large joints may be helpful, just as in rheumatoid arthritis.

Surgery is necessary in a few cases to correct deformity of the spine. Hip replacement can be beneficial if the hip joints are badly affected. Treatment of heart failure occurring as a result of the disease is given on page 52.

OVER-THE-COUNTER TREATMENT
*See **rheumatoid arthritis**, page 242.*

QUESTIONS TO ASK THE DOCTOR
■ Can I pass it on to my children?
■ What can I do to prevent rigidity of the spine?
■ Will physiotherapy help?
■ What sports can I play?

SIDE EFFECTS
*See **rheumatoid arthritis**, page 242.* Phenylbutazone may (rarely) cause heart failure and stop normal production of white blood cells in the bone marrow.

SELF-MANAGEMENT
*See **rheumatoid arthritis**, page 242.* However, maintaining mobility is of such importance that patients and those concerned with them should realize that:
■ More than 75 per cent of patients with ankylosing spondylitis can stay at work, moreover without taking a large amount of time off.
■ This is a chronic disease, and the long-term outcome depends largely on how much effort is put into exercise. Get into the habit of exercising regularly at home and continue these exercises for the rest of your life.
■ Physiotherapy is essential, both to prevent postural deformity, and to monitor progression of the disease.
■ Take up non-contact sports such as swimming. Your doctor will advise.

SELF-HELP IN AN ATTACK
*See **rheumatoid arthritis**, page 242* – the remedial action to be taken is identical.

Vertebrae which make up spine

Iliac bone of the pelvis

Sacro-iliac joint

Sacrum

Hip joint

Femur

The lower (lumbar) spine and pelvis, showing the joints which become inflamed in ankylosing spondylitis, including those between the vertebrae, and between the sacrum and iliac bones of the pelvis (the sacro-iliac joints).

CRAMP

WHAT IS CRAMP?

– Sudden painful spasm of muscles which control body movement. Mainly the calves, feet, thighs and less commonly the back, arms and hands are involved. Cramp occurs without warning and cannot be controlled. It lasts from a few seconds up to ten minutes, sometimes during sleep. The pain arises because the affected muscles 'lock up'. Though painful and unpleasant, cramp is not dangerous unless it occurs during activities such as swimming.

Writer's cramp affects those who use their hands for long periods performing delicate and intricate tasks. It is unlike the usual type of cramp and thought to be mainly the result of tension and other psychological conditions. It may last a long time.

CAUSES Not really understood: cramp can occur at any age, but is more common in the elderly. The problem may arise in some people because the body is deprived of fluids containing certain salts such as sodium or potassium. Other reasons may be injury to the muscle fibres and the nerves serving them, or medical conditions which prevent proper blood circulation. Certain drugs may also contribute. Some experts consider arthritis of the spine with sciatica may precipitate attacks, especially in the elderly. Cramp is also common in pregnancy, but usually does not signify any serious underlying problem.

PRESCRIPTION DRUGS

For bedtime cramp the most commonly prescribed drug is **quinine bisulphate.** The dose may vary, but it is usually 300 mg taken before going to bed. Other drugs given are **cyclandelate, oxerutin** and **inositol nicotinate BP.** For cramp after severe exercise in warm climates a doctor will suggest taking plenty of non-alcoholic fluid with added salt. Salt tablets may be advised for those susceptible to cramp who travel in hot climates.
How they work: Not fully understood, but quinine is thought to decrease muscle membrane excitability and hence prevent the muscle from going into spasm. The others are thought to help circulation in the muscles and to prevent the onset of cramp.

Muscles become more irritable when deprived of surrounding body fluid and salts, hence the need to take extra fluid and salts when excessive loss occurs.

OVER-THE-COUNTER TREATMENTS

Quinine can easily be taken as a glass of tonic water,

which contains the drug. Salt tablets are widely available; but consult your doctor before treating yourself: excessive salt can be dangerous. Proprietary anti-cramp preparations (such as Crampex) are also widely available: their value is unproven.

QUESTIONS TO ASK THE DOCTOR
■ Am I on any tablets which may cause cramp?
■ Do I need a treatment, or will my cramp just go?

SIDE EFFECTS
Quinine in the usually prescribed dose for night cramps has few side effects. Very occasionally nausea, vomiting, noises in the ear, abdominal pain, rashes, visual problems and allergy may occur: should you have any suspicion of these, stop taking it and report the symptoms to your doctor. **Cyclandelate** may cause nausea, flushing and dizziness with very high doses. Care has to be taken when these drugs are given to patients with certain heart complaints.

SELF-MANAGEMENT
Prevention
■ Avoid loss of body fluids by prolonged sweating, vomiting or diarrhoea. ■ Avoid risk of muscle stress by unaccustomed exercise when unfit. ■ Avoid extremes of temperature – cold can bring on an attack of cramp.

SELF-HELP IN AN ATTACK
■ Rub the muscle or apply a hot water bottle or ice pack. Or apply a firm bandage, but be sure not to cut off the circulation to the muscle. ■ Sudden cramp in a lower limb can often by cured by stretching the limb strongly or willing the opposite muscles to contract. For instance, if there is cramp in the calf, the foot should be pulled up and the leg straightened. ■ When cramp occurs in bed, try getting up and standing on the leg.
■ Analgesics such as paracetamol are usful for treating the residual pain after an attack.

Foot pulled up, leg straightened

Ear, nose and throat and eye

Ear, nose and throat problems are traditionally looked after by 'E.N.T.' surgeons – here we have also included problems with the eyes. Infection plays a large part in the common disorders mentioned here, many of which have great nuisance value.

DEAFNESS — 254-255

MIDDLE EAR INFECTIONS — 256-257

EXTERNAL EAR INFECTION — 258-259

HAY FEVER — 260-261

SINUSITIS — 262-263

CONDITIONS OF THE MOUTH — 264-265
including ulcers

LARYNGITIS AND CROUP — 266-267

RED-EYE AND DRY-EYE — 268-269

CHRONIC GLAUCOMA — 270-271

See also: *Influenza, page 138; common cold, page 134.*

NAMES YOU WILL HEAR
Anti-emetics
Chemical name: prochlorperazine;
trade names: Stemetil, Compazine,
Anti-Naus, Mitil, Vertigon. **Chemical
name:** cyclizine; **trade names:**
Marzine, Valoid. **Chemical name:**
cinnarizine; **trade name:** Stugeron.
Chemical name: promethazine
theoclate; **trade name:** Avomine.
Chemical name: meclozine; **trade
names:** Ancoloxin, Ancolan, Bonamine,
Navicalm.

**Drops for removal of wax from
ear**
Chemical name: turpentine oil
mixture; **trade name:** Cerumol.
Chemical name: docusate sodium;
trade names: Waxsol, Soliwax,
Molcer, Dioctyl.

WHAT IS DEAFNESS?

Partial or complete loss of hearing; in older patients especially, it may be associated with tinnitus (noises in the ears) and vertigo. **Vertigo** ('dizziness'), *see page 96,* is a feeling of movement, either of one's own body or of objects around one, and it is often more troublesome than the deafness itself.

CAUSES Obstruction in the canal leading into the ear; interference with the hearing apparatus within the ear; damage to the nerve from the ear to the brain (see diagram). The first can be a result of wax, or occasionally a foreign body, in the external ear canal. The second arises from damage to the ear drum, or disease such as ear infection in which fluid within the middle ear prevents the hearing mechanism from working properly. The last can be present from birth (as in children whose mothers have rubella during pregnancy); can develop suddenly due to damage to the nerve caused by meningitis or head injury; can develop gradually as part of the process of ageing.

PRESCRIPTION DRUGS

Anti-emetic drugs may help with the nausea associated with vertigo.
How they work: by acting on the brain, suppressing the stimulus to vomit.

The treatment of deafness depends, of course, on the cause. Wax in the ear can be removed by drops which liquify the wax. If this is inadequate, syringing may be necessary. **Middle ear infections** are treated in varying ways – *see page 256.* Damage to the ear drum or other parts of the hearing apparatus may be corrected by surgery. Lastly, hearing aids can restore a degree of hearing by increasing the sounds in the ear. Different types suit different forms of hearing loss; selecting the right one for the individual usually involves trial and error, and requires specialist help.

OVER-THE-COUNTER TREATMENTS

Anti-emetics such as Stugeron, and ear drops such as Cerumol, can be bought without a prescription; provided manufacturer's instructions are followed, self-treatment is appropriate.

QUESTIONS TO ASK THE DOCTOR

■ Will my hearing recover, stay the same, or get worse?
■ What can be done for the vertigo and tinnitus?

- What help is available to deaf people?
- Will a hearing aid help me?

SIDE EFFECTS

Anti-emetics cause drowsiness in many people and should not be taken when driving or working in a potentially dangerous environment. *See also **lung cancer**, page 202.*

Ear drops for removing wax can cause an allergic skin reaction: stop immediately if this occurs.

SELF-MANAGEMENT

One of the major causes of deafness in children can be prevented by immunization against rubella (German measles) before becoming pregnant. Hearing problems in young children are detected by screening tests at well baby clinics. Even milder cases need specialist help if schooling is not to suffer.

Severely or totally deaf people have to face up to communication problems without delay. Totally deaf people should learn lip-reading and finger-spelling as early as possible while hearing aids can help the partially hearing child or adult. Many partially hearing or deaf people underestimate their capabilities; self-help groups can help a patient acquire or regain confidence. Tinnitus may be less noticeable when the patient is mentally occupied.

Mechanical aids for the home are worth investigating: a flashing door bell light is available, for example.

If deafness has impaired balance, walking in the dark and working at heights should be avoided.

Hearing aids take some getting used to, but it is well worth persevering and having the aid regularly serviced.

PATIENTS' EXPERIENCES

"My deafness had been coming on gradually for a few years, but over the last year, since I retired, it has become much worse. I can no longer follow a conversation or watch television.

I had a hearing aid fitted a few years ago, but I found it very difficult to use. I went to see my doctor because of the noise in my ears, and problems with balance. Sometimes I would feel dizzy and sick. The consultation was difficult because he was busy and I couldn't understand what he was saying. He put me on some tablets to help with the nausea, but they made me sleepy, so I stopped taking them. They did not do much good, anyway. I got a different hearing aid later, and that helped for a few years.

I live alone and the deafness makes me more and more depressed. The constant noise in my ears is very disturbing; but at least if I make the effort to get out and do things, it takes my mind off the noise."

"My little boy aged three seemed to have become very naughty. He took no notice when I told him to behave. Also, he had become rather clumsy: he seemed to fall about more than usual. He had had a slight cold the week before.

I took him to the doctor who looked in his ears and diagnosed an ear infection. He gave him antibiotics and within a few days he was much better and his balance had improved.

The doctor asked me to take him back after a week to make sure that the fluid in his ears had cleared. It had, and it is obvious to me now that he was just not hearing properly when he had the ear infection."

Hearing apparatus in middle ear   Auditory nerve to brain

Organ of balance

External ear canal   Ear drum

Sound waves enter the external ear canal and hit the ear drum. This vibrates, causing the tiny bones of the hearing apparatus to vibrate too. This activates the auditory nerve, which conducts the sound message to the brain.

WHAT ARE EAR INFECTIONS?

When 'germs' from an infection of the nose and throat spread up the Eustachian tube to the middle ear (see diagram), it gets inflamed, causing severe ear ache, sometimes with dizziness, vomiting and a high temperature. In babies, who cannot complain of ear ache, the symptoms are vague: loss of appetite, vomiting, diarrhoea, fever, irritability. Sometimes the ear drum perforates under pressure, discharging green or yellow pus. The pain often goes away when this happens. The perforation nearly always heals, and hearing is unimpaired; but in view of the small risk of lasting deafness, doctors – and patients – need to monitor the condition carefully. The problem is commonest in children under ten: they are generally more susceptible to respiratory infections.

CAUSES Middle ear infections usually start a few days after a cold. Other causes include pressure changes (such as experienced when flying), enlarged adenoids (in young children), and diving into water (especially in children with colds). Some children are especially vulnerable: those with allergies, such as hay fever, and those born with a cleft palate.

PRESCRIPTION DRUGS

Antibiotics are often prescribed for all except the mildest degree of ear infection, although research has shown that most ear infections will clear up without them. Their use is sometimes justified by the need to prevent the serious complications: mastoiditis (rare) and chronic (persistent) discharging ear. The antibiotics most commonly used for this condition are listed.
How they work: by destroying the bacteria responsible for the more serious ear infections. However, they have no effect on the viruses which cause most of the milder forms of middle ear trouble.
Decongestants help to relieve blockage of the Eustachian tube; taken either as drops or spray applied up the nose, or as medicine or tablets taken by mouth.
How they work: by shrinking the swollen linings of the nose and Eustachian tube.
Antihistamines are often found in combination with decongestants, and are used whenever allergy is thought to be playing a part in the illness.
How they work: by reversing the effects of allergies.

OVER-THE-COUNTER TREATMENTS

Decongestants and antihistamines, usually in combination, are widely available, as of course are simple analgesics such as paracetamol. But if ear ache does not clear up with paracetamol and a decongestant, consult a doctor within a few days.

QUESTIONS TO ASK THE DOCTOR

■ Do I really need an antibiotic?
■ For how long should the antibiotic be taken?
■ Could the infection cause deafness?
■ What about swimming?
■ How can I get the most from these drops?

SIDE EFFECTS

Antibiotics are usually prescribed for seven days. Some people become allergic to certain antibiotics; this is shown by a rash, or itchy swelling of the face. More common side effects include diarrhoea, nausea, or feeling generally ill. *See also page 79.*

Decongestants taken by mouth, such as pseudo-ephedrine, can interfere with sleep, and children can also develop hallucinations and behaviour disturbance. Mild symptoms of this nature are probably quite common; they clear when the medicine is discontinued, and should not cause anxiety. Decongestant sprays or drops will irritate the nose if used for more than about one week, leading to further blockage and running (called vasomotor rhinitis). Patients with a history of high blood pressure should not take these drugs.

Most **antihistamines** (except newer types such as terfenadine) cause drowsiness, which can be an advantage in helping children to sleep at night. *See also* **cough**, *page 68* and **hay fever**, *page 260.*

SELF-MANAGEMENT

For mild ear ache in older children who have a cold, paracetamol and decongestant nose drops or medicine will often relieve the pain and fever and prevent a full-blown ear infection from developing. DO NOT PUT DROPS INTO THE EAR, as they will not help, and if the ear drum has perforated, will cause damage.

If ear ache persists for more than 24 hours, or becomes severe, consult your doctor.

Ideal position for instilling nose drops.

PATIENT'S EXPERIENCE
"My sisters are both deaf with perforated ear drums, so when my son got ear ache I took him straight to the doctor, who gave antibiotics and advised me to bring him back for more if it occurred again. Now he is ten, and he hasn't had any trouble for a whole year. We keep him off swimming whenever he has a cold. They checked his hearing at the clinic, but it was quite normal."

EXTERNAL EAR INFECTION

Astringent drops, antibiotics, anti-fungal drugs, steroids, wax-softeners

NAMES YOU WILL HEAR

Astringent drops
Chemical name: aluminium acetate; trade name: Aluminium Acetate Ear Drops.

Antibiotic drops/ointment
(* indicates steroid also present)
Chemical name: chloramphenicol; trade name: Chloromycetin. Chemical name: neomycin; trade names: Audicort*, Betnesol-N*, Neo-Cortef*, Otosporin*, Predsol-N*, Tri-adcortyl Otic*. Chemical name: framycetin; trade names: Framycort*, Framygen, Sofradex*, Soframycin. Chemical name: gentamicin; trade names: Cidomycin, Garamycin, Genticin, Gentisone HC*. Chemical name: tetracycline; trade name: Achromycin. Chemical name: oxytetracycline; trade name: Terra-Cortril*. Chemical name: clioquinol; trade name: Locorten-Vioform*.

Anti-fungal drops
Chemical name: co-trimazole; trade name: Canesten. Chemical name: nystatin; trade name: Tri-Adcortyl Otic*.

Antibiotic tablets/medicine
Chemical name: flucloxacillin; trade names: Floxapen, Flopen. Chemical name: erythromycin; trade names: Erythrocin, Erythromid, Ilotycin, EpMycin, Erostin, Emu-V, Ethryn, Eromel, Ilocap, Ilosone, Rythrocaps.

Steroid drops
Chemical name: betamethasone; trade names: Betnesol, Vista-Methasone. Chemical name: prednisolone; trade name: Predsol.

Wax-softening drops
Chemical name: dioctyl sodium sulphosuccinate; trade names: Dioctyl, Molcer, Soliwax, Waxsol.

WHAT IS EXTERNAL EAR INFECTION?

The external ear is simply a tube of skin lining the passage from the outside to the middle ear, which is separated from it by the ear drum. The outer part carries hairs and produces wax. Bacteria can enter the skin if it is broken, causing pain, swelling, and an offensive discharge. A boil can develop at the base of a hair, causing severe pain because the skin is closely attached to the bone, leaving little room for swelling.

CAUSES Irritation of the skin by accumulated wax, shampoo, water or a foreign body (such as an insect); or any pre-existing itchy skin condition, which causes scratching. Hot weather seems to encourage this condition, probably due to increased sweating and humidity.

PRESCRIPTION DRUGS

Astringent drops – aluminium acetate – are the simplest and often the only treatment necessary. They may either be applied as drops, or by soaking a strip of gauze which is inserted into the ear by a doctor or nurse.
How they work: by drying up inflamed tissues, so helping the natural healing process.
Antibiotics are usually applied as drops or ointment, but in severe cases will be given by mouth.
How they work: provided the bacteria responsible for the infection are sensitive to the particular antibiotic being used, and provided the drops can reach the infected skin, then the antibiotic should destroy those bacteria. Removal of dead skin and other matter from the ear canal, by syringing or mopping (a job for the doctor), is essential for the effective use of antibiotic drugs.
Anti-fungal drugs: Because some ear infections are caused by yeasts (Candida or thrush) often developing after treatment with antibiotics, anti-fungal drops may be prescribed.
How they work: in the same way as antibiotics, but only if the cause is this particular fungus or yeast.
Steroids: Antibiotic drops marked with a * in the NAMES YOU WILL HEAR list also contain one of these cortisone-like drugs, which reduce the irritation and swelling that often accompanies external ear infections.
How they work: steroids suppress the body's response to infection, injury and allergy. They are particularly effective in reducing the symptoms of eczema or dermatitis, which can occur in the ear.

Wax-softening drops will be prescribed to prepare the wax for syringing. Wax is a normal occurrence in the ear, and is only treated if it is completely blocking the ear canal, causing either deafness or pain and inflammation.

OVER-THE-COUNTER TREATMENTS
Drops for softening and removing wax are widely available. The simplest are the safest: olive oil, almond oil, glycerine or sodium bicarbonate are cheap, safe and effective. The softened wax will often flow out without the need for syringing. Proprietary ear drops, apart from those listed, can irritate the ear, and are best avoided.

QUESTIONS TO ASK THE DOCTOR
■ What is the best way to insert the ear drops or ointment?
■ For how long should I use the drops/ointment?
■ Is the infection contagious – can I pass it on?
■ What happens if I develop an allergy to the drops?

SIDE EFFECTS
Astringent drops cause mild, transient stinging, which is normal and to be expected. **Antibiotics** applied to the skin anywhere, including the ear canal, can cause an allergy. The irritation will get worse rather than better, and you might notice redness spreading out from the ear. If this happens, stop the treatment and report to your doctor. Some antibiotics, such as neomycin, gentamycin, and polymyxin, cause damage to the inner ear if applied to a perforated ear drum. If you know you have a perforation, always remind your doctor. **Steroid drops** can mask the effects of infection, and can lead to new infections developing. They should be used only for short periods, up to one week, and only under medical supervision.

SELF-MANAGEMENT
■ Take care to keep your ears dry, using disposable ear plugs or cotton wool smeared in vaseline to prevent water getting in while washing your hair or swimming.
■ DO NOT use cotton buds or anything else to try to remove wax. This usually pushes it further in; it can only be removed by syringing.
■ If you do suffer from a skin disease, seek your doctor's advice on the best preparation to use in your ears.
■ Avoid scratching your ears. It may cause an infection.

PATIENT'S EXPERIENCE
"My ears were producing a lot of wax, which I tried to remove with cotton-wool buds. One day, after I had washed my hair, I went completely deaf. I bought some wax-removing drops from the chemist, but they made my ears itchy. The next day, the whole side of my face was swollen, red and itching, so I had to go to the doctor. He said I had an infection of the outer ear, and also an allergy to the ear drops. The nurse syringed my ears when the infection had settled down – a lot of wax and some white stuff came out. The doctor prescribed some antihistamine tablets for the allergy. My doctor suggested I use a little warm olive oil in each ear if I felt them getting blocked, and that I should keep the water out when washing my hair."

Decongestants
Chemical name: xylometazoline hydrochloride; **trade names:** Otrivine Nasal Drops or Nasal Spray, Otrivine Paediatric Nasal Drops, Otrivine-Antistin, Otrix, Sinutab. **Chemical name:** antazoline; **trade names:** Antistin, Vasocona. **Chemical name:** oxymetazoline; **trade names:** Oxymetazoline Nasal Solution, Afrazine Nasal Drops or Nasal Spray, Afrazine Paediatric Nasal Drops, Drixine, Nafrine. **Chemical name:** ephedrine hydrochloride; **trade name:** Ephedrine Nose Drops.

Topical steroids
Chemical name: beclomethasone dipropionate; **trade name:** Beconase. **Chemical name:** betamethasone sodium phosphate; **trade name:** Betnesol. **Chemical name:** budesonide; **trade names:** Preferid, Rhinocort. **Chemical name:** flunisolide; **trade names:** Syntaris, Rhinalar.

Sodium cromoglycate
Chemical name: sodium cromoglycate; **trade names:** Rynacrom, Opticrom.

Oral antihistamines *(prescription-only types)*
Chemical name: astemizole; **trade name:** Hismanal. **Chemical name:** brompheniramine; **trade names:** Dimotane, Dimetane, Dimotapp. **Chemical name:** chlorpheniramine; **trade names:** Haymine, Piriton, Chlor-Tripolon, Histalon, Novopheniram, Allertex, Chlortrimeton, Histamed, Allergex, Bramahist Chloramine, Histaids, Teledrim. **Chemical name:** clemastine; **trade names:** Tavegil, Tavist, Trabest. **Chemical name:** mebhydrolin; **trade name:** Fabahistin. **Chemical name:** terfenadine; **trade name:** Triludan. **Chemical name:** trimeprazine; **trade names:** Vallergan, Panectyl. **Chemical name:** triprolidine; **trade names:** Actidil, Pro-Actidil.

Allergent extract vaccine
Chemical name: alum precipitated extracts from aqueous pyridine solutions; **trade names:** Alavac-P,

WHAT IS HAY FEVER?
– An allergic reaction causing sneezing, watering and irritation of the eyes and nose, and obstruction of the nose. It is common in adults aged 15-45 years; the symptoms tend to recur annually during the grass pollination season.

CAUSES Inhaled allergens, usually grass or tree pollens and moulds. The reaction is mediated by chemicals such as histamines which are produced in 'mast cells' in the conjunctiva, and the lining of the nose, soon after exposure to pollen.

PRESCRIPTION DRUGS
Local applications
Decongestant eye drops give only temporary relief; likewise nose drops, indeed they can make symptoms worse if used for long periods. See SIDE EFFECTS. Neither are therefore the first choice of treatment.
How they work: *see sinusitis, page 262.*
Steroids and **sodium cromoglycate** are available as nasal sprays and eye drops. Start sodium cromoglycate prefereably before the hay fever season begins, to prevent attacks. Steroid nasal sprays are effective in reducing the symptoms of an attack. These drugs are usually taken two to four times a day, and as their effect is cumulative, they need to be continued several weeks, or even months.
How they work: by stabilizing mast cells, thus stopping the allergic reaction. Cromoglycate only works to prevent future attacks, not to help during an acute episode.

Oral drugs
Antihistamine tablets help both eye and nose symptoms. They are usually used to stop attacks in courses lasting a few days, but they may also be used continuously.
How they work: by preventing released histamine access to its receptor. Antihistamines occupy the same receptor as histamine, thus preventing histamine having its effects.
Steroids are a powerful expedient for very severe attacks, or if an immediate response is essential. Relief of symptoms can be quite dramatic, but they are used for short periods only.
How they work: by blocking both allergic and inflammatory reactions.
Desensitization injections can be given in courses before the hay fever season starts. They work by slowly

acclimatizing the body to the various allergens and thus reducing the reaction when next exposed.

OVER-THE-COUNTER TREATMENTS
Many of the nasal decongestants, antihistamines and sodium cromoglycate preparations can be bought over the counter. Steroids and steroid preparations are only available on prescription. In all but the most severe attacks, self-treatment is appropriate. See SELF-HELP IN AN ATTACK.

QUESTIONS TO ASK THE DOCTOR
■ How often should I take the treatment, and for how long?
■ Can the treatment prevent attacks, or does it only treat them?
■ Can I treat myself in future attacks?
■ Can I have the type of antihistamine that causes least drowsiness?

SIDE EFFECTS
Decongestants: prolonged use – typically more than two weeks continuously – can damage the lining of the nose. Also, stopping them can cause a rebound effect: the symptoms not only recur, but are actually worse than if the drops had not been used at all.
Topical cromoglycate and **steroid preparations** have no significant side effects.
Antihistamines: The main side effect is drowsiness which can make driving or operating machinery dangerous (the effect is additive with alcohol). Some of the newer antihistamines, for example terfenadine, cause less drowsiness. Chlorpheniramine, by contrast, can make some people very drowsy. Other effects include dry mouth and blurred vision.
Steroids by mouth have many serious side effects if used in large doses for several weeks *see* **anaemia,** *page 224;* short courses, seven to ten days, are safe and have few side effects.

Desensitization injections have the risk of a rare but grave side effect called anaphylactic (allergic) reaction. It can result in collapse or even death, and for this reason is no longer routinely recommended.

SELF-MANAGEMENT
■ Avoid exposure to pollen: stay indoors, particularly on hot days, and when the pollen count is high. ■ Sufferers should particularly avoid freshly mown grass and hay fields.

Allpyral-G, Conjuvac, Norisen Grass, Pollinex, Spectralgen.

Oral steroid
Chemical name: prednisolone; **trade names:** Codelsol, Delta Phoricol, Deltacortril, Deltalone, Deltastab, Precortisyl, Prednesol, Sintisone, Nisolone, Delta-Cortef, Deltasolone, Prelone, Lenisolone, Meticortilone, Predeltilone.

PATIENT'S EXPERIENCE
"My hay fever used to make me feel desperate – gasping for air, swollen eyes and face, blocked nose, throat and chest. I often wondered whether to call a doctor. I used a decongestant spray bought from the chemist: it gave real relief – but only for about five minutes.

Then, this spring, I went to the allergy clinic I had heard about at the local hospital. The specialist advised me to stop using the spray immediately: he told me it could be making the symptoms worse. I did what he said. So far this summer the symptoms have been much less aggravating than usual: maybe it's partly because there is less pollen around, but the improvement is so dramatic that I suspect dropping the spray has helped. The specialist said that my GP could prescribe the sodium cromoglycate spray just before the pollen count rises next spring."

IN AN ATTACK
Go indoors if possible. Avoid bright sunlight: it puts extra strain on already irritated and watering eyes. Dark glasses can help. During a mild attack, try topical steroids or cromoglycate drops or sprays. If the symptoms are more severe, or you want more effective relief, start yourself on antihistamine tablets straight away and continue for several days. Both these preparations can be used simultaneously if necessary. With very severe attacks, or when attacks are so frequent that they warrant continuous treatment, consult a doctor.

NAMES YOU WILL HEAR
Decongestants *(oral)*
Chemical name: pseudoephedrine hydrochloride; **trade names:** Sudafed, Sudelix, Drixora, Repetabs, Eltor.

Decongestants *(nasal)*
Chemical name: xylometazoline; **trade names:** Otrivine, Otrix, Otrivin. *See also* **hay fever,** *page 000.*

Oral antihistamines
(Prescription-only types)
Chemical name: astemizole; **trade name:** Hismanol. **Chemical name:** brompheniramine; **trade names:** Dimotane, Dimetane. **Chemical name:** chlorpheniramine; **trade names:** Piriton, Allergex. **Chemical name:** clemastine; **trade names:** Tevegil, Tavest, Trabest. **Chemical name:** mebhydrolin; **trade name:** Fabahistin. **Chemical name:** terfenadine; **trade name:** Triludan. **Chemical name:** trimeprazine tartrate; **trade names:** Vallergan, Panectyl. **Chemical name:** triprolidine; **trade names:** Actidil, Pro-Actidil.

Antibiotics
Chemical name: phenoxymethyl penicillin, penicillin-V; **trade names:** Crystapen V, Distaquaine V-K, Stabillin V-K, V-Cil-K, Abbocillin-VK, Bramcillin, Cilicaine VK, Compocillin VK, Crystapen VK, Falcopen VK, LPV, Pfipen V, Propen VK, PVK, PVO, Rocilin, Viraxacillin-V, Ledercillin VK, Nadopen-V, Novopen-VK, PVF K, V-Cillin K, VC-K, Copen, Darocillin, Deltacillin, Fenoxypen, Incil-VK, Jatacillin, Novo-VK, Nutracillin. **Chemical name:** ampicillin; **trade names:** Ampifen, Penbritin, Pentrexyl, Vidopen, Austrapen, Bristin, Amcill, Ampicin, Ampilean, Biosan, Ampil, Famicilin, Pentrex, Petercillin, Synthecillin. **Chemical name:** amoxycillin sodium; **trade names:** Amoxil, Moxacin, Moxilean, Novamoxin, Penamox, Polymox. **Chemical name:** erythromycin; **trade names:** Erythrocin, Erythromid, Ilotycin, Frostin, Emu-V, Ethryn, Eromel, Ilocap, Ilosone, Rythrocaps. **Chemical name:** doxycycline; **trade names:** Vibramycin, Doxin.

WHAT IS SINUSITIS?

The sinuses are spaces in the bones of the face and forehead, lined by a form of skin similar to that on the inside of the nose, and connected to the nose by small openings or passages. True sinusitis is an infection of one or more of these spaces, which occurs when the opening becomes blocked due to swelling of the lining, as happens frequently during a cold. Bacteria invade the lining of the sinus and the bone itself. The spaces fill with yellow or green pus, causing severe pain and a high temperature; you feel very ill indeed.

The condition commonly called ''sinusitis'', or just ''sinus'', is in fact a less severe form of true sinusitis: one or more sinuses become blocked, and may fill with mucus, causing discomfort, often worse on bending.

CAUSES anything which leads to blockage of the sinus openings, but the common cold is the most usual.

PRESCRIPTION DRUGS

Decongestants: the first line of treatment; the drops or sprays should not be used for more than five days, since they eventually worsen the congestion.
How they work: by shrinking the swelling inside the nose, allowing the mucus or pus to drain out. See also SIDE EFFECTS.
Antihistamines: these are often found in combination with decongestants in medicines such as Actifed or Dimotapp.
How they work: by reversing the effects of allergies. Thus they may be helpful in sinus blockage caused by hay fever, or allergy to dust or animals.
Antibiotics: commonly prescribed, but probably unnecessary for the milder forms of sinus pain as described above. Many varieties: those most commonly used for sinusitis are listed.
How they work: by destroying certain bacteria, but not the viruses that cause colds and flu. In true sinusitis they stop the infection, relieving pain and fever.

OVER-THE-COUNTER TREATMENTS

Decongestants, both nasal and oral, are widely available, and often advertized on TV. Combination medicines with antihistamines are ever more common. Provided the side effects are noted, self-treatment with these preparations is entirely appropriate in mild cases.

QUESTIONS TO ASK THE DOCTOR

■ How long should I take the prescribed medicine(s)?

- Can I take simple pain killers as well?
- Can I drive my car, or drink alcohol?

SIDE EFFECTS

Decongestants taken by mouth, such as pseudo-ephedrine, can interfere with sleep, and in children can also cause hallucinations and behaviour disturbance. Mild symptoms of this nature are probably quite common; they clear when the medicine is discontinued, and should not cause anxiety. Decongestant sprays or drops will irritate the nose if used for more than about one week, leading to further blockage and running (called vasomotor rhinitis). Patients with a history of high blood pressure should not be given these drugs. Most **antihistamines** cause drowsiness, and imapair co-ordination. Preferably don't drive, or operate machinery when on these drugs: concentration is significantly impaired. One or two of the newer antihistamines are relatively free of this effect (eg Terfanedine or Triludan). **Antibiotics** are usually prescribed for five to ten days. Some people become allergic to certain antibiotics and develop a rash or itchy swelling of the face. These should be reported at once to your doctor. More commonly side effects include diarrhoea, nausea, or feeling generally ill. *See also* **pneumonia** *and* **pleurisy,** *page 78.* Women taking ampicillin, or other broad spectrum antibiotics, may develop thrush.

SELF-MANAGEMENT

Because the initial cause of an attack of true sinusitis is obstruction of the openings into the nose, treating a blocked nose by simple steam inhalation (see margin), or carefully sniffing cold water (with a little salt dissolved in it), or using a decongestant spray for not more than three or four days may prevent sinusitis.

SELF-HELP IN AN ATTACK

- Whenever your nose feels blocked, try to identify the cause – a cold (virus infection), an allergy such as hay fever, or an irritant.
- Use decongestant drops or nasal spray three or four times a day for three or four days only; or, if you prefer, a decongestant tablet or medicine. (Avoid tablets or medicine if you are pregnant – see SIDE EFFECTS.) Use drops as shown in the diagram.
- Fresh air often helps. Avoid hot, dry atmospheres, central heating and air conditioning.
- Simple analgesics, aspirin or paracetamol, may be taken to give pain relief three or four times a day.

Cut away diagram of the face to show the two main sinuses, and their connections with the nose.

Maxillary sinus

Frontal sinus

STEAM INHALATION
Sit at a table with a jug of water that has only just boiled (take due care). Place a towel over your head and the jug, and breathe in the steam for five to ten minutes. Try to breathe through your nose. Repeat as often as you feel the exercise is useful. Preparations to add to the water for inhalation are widely available, but of unproven worth – apart from their pleasant smell. The real value is in the steam, which liquifies the excess mucus.

Antiseptic mouthwashes, low-potency steroids, iron, antibiotics, anti-fungals.

WHAT ARE MOUTH DISORDERS?

– Three distinct types of problem occur:

Mouth ulcers, from which most people suffer from time to time, are areas of soreness and swelling on the inside of the mouth, often associated with infection. Though fairly painful, they are not sufficiently so to prevent eating. There are, however, many kinds of mouth ulcer, and even the simplest may occasionally be associated with minor degrees of anaemia and similar conditions. It is therefore essential to mention any persistent mouth ulcer to a dentist or doctor. If you are told that it is simple ulceration, then self-treatment is appropriate. Any ulcer which lasts for more than two weeks without showing signs of healing should have expert attention.

A sore mouth has many causes, some obvious – such as the fitting of new dentures – and some less so. If you have a sore mouth or tongue which lasts for more than a week or two for no obvious reason, consult a dentist or doctor. If there is no clear reason for the problem, an investigation such as a blood test may be advised. Many diseases which affect the skin also appear in the mouth, sometimes before the skin is seen to be involved. You may need a biopsy – the removal of a small section of the mouth lining (a local anaesthetic eliminates any pain) for microscopic examination. This does not necessarily mean that some sinister disease is suspected. In a few patients, usually women at or around the time of the menopause, no cause is ever found for the complaint.

Thrush is an infection of the mouth by a fungus. It is usually present in healthy mouths, but becomes active when an individual is weakened by illness, and appears as white flecks on the lining of the mouth; it is usually moderately sore. Thrush may occur also in young or old patients with no other significant illness, and in patients taking certain drugs – particularly steroids and, sometimes, antibiotics.

PRESCRIPTION DRUGS

Antiseptic mouthwashes will be suggested for mild ulceration.

Low-potency steroids, given as lozenges, may be suggested for more severe mouth ulceration. Bear in mind that whatever the treatment, there is no cure for mouth ulcers; the best you can hope for is improvement until they clear of their own accord.

Iron tablets may be given if a sore mouth is caused by anaemia *(see page 224)*. Since a sore mouth can be caused by a number of conditions, treatments vary widely. **Antifungal preparations** and antibiotics are prescribed for thrush; they are usually given as lozenges, gels, creams, or suspensions for use in and around the mouth. Only occasionally will they be in a form designed to be swallowed.

OVER-THE-COUNTER TREATMENTS
There is an enormous range of mouthwashes, pastilles and lozenges which can effectively relieve these complaints. However, it is essential to have any persistent ulceration or soreness checked out by a doctor/dentist rather than persist with self-treatment.

QUESTIONS TO ASK A DOCTOR OR DENTIST
■ How often should I use the mouthwash/lozenges?
■ How long should I use the mouthwash/lozenges?
■ Should I keep on using them when my mouth is better?
■ What should I do if the treatment seems to be making my mouth worse?
■ Is the treatment a permanent cure?

SIDE EFFECTS
Mouthwashes and iron tablets have no significant side effects; low-potency topical steroids, used short-term, have none either. For *antibiotics* and *antifungals, see pages 79 and 285.*

SELF MANAGEMENT
■ Oral hygiene is enhanced by regular brushing of the teeth in the correct fashion, with a toothbrush of the size advised for you individually. Ask your dentist. ■ Additional oral hygiene, again on the advice of a dentist, may be necessary for people with disorders of the structure – gums, bone and other tissue – supporting the teeth. Measures include use of dental floss and wooden picks for removing plaque.

Plaque – bacterial deposits – is revealed by chewing a disclosing tablet. This procedure can be an invaluable aid to maintaining a clean mouth and avoiding mouth disorders.

LARYNGITIS AND CROUP

Local anaesthetic lozenges, analgesics, cough suppressants antibiotics

NAMES YOU WILL HEAR

Antibiotics
Chemical name: amoxicillin sodium; trade names: Amoxil, Moxacin, Moxilean, Novamoxin, Penamox, Polymox. Chemical name: co-trimoxazole; trade names: Bactrim, Fectrim, Nodilon, Septrim. Chemical name: erythromycin; trade names: Arpimycin, Erycen, Erymax, Erythroped, Retcin, Erythrocin, Erythromid, Ilotycin, EpMycin, Erostin, Emu-V, Ethryn, Eromel, Ilocap, Ilosone, Rythrocaps.

Local analgesics
Chemical name: benzocaine; trade names: AAA Spray, Tyrozets, Benzocaine. Chemical name: benzocaine and dequalinium chloride; trade name: Dequacaine.

Analgesics
Chemical name: paracetamol; trade names: Panadol, Pamol, Calpol, Tylenon, Paracin, Parmol, Panado, Ceetamol, Atosol, Exctol, Tylenol, Ennagesic, Ilvamol. Chemical name: aspirin; trade names: Aspirin, Astrin, Bi-Prin. See also **pain**, page 106.

Cough suppressants
Chemical name: codeine phosphate; trade names: Codeine Linctus, Codeine Syrup, Dimotane Co, Galcodine, Phensedyl, Tercoda, Terpoin, Uniflu. Chemical name: pholcodine tartrate; trade names: Dia-Tuss, Duro-Tuss, Pholtex, Copholco, Copholcoids, Davenol, Expulin, Galenphol, Pavacol D, Pholcomed, Rinurel.

WHAT IS LARYNGITIS?

- An inflammation of the voice box (larynx) resulting in hoarseness or total loss of voice. Acute laryngitis comes on suddenly and lasts a few days. It is usually associated with a sore throat and sometimes there is a dry cough.

Acute laryngitis can cause croup in young children. Swelling of the air passage results in obstruction to breathing – the airways are relatively narrower in young children. The child has a hoarse cry and makes a noisy sound (stridor) when breathing in. If the obstruction is severe, the child will start to breathe rapidly, with straining of the breathing muscles.

Chronic laryngitis comes on more gradually and lasts a longer time. It is usually not painful.

CAUSES Acute laryngitis is usually caused by a viral infection such as the common cold, influenza or measles. Chronic laryngitis may be caused by faulty voice production and shouting, habitual over-indulgence in alcohol or tobacco, or chronic sinus infection. Hoarseness may also be caused by nodules or tumors on the vocal cords.

PRESCRIPTION DRUGS

Antibiotics are usually unnecessary in the treatment of acute laryngitis, as the cause is most often a virus, but they may be used in the treatment of associated bacterial infection such as sinusitis or ear infection. For details of these antibiotics, see **pneumonia and pleurisy**, page 78.

OVER-THE-COUNTER TREATMENTS

A **local anaesthetic** in the form of a lozenge will ease the sore throat by decreasing the conduction of nerve impulses near the site of application, so making the throat less sensitive.

Analgesics such as aspirin and paracetamol will also help the sore throat and the general symptoms associated with acute laryngitis. See **common cold**, page 134.

Cough suppressants will suppress the cough. Laryngitis is one of the few good reasons for the use of cough suppressants. The cough is usually irritating and non-productive, and persistent coughing may further inflame the larynx. See **cough**, page 68.

QUESTIONS TO ASK THE DOCTOR

■ How long will it last?
■ Will stopping smoking help?

- Will resting my voice help?
- Will antibiotics help?
- (If a baby has croup)
  How should I treat the high temperature?
  How can I stop the hoarse cough?
  Is the fast breathing a danger sign?
  What danger signs should I look for?

SIDE EFFECTS
Antibiotics: *see **pneumonia and pleurisy**, page 78.*
Local anaesthetics are generally very safe. Occasionally they cause an allergic reaction which results in mild ir-ritation of the mouth.
Analgesics: *see **common cold**, page 134.*
Cough suppressants: *see **cough**, page 68.*

SELF-MANAGEMENT
■ The usual cause of laryngitis and croup is the com-mon cold; *see the advice on page 134.*
■ If you have laryngitis, rest your voice: this really is important – talking will aggravate the condition.
■ Treat your sore throat regularly with analgesics, either in the form of anaesthetic lozenges or tablets (for example aspirin or paracetamol). If you are not sure which is best, *see **common cold**, page 134.* Try gargling soluble paracetamol or aspirin.
■ If there is any difficulty in breathing associated with hoarseness, especially in a child, consult your doctor at once.
■ Hoarseness which persists for more than three weeks should be investigated by your doctor.

TREATING CROUP
Croup can usually be treated at home if it is mild.
1 It is important to control the temperature *(see **common cold**, page 134):* the condition worsens if the child is hot, irritable and crying.
2 Increase the humidity in the child's room, both to minimize the problem, and to treat the acute attack. Simply boil a kettle, with the windows and doors clos-ed, or sit the child in a steamy bathroom.
3 Encourage the child to drink clear fluids: dehydration can occur as a result of rapid breathing and sweating due to high temperature.
4 Keep the child calm: croup becomes much worse as soon as the child starts to cry.
5 If a child is breathing fast (chest heaving more than 50 times a minute), or having difficulty breathing, call a doctor.

WHAT IS RED EYE?
– A general term for several distinct eye conditions:

CONJUNCTIVITIS
– Gritty, irritable eyes with discharge during the day
and stickiness in the morning.

CAUSE Usually a bacterial infection, but sometimes a
virus. Viral conjunctivitis often occurs in epidemics.

PRESCRIPTION DRUGS
Antibiotics: many are available; the commonest is
chloramphenicol. All may be given as drops or ointment
– drops should be used two-hourly, ointment four times
a day. A seven-day course should clear a bacterial infection. Your doctor will tell you to pull down the lower
lid and apply one to two drops or a $\frac{1}{2}$-inch (1.5 cm)
squeeze of ointment to the inside of the lid.
How they work: by killing bacteria. There is no treatment
for viral conjunctivitis, but it clears in 14–21 days.

BLEPHRITIS
– Red, sore, itchy eyelids. The condition is usually
longstanding (chronic). Two types occur: bacterial,
with pus and ulceration along the lid margins; and
squamous, with flakes of skin amongst the eyelashes.
CAUSES Bacterial blepharitis is due to the bacterium
staphylococcus and tends to wax and wane.
Squamous blepharitis is a manifestation of a skin
disease known as seborrhoeic dermatitis – the
eyebrows and scalp are usually involved as well.
Secondary bacterial infection can occur in squamous
blepharitis.

PRESCRIPTION DRUGS
Antibiotics: Ointment applied to the lid margins four
times a day should clear a flare-up of bacterial
blepharitis, but will not prevent a recurrence. Drops are
of no value. Occasionally, antibiotics may be given.

OVER-THE-COUNTER TREATMENTS
Medicated shampoos: treating the scalp and eyebrows
with one of these will improve squamous blepharitis
when combined with lid hygiene.

CORNEAL ABRASION AND FOREIGN BODIES
Any injury or foreign body can scratch the cornea, the
front of the eye. Your doctor will remove the foreign
body and give antibiotics against secondary infection.

A corneal abrasion heals over two to three days in much the same way as a scratch or graze on the skin, and only rarely causes long-term damage. During the healing process, however, it feels as if there is still something in the eye and it hurts to look at bright lights. Wear dark glasses and rest; stop the antibiotic when the sensation clears.

QUESTIONS TO ASK THE DOCTOR
■ Should I cover my eye?
■ Is my eye contagious? Can I protect the rest of the family from catching it? Should I stay away from work?

SIDE EFFECTS
Antibiotic ointment blurrs the vision for about 30 minutes, so don't drive until this has cleared. All eye treatments can occasionally cause allergy, ointment more commonly than drops. The allergy is to the preservatives or base rather than the active ingredient and appears as swollen red lids and conjunctiva. It can be dramatic, but clears once treatment is stopped.

SELF-MANAGEMENT
Do not use over-the-counter eye treatments unless first advised by a doctor. At best, they have no effect on the underlying condition and frequently cause an allergic reaction. In blepharitis, lid hygiene is the mainstay of control. Every morning, clean the eyelids with cotton wool and warm water ensuring that all crusts and flakes are removed from the margins. If necessary, use a cotton-bud – rub it along the lash bases. Repeat as often as necessary through the day. In a flare-up, increase cleaning to four times a day and apply ointment.

OTHER CAUSES OF A RED EYE
These include acute glaucoma *(see page 270)*, acute iritis, corneal ulcer and corneal abscess. They are all uncommon and very painful with marked blurring of vision. If these occur with a red eye, see your doctor.

DRY EYE
This common problem occurs usually with age and causes a number of troublesome symptoms including itching, burning, discomfort, heaviness of the lids, frontal headaches and transient blurring of vision. It is not painful and the eye does not go red except in severe cases. It is worse in smoky or dry atmospheres and in the evening.

CAUSE Tear production falls below a level at which the lids can adequately wet the cornea.

Treatment Artificial tears usually contain hypromellose. Commonly used brands are Ilube, Isopto Tears and Tears Naturale. Other artificial tears include SnoTears, Liquifilm and Lacrilube.

Self-help Understanding the condition: if tears are insufficient, dry spots occur. These cause the symptoms, which come on over four to six hours and last for about 24 hours. Instil the artificial tears regularly and frequently enough to ensure wetting at all times: **1** Put the drops in every two hours to start with. **2** If the symptoms are going to clear, this will take at least a day, so don't give up. **3** If, after a few days, there is no improvement, increase the drops to hourly or even half-hourly: there are no side effects. **4** When there has been an improvement, gradually reduce the frequency every other day to a level which keeps the eyes comfortable: use trial and error.

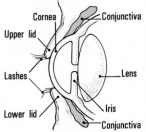

Cornea — Conjunctiva
Upper lid
Lashes — Lens
Lower lid — Iris
— Conjunctiva

The lids *are in contact with the cornea and spread tears over its surface by blinking. The under surface of each lid is covered with conjunctiva which loosely spreads out above and below the eye to form potential spaces. Ointment or drops can be applied into the lower of these spaces by gently pulling down the lower lid.*

WHAT IS CHRONIC GLAUCOMA?

– Gradual, painless rise of pressure in the eyeball causing loss of vision over several years. It starts as islands of reduced vision away from central field. These islands slowly enlarge, but are not usually noticed until the late stages when only a small area of central vision is left (tunnel vision) before blindness takes over.

Acute glaucoma is by contrast usually sudden in onset, very painful, with altered vision and a red eye.

CAUSE Inability of the intraocular fluid, the aqueous, to escape from the eye quickly enough. The intraocular pressure rises gradually until it is high enough to cause damage to the optic nerve. The optic nerve carries the nervous messages of sight from the eye to the brain and when it is completely destroyed, blindness results.

PRESCRIPTION DRUGS

Antiglaucoma drugs are usually given as drops, occasionally as ointment. They are often used in combination to achieve better control, and are taken for life.

Beta-blockers: Timolol is the commonest, given as drops twice a day.

Sympathomimetics are also used twice a day mainly in people with chest disease, who may suffer potentially serious side effects if given beta-blockers.

Pilocarpine drops are used three or four times a day and often added to timolol or adrenaline.

Acetazolamide is taken as tablets two or four times a day; not often used due to side effects.

If these drugs do not control the pressure, a minor operation may be necessary to create a new drainage channel: this is known as a trabeculectomy.

How they work: They all lower the intraocular pressure by reducing the production of aqueous, except pilocarpine, which allows it to escape more easily.

OVER-THE-COUNTER TREATMENTS

None.

QUESTIONS TO ASK THE DOCTOR

■ How often should I take the drops?
■ What happens if I miss out the drops once or twice?
■ What strength should I use?
■ What happens if the drops don't work?
■ What are the side effects?

SIDE EFFECTS

Beta-blockers usually have no side effects; however they can cause breathlessness. If this happens, stop them immediately and report it to your doctor.

Sympathomimetics: adrenaline causes eye redness in many people; dipivefrin does not and is thus more widely used.

Pilocarpine may cause headache for 30 minutes after use, but this problem usually fades in a week. It makes the pupil constrict, and can dim the vision particularly where there is also a cataract. It also paralyses the eye's ability to focus and may make life very difficult for younger people.

Acetazolamide has many side effects: numbness and tingling in the fingers and toes, lethargy, loss of appetite, nausea, weight loss and confusion. Occasional but serious side effects are diabetes and kidney stones. Use is rarely justified, except in people who happen not to be prone to these effects.

SELF-MANAGEMENT

■ Take the drops and tablets regularly to keep the pressure normal throughout the day. This way you will slow down or halt progress of the disease.

■ Take the treatment as usual on the day you attend the clinic so the specialist can get an idea of what the pressure is between visits.

■ If you are taking more than one type of drop, leave five to ten minutes between each: this prevents the first being washed away before it can work.

■ Glaucoma runs in families, so if you are told you have it, inform all close blood relatives. Parents, brothers and sisters over 40 should visit an optician for a check.

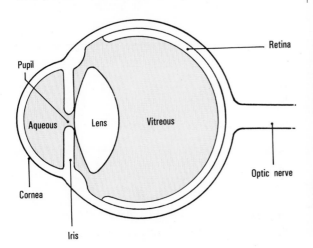

Light passes through the cornea, pupil and lens and focuses on the retina. The retina converts the image into nervous impulses which travel down the optic nerve to the brain. A degree of intraocular pressure is essential to give the ocular structures their support. But the eye's interior is essentially a non-expandable space, and if pressure in the aqueous builds up, as in glaucoma, this is transmitted all over the eye, which then becomes tight and hard. This in turn damages the optic nerve, which leads off to the brain at the back of the eye, but has numerous endings in the retina.

Skin and hair

The skin is probably the largest organ in the body and has a number of functions. To keep working well, it is constantly replaced – in fact everyone's skin is totally replaced every two to three weeks. The old skin falls off as flakes of dry skin which are rarely seen but which account for much of the dust in houses. Hair is a specialized form of skin.

ACNE	**274-277**
SUNBURN	**278-279**
ECZEMA	**280-281**
VIRAL WARTS	**282-283**
FUNGAL INFECTIONS	**284-285**
SKIN PARASITES	**286-287**
BITES AND STINGS	**288-289**
PSORIASIS	**290-291**
SKIN CANCERS	**292-293**

See also: *Shingles, page 140; middle and external ear infections, page 256.*

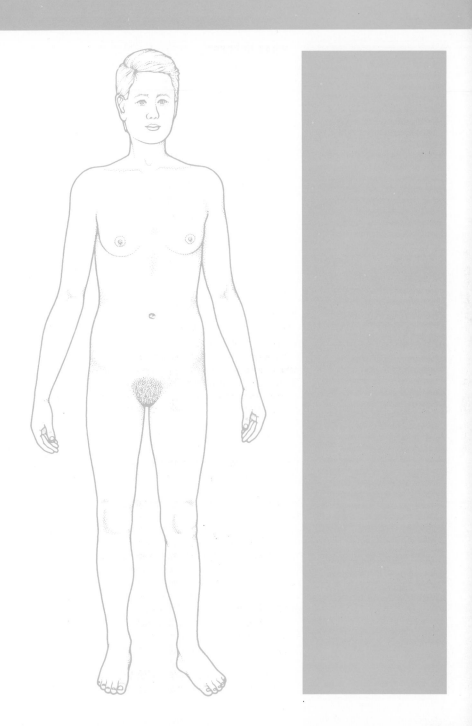

NAMES YOU WILL HEAR
Selected Commercial Preparations
Topical agents
Chemical name: benzoyl peroxide preparations; **trade names:** Acetoxyl, Acnegel, Benoxyl, Benzagel, Debroxide, Nericur, Panoxyl Aquagel, Quinoderm, Theraderm. **Chemical name:** tretinoin. retin A; **trade name:** Retin-A. **Chemical name:** resorcinol/salicylic acid/sulphur preparations; **trade names:** Dome-Acne, Eskamel. **Chemical name:** aluminium oxide in detergent paste; **trade name:** Brasivol. **Chemical name:** corticosteroid combinations; **trade names:** Actinac, Medrone, Neomedrone, Quinoderm HC.

Others
Topical antibiotics
Chemical name: tetracycline for topical solution; **trade name:** usually prescribed by chemical name.

Oral antibiotics
Chemical name: oxytetracycline; **trade names:** Bramcycline, Betacycline. **Chemical name:** erythromycin; **trade names:** Arpimycin, Erycen, Erymax, Erythroped, Retcin, Erythrocin, Erythromid, Ilotycin, EpMycin, Erostin, Emu-V, Ethryn, Eromel, Ilocap, Ilosone, Rythrocaps. **Chemical name:** co-trimoxazole; **trade names:** Bactrim, Fectrim, Nodilon, Septrim. **Chemical name:** minocycline; **trade names:** Minocin, Minomycin, Ultramycin. **Chemical name:** doxycycline; **trade names:** Vibramycin, Dioxin.

Hormone therapy – 'the Diane' pill
Chemical name: isotretinon or 13-cis retinoic acid; **trade name:** Roaccutane.

Acne soaps and face cleansers
Acne Aid, Biactol, Clearasil, Dome-Acne Cleanser, Hibiscrub, Phiso-Med, Ionax Scrub.

WHAT IS ACNE?

– Inflammation of the skin involving the sebaceous or grease glands. It occurs in areas of skin rich in those glands: the face, back and upper chest.

Nearly all teenagers have acne, though the severity varies enormously. Surprisingly, some girls do not develop it until their early 20s; though mild, it may unfortunately persist until the mid to late 30s.

CAUSES The chain of events which lead to acne are understood, but not the root cause(s). At puberty, the skin becomes especially greasy (sebhorrhoea); the increased flow of grease (sebum) irritates the lining of the grease duct (see diagram) so that debris is produced. This builds up, blocking the duct opening. The debris may be pushed out by the sebum (blackhead); or the opening may remain blocked (whitehead) so that the sebum accumulates in the channel, ruptures its lining and escapes into the skin, causing the inflammation. The stagnation of the sebum leads to a change in the bacteria living in the sebaceous duct which produce substances which aggravate the inflammation produced by the duct rupture.

It is not infectious, and strictly speaking, it is not inherited: just because a father had severe acne, it does not mean his son will. However, there are unusually severe variants which do tend to run in families.

Ten per cent of teenagers have no acne at all, and 30 per cent have a few spots at odd times – 'physiological' (almost normal) acne and require no treatment. About 40 per cent have mild acne with mostly blocked pores (blackheads and whiteheads) and a few red- (papules) and yellow-headed (pustules) spots. About 20 per cent have moderate or severe acne with many papules and pustules which require prescription treatment with both topical agents and oral antibiotics.

Dermatologists see most patients at 12-14 years when the acne is just starting and then they are not sure what it is; at 16 (females) or 18 (males) when the acne is at its peak and most stubborn; and in early 20s when it should have gone, but has not.

TREATMENT

Topical agents (ie applied to the skin) are largely based on **benzoyl peroxide.** They can be successful in treating mild to moderate acne, clearing both blackheads and whiteheads and papules and pustules. The preparation needs to be applied to the whole acne-prone area, not just the individual spots. In some preparations, benzoyl

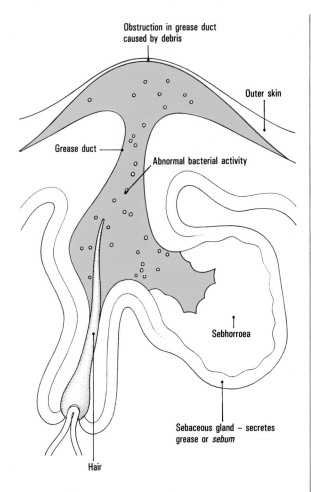

Obstruction in grease duct caused by debris

Outer skin

Grease duct

Abnormal bacterial activity

Sebhorroea

Sebaceous gland – secretes grease or *sebum*

Hair

peroxide is combined with a topical steroid to settle the inflammation, and an antibiotic.

How they work: by relieving the blockage of the sebaceous ducts and destroying the bacteria which live in the ducts. Other topical agents are abrasives (which is based on resocinol), sulphur, salicylic acid and aluminium oxide.

Acne soaps and antiseptic face washes are also useful. *See* **OVER-THE-COUNTER TREATMENTS.**

How they work: by relieving the obstruction in the sebaceous ducts.

Oral antibiotics are the mainstay for moderate or severe acne. They take time to work, and need to be taken for three to six months to produce maximum improvement. Unfortunately, acne frequently recurs on discontinuing the antibiotics. Often a low dose has to be continued on a long-term basis. A change from one type of antibiotic to another may give further improvement.

How they work: by killing bacteria in the ducts, so preventing inflammatory damage to the acne. They do not help get rid of blackheads and whiteheads – in which there is no inflammation.

In recent years, research has been directed at finding drugs to deal with the underlying problem of acne – greasiness of the skin. Two drugs are useful:

The Diane pill is a hormone preparation which reduces the sebhorrhoea by 30 per cent. It takes six to 12 months to produce the best result, and does not produce a long-term cure. It is also an effective contraceptive pill, but contains a high dose of oestrogen – see **SIDE EFFECTS.** However, the Diane pill is more effective than antibiotics, and is a worthwhile alternative, especially in the older teenager or female in her 20s who also requires contraceptive cover.

Isotretinoin or **13-cis retinoic acid** is a synthetic form of vitamin A, reserved for the most severe forms of acne and confined to hospital pharmacies. It can reduce seborrhoea by 90 per cent and improves the acne by 70 per cent within four months. There is a 1:2 chance of a long-term remission of over two years. However, it is an uncomfortable drug to take – see **SIDE EFFECTS.**

Most patients notice that their acne improves in the summer and artificial sunlight (ultraviolet light) therapy is sometimes prescribed. There are long-term problems with this therapy *(see **skin cancers,** page 292)* so it is only given in short courses.

As a general rule, diet has no part to play in the treatment of acne, though certain individuals may have exacerbations after eating specific foods such as chocolate.

OVER-THE-COUNTER TREATMENTS

Many of these contain benzoyl peroxide (examine the packet) and are genuinely useful for mild to moderate acne. Self-treatment with acne soaps and face washes (often containing abrasives) is also appropriate for mild to moderate acne. Don't be misled by the advertisements: no tretament can perform miracles, and all need to be used with persistence, and according to the directions. Perhaps the key point about commercial preparations is their expense.

QUESTIONS TO ASK THE DOCTOR
■ How long should I use this treatment for?
■ Should I be on any particular diet?

SIDE EFFECTS
Benzoyl peroxide causes redness and dryness, better tolerated if application is gradually increased from two hours each evening during the first week to (subsequently) morning and evening applications.

Antibiotics may cause gastro-intestinal upset (nausea or diarrhoea) and vaginal thrush infections.

The Diane pill can cause weight gain, breast tenderness, headaches, altered libido and increased blood pressure. *See also* **contraception,** *page 178.*

Isotretinoin causes dry, cracked lips, dry eyes, a dry nose and nose bleeds, dry rashes on the hands, headaches and joint pains. It can also damage the foetus, and is thus prescribed with extreme caution to females.

SELF-MANAGEMENT
■ Acne can cause scars. The commonest are tiny pits in the surface of the cheeks known as icepick scars. Not so well recognized are flat white blemishes over the back. Occasionally thick, raised, overgrown scars called keloids occur on the chest and shoulders. Plastic surgery can make good the damage but the only satisfactory answer to scarring is lasting and purposeful treatment of the acne.

■ Career prospects: acne becomes worse in hot humid environments, especially the Far East. The armed forces used to be very reluctant to take teenagers with moderately severe acne, though the use of isotretinoin is changing this attitude. A hot humid kitchen is similarly not to be recommended. Prejudice against skin disease, unjust as it may be, is prevalent and acne sufferers are probably best advised not to court disappointment by applying for jobs with a high public profile while their acne problem lasts.

■ Accept – realistically, but optimistically, that acne is part of being a teenager. Don't be cynical of the value of skin cleansing, diet and UV treatment as recommended by a doctor: in moderate or severe cases, these are an essential back-up to the mainstay drug treatments.

■ Don't use heavy oil-based cosmetics. Water-based and light powdered cosmetics are however harmless and indeed have an essential role in hiding the more unsightly acne.

DOCTOR'S EXPERIENCE
"Phillip, a 14-year-old who had had acne since he was nine, was teased continuously at school and often stayed at home locked in his bedroom. His family doctor tried various antibiotics, and sun-lamp treatment, for three years with no success. At that stage he was referred to the skin specialist at the local hospital and started on isotretinoin. His lips cracked, and his face and hands became dry and scaly. He was inclined to give up – but then the acne began to improve, and so he persisted with the treatment. The drug was stopped after four months, but the acne continued to clear. Three years later he is still free of spots."

SUNBURN

Steroid creams
Chemical name:
hydrocortisone/hydrocortisone-acetate;
trade names: Dioderm, Dome-Cort
Cream, Cort-Dome Cream, Efcortelan,
Hydrocortisyl, Hydrocortistab, Emo-
Cort, Hydro-Cortilean, Unicort,
Carimol, Hydro-Cortemel, Egocort,
Cortef, Derma-Cort 'O', Hydrocortisyl,
Hydrosone, Squibb-HC.

Antihistamines
Chemical name: chlorpheniramine;
trade names: Haymine, Piriton, Chlor-
Tripolon, Histalon, Novopheniram,
Allertex, Chlortrimeton, Histamed,
Allergex, Bramahist Chloramin,
Histaids, Teledrim. **Chemical name:**
promethazine; **trade names:**
Phenergan, Histantil, Lenazine, Prohist,
Progan. **Chemical name:** trimeprazine;
trade names Vallergan, Panectyl.
*See also **pain**, page 106, for
analgesics.*

WHAT IS SUNBURN?

– Inflammation of the skin caused by exposure to sun
rays of a certain wavelength technically known as middle wave ultraviolet light or UVB. UVA is by contrast the
tanning element in sunlight. Sunlight has three effects
on skin:

1 Initial redness (erythema) which occurs while in the
sun but soon disappears. This is followed two to four
hours later by a second phase of erythema which lasts
for about 48 hours. These is associated with a variable
degree of inflammation, pain, heat and blistering.

2 Tanning, which follows the second phase of
erythema, is a protective response by the skin, mainly
the result of increased production of the brown pigment
melanin. Dark skin is rich in melanin, and so can cope
more easily than pale skin with strong sunlight.

3 Skin cancer – *see page 292*.

Some drugs, such as tetracyclines, culphonamides,
chlorothiazidesand phenothiazines increase sensitivity
to sunlight. If you are on regular medication, ask your
doctor before sunbathing.

CAUSES There are three important factors which determine how sunburnt you become: the degree of pigmentation prior to exposure; duration of exposure; the
strength of the sun. The more vertical the sun's rays,
the more damage to the skin. Exposure at midday,
when the sun is at its highest, is the most damaging.

TREATMENT

Self-management (see below) is of course the answer
to most sunburn. If a doctor sees a really serious case,
the options are:

Analgesics: aspirin and paracetamol, *see **pain**, page 106*,
are the first choice for moderate or mild cases;
paracetamol plus codeine preparations are effective in
more severe cases.

How they work: *see **pain**, page 106*.

Antihistamines: If the problem is itching more than pain,
these may be useful.

How they work: in this context, mainly a sedative effect.

OVER-THE-COUNTER TREATMENTS

For protection: **Sunscreens** contain aminobenzoic acid or
amyl dimethyl aminobenzoate, essentially their only active ingredient. It 'filters out' a proportion of the harmful
rays; burning can still occur. The sun protection factor
(SPF) gives an indication of the degree of protection offered. The higher the SPF, the greater the protection.

For treatment: Calamine lotion is an effective anti-itch and cooling preparation. It has several active ingredients including calamine, zinc oxide and glycerol. There no side effects and it can be used as often as desired.

Low-strength **steroid creams** (1 per cent hydrocortisone) are now available over-the-counter in some countries. See **SIDE EFFECTS**.

Simple analgesics and also antihistamines are widely available from chemists.

Some natural oils (for example coconut oil) and indeed some commercial preparations are claimed to promote tanning, and indeed may appear to do so; but there is no scientific basis for the claim.

QUESTIONS TO ASK THE DOCTOR

■ Will the tablets I taking on a regular basis make me more likely to get sunburn?
■ What do I do if blisters develop?
■ How long will it take to subside?
■ Can I drink alcohol with tablets containing antihistamine or codeine?

SIDE EFFECTS

Analgesics: *See pain, page 106.*

Steroid creams, which might be used for severe sunburn, are low-strength, and sunburn is a short-lived condition. The serious long-term side effects of their use *(see eczema, page 280)* are not an issue here.

Antihistamines increase the sedative effects of alcohol, so holiday drinking needs to be moderated; avoid driving or using machinery.

COMMONSENSE PRECAUTIONS

■ Don't sunbathe, or expose your bare skin, for long periods at the start of a holiday. Build up exposure gradually over a period of days, starting with half an hour to an hour, and increase exposure by no more than 45 minutes daily. Individuals can take widely varying degrees of exposure. As a guide, stop sunbathing as soon as you feel the hot 'pricking' sensation of the sun on your skin.
■ Avoid sunbathing when the sun is highest.
■ If your skin is fair, use a sunscreen.
■ If swimming or snorkelling, your back may get badly burned, despite its feeling cool in the water. You can also get sunburned through tights.
■ A sun-bed can cause sunburn (even though most of its light is UVA, the tanning part of ultraviolet light).

ONCE YOU ARE SUNBURNT ...
■ Avoid further exposure.
■ Towels soaked in cold water applied gently over the affected areas may help to reduce the inflammation.
■ Calamine lotion has a soothing effect.
■ Take simple painkillers.
■ Local steroid cream may help short-term.
■ Take plenty of rest.
■ Moisturisers used daily will help to prevent the skin becoming excessively dry and also help to minimize peeling.

WHAT IS ECZEMA?

– An itchy rash in which the skin is typically red and may develop small blisters which are then scratched, leaving raw areas. In long-standing eczema, the skin becomes thickened and the normal skin markings may be accentuated. There are five main types:

1 Atopic eczema usually starts in childhood and in some cases is associated with asthma and hay fever. There is often a family history of one or more of these conditions. In children it typically affects the face, the elbow creases, and behind the knees. In adults the common areas are the face, neck and elbow creases. In about 85 per cent of children with infantile eczema, the rash clears spontaneously during childhood. In a small number of individuals atopic eczema may be provoked by allergy to foods or to the house dust mite. **2 Seborrhoeic eczema** causes flaking and itchiness of the scalp, face, eyebrows and eyelids, sometimes with a rash on the chest, under the arms, and in the groin. **3 Discoid eczema** usually occurs after middle-age and causes circular itchy patches, often scattered on the limbs. **4 Varicose eczema** occurs on the lower legs in association with varicose veins and leg ulcers. **5 Contact eczema** is caused by sensitivity to substances which touch the skin. This may be due to allergy, for instance to metals such as nickel which is found in costume jewellery; or to chronic irritation, for example detergents causing 'housewive's hand'. This type of the rash may spread.

PRESCRIPTION DRUGS

Steroid ointments and **creams** reduce the amount of inflammation in the skin and heal the eczema. The weakest possible preparation should be used for maintenance treatment, but in acute exacerbations, strong steroids may be required for a short time. When the skin is dry, the steroid drugs in ointment form, which are greasy, are much better absorbed than creams. Sometimes preparations which combine a steroid with an antibiotic are used if the eczema has become infected.
How they work: by blocking the inflammatory reaction.
Tar preparations *(see psoriasis, page 290)* are sometimes used in the treatment of long-standing eczema: they can reduce the itching and inflammation.
Antihistamines reduce itching and have a sedative effect. Taken before bed, they can promote sound sleep.

OVER-THE-COUNTER TREATMENTS

Moisturizers and bath oils are commonly available and

essential in the treatment of atopic eczema in which the skin is usually very dry. They should be used freely and frequently. In sebhorrhoeic eczema, antidandruff shampoos benefit an itchy, flaking scalp. Low potency steroid creams are available in most chemists.

QUESTIONS TO ASK THE DOCTOR
■ For how long should the treatment be continued?
■ Which preparation is the moisturizer, and which the topical steroid?
■ Will the treatment cause staining?

SIDE EFFECTS
Strong topical steroids, used for long periods, cause thinning of the skin and easy bruising. This thinning occurs particularly under the arms and in the groin, where stretch marks may develop. Strong steroids can also eventually cause redness and a rash on the face. Stunting of growth may occur if potent steroids are used in childhood for extended periods. However, most of these side effects are caused by abuse and/or overuse: strong steroids are extremely valuable when used strictly as prescribed. Steroid creams and ointments should always be applied sparingly and rubbed well in. **Antihistamines** cause drowsiness; patients taking them should not drive or operate machinery. They have an additive effect with alcohol, and can also cause dryness of the mouth, blurred vision, and difficulty urinating.

SELF-MANAGEMENT
■ Atopic eczema usually causes a very dry skin; regular use of moisturizers is essential.
■ Soaps and detergents such as bubble baths can irritate eczema, and should be avoided.
■ Children with eczema are more comfortable in cotton clothing. Wool next to the skin increases itchiness.
■ Clothing, especially bedclothes, should be cool and loose; itchiness tends to be worse if the body is hot.
■ Adults with a history of eczema should always protect their hands from the effects of water and detergents by wearing gloves when doing the washing-up and other chores.
■ Parents of children with eczema should warn them against occupations which can damage the skin, and particularly the hands. These include hairdressing and garage repair work.
■ Varicose veins and varicose eczema are helped by the use of support tights or bandages which also help to prevent ulcers forming on the leg.

Antihistamines
Chemical name: promethazine: **trade names:** Phenergan, Avomine, Progan, Prothazine, Histantil, Lenazine, Prohist, Profan. **Chemical name:** trimeprazine tartrate; **trade names:** Vallergan, Panectyl. See also **hay fever,** page 260.

Moisturizers
Aqueous Cream; Emulsifying Ointment; Alpha Keri Bath Oil; Balneam Bath Oil; Oilatum Emollient; Boots E45 Cream; Unguentum Merck; Ultrabase Cream; Aquadrate: Aveeno Bath Emollient; Emulsiderm.

Shampoos
Polytar Liquid, Ceanel Concentrate, Selsun Shampoo.

PATIENT'S EXPERIENCE
"I had eczema behind my knees as a child, but grew out of it when I was about seven years old. I had almost forgotten I had had it – until just after my first baby was born. My hands became extremely red and sore, and the skin started splitting and peeling off. I had been doing a lot of washing with all the nappies and the baby's clothes, but have never worn rubber gloves – I don't like their clammy feel. My doctor told me I should stop using soap on my hands and always wear rubber or plastic gloves when doing wet work, particularly rinsing out the nappies after they had been soaking in detergent. I started to use a moisturizer regularly on my hands, and followed the advice about gloves. It was worth the effort: my hands soon started to heal."

AVOIDING ALLERGENS
Atopic eczema sufferers, particularly those who have asthma as well, should keep their bedrooms as dust-free as possible in order to minimize allergic reaction to the house-dust mite. See **asthma,** page 74. Likewise, avoid contact with any other substance which happens to cause a reaction, including metal jewellery.

NAMES YOU WILL HEAR
Chemical name: formaldehyde 3% solution; **trade name:** usually prescribed by chemical name.
Chemical name: 1.5% formaldehyde in gel; **trade name:** Veracur.
Chemical name: salicylic acid (sometimes combined with lactic acid), salicylic acid plasters (20-40%) and salicylic acid collodion (12%), a sticky preparation applied to warts on hands of feet; **trade names:** Verrugon, Salactol, Duofilm, Cuplex (latter also contains copper acetate). **Chemical name:** glutaraldehyde 10%; **trade names:** Glutarol, Diswart, Verucasep. **Chemical name:** benzalkonium chloride-bromine; **trade name:** Callusolve. **Chemical name:** podophyllin; **trade name:** usually prescribed by chemical name; used in variety of strengths and applications prepared by the pharmacist. **Chemical name:** 20% podophyllin, 25% salicylic acid; **trade name:** Posalfilin. **Chemical name:** inosine pranobex; **trade name:** Immunovir.

WHAT DO VIRAL WARTS LOOK LIKE?

Appearances differ, but they usually present as raised, skin-coloured, thickenings of skin. They may take the form of small nodules, as on the hand, otherwise known as common warts, or small flat lesions, known as planar warts. On the soles of the feet, warts appear as hard nodules, similar to calluses, or as multi-faceted, flatter lesions, known as mosaic warts. These are also known as plantar warts, or verrucae. Because they are weight-bearing, they tend to grow in, rather than out.

Genital warts (and occasionally other types), project out from the skin, with a feathery or cauliflower-like, pedunculated appearance. Ano-genital warts tend to be small and multiple, and may occur in massive crops. Elsewhere on the body projecting warts are often described as filiform.

WHO GETS VIRAL WARTS?

Virtually everyone, but some are more prone than others. Common warts and plantar warts are most frequent in children. As immunity develops, the warts resolve. The vast majority of people with warts do not have a defect of immunity, but those with altered immunity, for example, atopic eczema sufferers, may be more severely affected. People receiving immune-suppressing drugs, and AIDS patients, run the more serious risk of developing florid wart infections. The sexually promiscuous are more likely to get ano-genital warts. Whether warts are contagious depends on the site and type of wart: common hand and planar warts are not particularly so and as the virus is prevalent it is likely that those without resistance will eventually get warts and those with immunity will not. There is no reason for children to avoid contact with other children who have hand or plantar warts: banning children with plantar warts from swimming is unnecessary.

In general, there is no known link between common warts or plantar warts and cancer. In females with genital warts involving the cervix there is an increased risk of cancer of the cervix. Large warty lesions, particularly in the elderly, may be skin tumours, not viral warts: seek medical advice.

CAUSES Papilloma-viruses: over 40 different forms have been identified and many are specific to certain types of infection. The virus locally takes over division of skin cells, reproducing itself.

Most people recognize viral warts without much difficulty. However, there may occasionally be doubt about diagnosis, in which case the family doctor is the best person to consult initially.

TREATMENT

Common and plantar warts in children are best left untreated unless they are causing problems; they often resolve spontaneously in a few years. If required, **topical salicylic acid, glutaraldehyde, formaldehyde** or **lactic acid preparations** can be used, but are best avoided on the face and in the ano-genital region.

In older patients, freezing with liquid nitrogen is often appropriate, but this is painful and can cause blistering. Warts on the soles, which have become thickened, should either be pared down with a sterile blade or rubbed down with an abrasive emery board before treatment. Then one of the above mentioned preparations can be applied; salicylic acid plasters are particularly useful at this site; alternatively, a **podophyllin compound** can be used. If these are unsuccessful, freezing and other destructive methods may be tried.

Genital and peri-anal warts are infectious: patients and their sexual partners should be examined in a specialist department. Females may require an internal examination for warts. Podophyllin 5-25% is commonly used externally: it is washed off after four to six hours and is normally started at low concentration, then built up. Some stinging and discomfort can occur, and if severe it should be stopped. Podophyllin should not be used during pregnancy. Freezing and/or surgery are further options.

Laser therapy has proved useful in treating certain cases of ano-genital and cervical warts. A new immunity-modulating drug, **inosine pranobex**, appears to be helpful in severe cases of genital warts.

OVER-THE-COUNTER TREATMENTS

These can be helpful, but avoid use on the face or ano-genital regions.

QUESTIONS TO ASK THE DOCTOR

■ Is it a viral wart, and does it need to be treated?
■ Is it infectious? Do I need to see a specialist?

SELF-MANAGEMENT

■ Common and plantar warts do not require treatment unless they cause discomfort. Don't share razors.
■ Don't place undue faith in old wives' tales for curing warts, even if they do seem to work: many viral warts have a tendency to resolve of their own accord.

PATIENT'S EXPERIENCE

"I first developed warts on my fingers when I was eleven years old. My mother used all sorts of things on them from the chemist, but they didn't make much difference. I was taken to my family doctor, who suggested that they were left alone; my mother was not very happy with this. The doctor gave me some liquid to apply from a bottle: it worked on a few of the warts, but I was still getting new ones. My parents were getting impatient, and asked the doctor if I could see a specialist. When I saw him, he explained that the warts would go in due course, but that he could not say when. As I had been teased at school, my mother insisted that something was done. The doctor, who was a dermatologist, said that we could have some liquid to apply to them, but this was the same as our doctor had given me. Alternatively, he said they could be frozen, but he was not very keen on this: he said it would sting and often required many freezings. In the end, my mother got her way and the warts were frozen with a spray of cold gas. It hurt; when I got home my finger was throbbing with blisters where the warts had been frozen. Several of the warts dropped off, but when I went back to the doctor they had started to grow back again. I told the doctor I didn't want any more freezing and he agreed. New warts stopped coming after six months; the old warts started to go after a year and they had all gone in two years.

Two years later I got warts on my feet. The doctor gave us some formaldehyde solution to soak my feet in; after drying, we had to rub the hard, thickened areas with an emery board. Salicylic acid plasters were then put on and this was repeated every evening. The warts went after about six months and I haven't had any trouble since."

WHAT IS A FUNGAL INFECTION?

– A tiny living organism which grows in long strands. It can live as mould on cheese, or indeed mould in a damp house; and some varieties prefer to live on human skin. In doing so they cause infections such as athletes' foot, ringworm, 'groin itch' and thrush. Usually they affect the top layers of skin only, making it dry, scaly and likely to flake off. The skin may be slightly itchy. The fungi thrive on warm, moist skin, so are commoner under the arms, beneath the breasts, in the groin and in the mouth. But different fungi have different patterns of growth and prefer particular sites, including hair, skin, nails, mouth and vagina. Fungal infections are rarely serious or life-threatening, but they do sometimes take a long time to clear up.

CAUSES *Candida* (thrush) normally lives in small numbers in the gut. Sometimes for no reason at all, and sometimes if an individual is run down, it multiplies and causes infection. Taking antibiotics for other bacterial infections also makes one more vulnerable to thrush: *see* **pneumonia and pleurisy,** *page 78.*

People who have diseases which decrease the body's defences (for example, leukaemia and AIDS) are also vulnerable to thrush. Babies may also develop thrush in the form of a nappy rash.

Athletes' foot and ringworm are usually caught from other people. Occasionally humans catch fungal infections from animals, for example cats and cattle, and these can also cause extensive rashes which take time to clear up.

If you or your doctor are uncertain whether the rash is fungal, it may be necessary to scrape off a sample of cells from the skin for examination.

PRESCRIPTION TREATMENTS

Lotions, creams, sprays or ointments are given according to the individual's needs and the type of infection. Creams wash off most easily and are easier to put on. Ointments are greasy and keep air off the affected area. Lotions are liquid and are particularly helpful when a large area of skin is affected or when the skin needs cooling because it is hot and inflamed. Dusting powders help to dry up wet rashes like athletes' foot, but will not cure the infection because they cannot penetrate the layers of affected skin.

Irridazole creams are the commonest treatments, for example miconazole, econazole and clotrimazole. Depending on the severity of the infection, all of these may have to be used for at least four weeks and often much longer to penetrate all the layers of skin and kill off all the fungi.

Whitfield's Ointment and **Castellani's Paint** are long-established and quite effective treatments, but increasingly superceded by the creams mentioned above which are easier to apply and more widely available.

Infections of the nails can be a particularly severe problem because replacement of infected tissue is slow. Long-term treatments such as **griseofulvia** and **ketoconazole** tablets may be necessary for up to a year.

QUESTIONS TO ASK THE DOCTOR
■ How do I know that I have a fungal infection and not eczema or psoriasis?
■ What will happen if I stop treatment too soon?

SIDE EFFECTS
Sometimes the skin will develop a secondary infection – another organism will take advantage while the skin's defences are poor. If the skin becomes bright red and tight around the rash, a bacterial infection may be developing and a course of antibiotics may be required: see a doctor.

Some people develop an allergy to the cream they are using: a different rash develops. Stop applying it immediately and see a doctor. **Ketoconazole** will only be prescribed by a specialist because it sometimes impairs liver function.

SELF-MANAGEMENT
Try to prevent warm, moist skin conditions by:
■ Washing regularly – particularly groin, armpits, feet and hair.
■ Drying the skin carefully – especially between the toes.
■ Avoiding shoes which make the feet sweat or which have no ventilation. Similarly avoid tight jeans.
■ If you do have naturally sweaty feet, use antifungal dusting powder.
■ Avoid walking in wet areas in bare feet.

Also:
■ Eat well to keep up the body's defences.
■ If you suffer from a condition which weakens your resistance to infection, for example diabetes, look after skin and feet and stick to any recommended diet.
■ Avoid close contact with animals or with people who have fungal infections.

WHAT ARE PARASITES?

– In the medical context, they are a number of different mites which live on human skin or hair, many of which do no harm. **Scabies** burrow their way under the skin and lay their eggs. These hatch out after two to three weeks and make the skin around them itchy and red. Areas affected are the hands (between the fingers), insides of the wrists, the elbows, the genital area, the arms and the feet. **Nits** prefer the hair, laying little white eggs which stick to the hairs and make the scalp itchy; do not confuse with dandruff, which can be shaken off. **Crabs** live on pubic hair – tiny whitish specks, accompanied by their white eggs as well. **Body lice** are a less common sort of parasite which cause itching all over the body and can be found in seams of clothes.

All parasites are transmitted by close contact with someone else who is infected: indeed one can catch head lice by using another person's comb or hat. People who live in poor housing or who have poor washing facilities are more vulnerable because of overcrowding. People who catch scabies are not necessarily dirty: it is easy for anyone to contract them.

Pubic lice are usually transmitted by sexual or very close bodily contact. If you have pubic lice, you may have some other sexually transmitted disease too, so have a check-up. Your doctor or a sexually transmitted disease clinic can arrange the tests.

PRESCRIPTION TREATMENTS

The lotions listed under NAMES YOU WILL HEAR for scabies, crabs and lice are applied all over the body except on head and neck. The lotion is put on after a bath and then washed off after the time stated in the instructions. The itching may continue for a while after the treatment.

Crotamiton cream – Eurax – can help relieve the itching before the treatment has had its effect.

For nits a lotion or a shampoo is applied all over the hair: keep it away from eyes and mouth. A nit comb may also be useful.

How the treatments work: by killing both mites and eggs.

OVER-THE-COUNTER TREATMENTS

Most of the treatments listed under NAMES YOU WILL HEAR are available from chemists without prescription, including nit combs, Sueol M, Quellada and Prioderm. Self-treatment is fine – just follow the directions carefully. And remember that scabies can persist even after the treatment; if this happens, see a doctor.

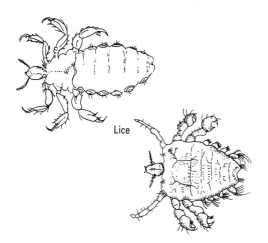

Lice

QUESTIONS TO ASK THE DOCTOR
- For how long will I be infectious?
- Can I get it again?

SIDE EFFECTS
Some people's skin can be irritated by these lotions; and sometimes infected yellow spots develop on top of the rash: a doctor may then need to prescribe antibiotics. **Malathion** and **carbaryl,** containing alcohol, are inflammable. Having applied either of them to the hair, after washing it, NEVER DRY THE HAIR BY A FIRE OR WITH AN ELECTRIC HAIR DRYER. There is a small, but real risk of the hair catching alight.

SELF-MANAGEMENT
- Immediately after using the treatment, wash all clothes and sheets which have been in use. Wash combs and brushes if the problem has been hair lice.
- Anyone who has been in close bodily contact with an infested person should also have treatment – children, parents and sexual partners. It is not necessary to shave the head if there have been nits, but cutting hair shorter is helpful.

SELF-HELP
To prevent infection:
- Have a bath as often as possible.
- Change clothes every day.
- Do not use other people's combs/brushes.
- Change bed clothes regularly.

BITES AND STINGS

Tetanus toxoid, antibiotics, rabies vaccine, calamine lotion, antihistamines, adrenaline,

NAMES YOU WILL HEAR

Chemical name: tetanus toxoid; **trade name:** Adsorbed Tetanus Vaccine. **Chemical name:** rabies vaccine; **trade name:** Merieux Rabies Vaccine. **Chemical name:** adrenaline; **trade name:** Adrenaline Injection.

Antibiotics
Chemical name: benzylpenicillin; **trade name:** Crystapen. **Chemical name:** amoxycillin sodium; **trade names:** Amoxil, Moxacin, Moxilean, Novamoxin, Penamox, Polmox. **Chemical name:** erythromycin; **trade names:** Arpimycin, Erycen, Erymax, Erythroped, Retcin, Erythrocin, Erythromid, Illotycin, EpMycin, Erostin, Emu-V, Ethryn, Eromel, Ilocap, Ilosone, Rythrocaps.

Local antihistamines
Chemical name: mepyramine maleate; **trade name:** Anthisan.

Oral antihistamines
Chemical name: promethazine; **trade names:** Phenergan, Avomine, Progan, Prothazine, Histantil, Lenazine, Prohist, Profan. **Chemical name:** chlorpheniramine; **trade names:** Haymine, Piriton, Chlor-Tripolon, Histalon, Novopheniram, Allertex, Chlortrimeton, Histamed, Allergex, Bramahist Chloramin, Histaids, Teledrim.

Steroids
Chemical name: hydrocortisone; **trade names:** Dioderm, Dome-Cort Cream, Cort-Dome Cream, Efcortelan, Hydrocortisyl, Hydrocortistab, Emo-Cort, Hydro-Cortilean, Unicort, Carimol, Hydro-Cortemel, Egocort, Cortef, Derma-Cort 'O', Hydrocortisyl, Hydrosone, Squibb-HC.

Analgesics
Chemical name: paracetamol; **trade names:** Panadol, Pamol, Calpol, Tylenon, Paracin, Parmol, Panado, Ceetamol, Atosol, Exctol, Tylenol, Ennagesic, Ilvamol. **Chemical name:** aspirin; **trade names:** Aspirin, Astrin, Bi-Prin. See also **pain,** page 106.

DIFFERENT TYPES, DIFFERENT PROBLEMS

■ **Animal bites** – typically by dogs, monkeys and humans – can be serious: bacteria introduced into the wound may cause severe infection. ■ **Insect bites:** reaction to all of these is similar and varies only in degree. The insect injects a substance into the skin which causes irritation and slight redness and swelling. Complications occur if the bite is scratched, breaking the skin so that bacteria enter and cause infection. ■ **Insect stings** by bees, wasps or hornets can be painful and unpleasant. The symptoms gradually improve over a few hours. Allergy to a specific sting produces a severe reaction, sometimes life-threatening. ■ **Snake bites** inject a poison into the body. There may be severe local pain, swelling and bleeding into the skin; also agitation, abdominal pain, diarrhoea and vomiting. Most people recover from adder bites: those at risk are very weak individuals who receive a large amount of venom. Tropical snake bites may, of course, be lethal.

PRESCRIPTION DRUGS

Animal bites: The chief danger is contracting tetanus, a potentially fatal condition affecting the nerves and inducing muscle spasm. **Tetanus toxoid** will prevent it if given by injection within a few days of a bite, and it should be given for any animal bites if the patient has not received the immunization within the last five years. Most infants receive it automatically, and most children on starting and leaving school. **Antibiotics** are not given routinely for dog bites, but they are always given for monkey and human bites, which almost always become infected. **Rabies vaccine** may be given to people at high risk, eg those working in quarantine stations.

Insect bites and stings: Calamine lotion is, all told, the most useful agent for soothing the irritation of insect bites. **Antihistamines** can be taken as tablets to decrease irritation. Given by injection, they will promptly alleviate allergic reactions to stings. **Adrenaline** and **steroids,** also given by injection, are used to treat severe allergic reactions. Antihistamine creams are available, but may cause allergic reactions and are not recommended.
Snake bites: Analgesics are usually necessary: aspirin or paracetamol are appropriate. There is a specific **anti-venom** for adder, and other, snake bites, given by drip; but it is only used if symptoms are severe.

QUESTIONS TO ASK THE DOCTOR
■ Is tetanus toxoid necessary?

■ Having had an allergic reaction to a sting, should I now always carry an antihistamine tablet?
■ (After a snake bite): Is an anti-venom injection necessary?

SIDE EFFECTS

Tetanus toxoid injection can cause pain and redness at the injection site, but this is not usually very severe and subsides within a few days. A lump may remain at the site for a few weeks. Allergy is rare. **Antibiotics:** *see pneumonia and pleurisy, page 78.* **Rabies vaccine** can cause allergic reactions. **Calamine lotion** has no side effects.

Antihistamine creams and **ointments** commonly cause allergic rashes: calamine lotion, or antihistamine tablets are generally preferred. Antihistamines by mouth do have side effects: *see **hay fever**, page 260.* Antihistamines should not be taken during pregnancy: *see page 184.* Adrenaline can cause tremor, dry mouth, rapid heart rate and irregular heart rhythm. These effects are related to the dose and are quickly reversible; even so, the drug should not be used in elderly patients and those with heart disease, except in life-threatening conditions.

Steroids do not have significant side effects when used for short periods, as in the case of allergic reactions. **Analgesics:** *see **pain**, page 106.*
Snake anti-venom may itself cause a severe allergic reaction, leading to wheezing, swelling of the throat and shock. Thus anti-venom is usually given in hospital.

SELF-MANAGEMENT

Animal bites:

■ Clean the wound and cover with clean dressing. ■ See a doctor if the wound requires stitching, or if the patient has not had a tetanus toxoid injection within the last five years. ■ Consider whether there is a rabies risk. If so, see a doctor as soon as possible.

Insect bites and stings:

■ Prevent bites by wearing trousers and a long-sleeved shirt. Use insect repellant, and a mosquito net, particularly in areas where malaria is common. ■ Remove a bee's needle-like sting by scraping across the skin with a blade. Forceps will squeeze more venom into the wound. ■ Patients allergic to bee stings should carry a card or wear a Medic-alert bracelet. They should also carry an antihistamine tablet with them at all times and take it immediately if stung: the dangerous effects usually occur within half an hour of being stung.

Local anaesthetic
Chemical name: lignocaine hydrochloride with adrenaline injection; trade name: Lignocaine and Adrenaline Injection.

Antivenoms
Chemical name: snake venom antiserum; trade names: Zagreb Antivenom. Other countries have specific and polyvalent antiserum against local venomous snakes, spiders and scorpions.

Calamine
Chemical names: calamine, zinc oxide glycerol; trade name: Calamine Lotion.

PATIENT'S EXPERIENCE

"My daughter aged 11 was bitten by a pet monkey. The bite was not very big, but it was on her face and I was worried about a scar. We took her to the doctor, who cleaned the cut carefully and put a stitch in. He said that she needed a tetanus toxoid injection as she had not had one for more than five years. She also needed antibiotics: apparently monkey bites are likely to become infected. He asked me to take her back to see him two days later, to check for infection. If it was infected, the stitch would have to come out. In fact, the cut healed with hardly a mark."

SNAKE BITES

■ Check whether the fangs have pierced the skin. ■ Try to identify the snake – usually not easy. ■ Do not incise the wound or use a tourniquet. ■ Wipe the wound area and flush it with plenty of water. ■ Keep the bitten limb absolutely still. Any movement will spread the venom. ■ Keep the patient calm and still, and get them to hospital.

PSORIASIS

NAMES YOU WILL HEAR

Chemical names: coal tar, as paste or paint, coal tar and salicylic acid ointment, liquor picis carbonis; **trade names:** Alphosyl, Carbo-Dome, Clinitar, Gelcotar, Ionil T, Polytar Emollient & Liquid, Psoriderm, Psorigel, Pragamatar, Polytar, Gelcotar, Tarbonis, Polytar. Note: these products are not necessarily exact counterparts – different combinations are used in different countries. Goeckerman regime is a term encountered in English worldwide for a combination of UVB light and tar treatment. **Chemical name:** dithranol or anthralin – often made up in stiff paste called Lassar's Paste; **trade names:** Anthranol, Dithrocream, Psorodrate. Ingram regime is a term encountered in English worldwide for a combination of UVB and dithranol treatment. Short contact therapy is the term for dithranol treatment left on for only a short period.

Topical steroids

Chemical names: hydrocortisone (often called HCl), betamethasonesters, fluocinolone acetonide and many more; **trade names:** numerous and confusing – slight modifications of chemical name and concentration make significant differences in potency.

Retinoids

Chemical name: etretinate; **trade names:** either Tigason or Tegison.

Cytotoxics

Chemical names: methotrexate and hydroxyurea; **trade names:** the chemical names tend to be used instead.

WHAT IS PSORIASIS?

A skin condition which usually appears as raised red patches, often covered by silvery white scales. These plaques vary in size and can occur at almost any site, but commonly involve elbows, knees and scalp. The nails may also be affected.

Different terms are used for psoriasis in its different appearances and distributions. Guttate psoriasis is common in children and may follow a sore throat. Pustular (blistering) forms of psoriasis are more stubborn and serious.

Psoriasis cannot be caught off someone else. There is no way of predicting how the disease will progress. Diet does not usually influence it. It can start at any age, and has phases of exacerbation, improvement and remission, which may be related to stress.

CAUSES The root cause is unknown. There is an excess local turnover of skin cells; it may be inherited.

PRESCRIPTION DRUGS

There is no cure: treatment is aimed at reducing the number of plaques. It is not always possible to achieve complete clearance. In mild to moderate psoriasis, topical therapies (applied to the skin) are the mainstay.
Tar, though messy in its crude form, is now available in more useful preparations. They are applied directly to the skin, used in the bath, or as a shampoo. In extensive cases, tar can be combined with ultraviolet light.
Dithranol, another topical therapy, is effective in clearing even severe psoriasis. It is best avoided in delicate skin areas, especially the face. Dithranol is also combined with ultraviolet light for severe cases.
Topical steroids vary in potency. Mild to moderate potency topical steroids require long-term use to maintain an improvement; but this can cause side effects. They are often used in small amounts to treat delicate skin areas. Potent steroids may be used on small areas of stubborn psoriasis. Topical steroids may be diluted with moisturizers, tar or salicyclic acid.
Salicyclic acid, a descaling agent, may be mixed with other preparations to enhance efficacy.

Ultraviolet light helps psoriasis.
Retinoids: Etretinate, a drug derived from vitamin A, is particularly useful in severe forms, and may be combined with ultraviolet light therapy.
Cytotoxics: Methotrexate and hydroxyurea have a role in problem cases.
How they work: Most of the drugs mentioned act by

limiting the rate at which skin cells are produced. Some of the additional treatments, or components of the treatments, are moisturizing or de-scaling agents.

OVER-THE-COUNTER TREATMENTS
See **SELF-MANAGEMENT**.

QUESTIONS TO ASK THE DOCTOR
■ Where is the treatment to be used?
■ How often and how long should I use it?
■ What should I do if the treatment burns or irritates?

SIDE EFFECTS
Tar and **dithranol** may stain the skin transiently and the clothing permanently. Dithranol may burn the skin.
Topical steroids can cause skin thinning, and other important side effects such as fluid retention *(see page 281)*. If used excessively, they cause rebound of psoriasis on stopping the steroid treatment.
Ultraviolet light therapy may increase the risk of skin tumours if prolonged. Take care to avoid burning.
Etretinate: Dryness and cracking of the lips are common, as is also a small increase in hair loss. Etretinate also causes foetal abnormalities if pregnancy occurs during therapy or for up to a year after stopping (all psoriasis drugs taken by mouth are avoided in pregnancy). Elevation of blood fats and liver and bone problems can also occur. **Methotrexate** and **hydroxyrea** can cause bone marrow damage, the former liver problems.

Side effects of the last three drug types are potentially grave; so drug administration is carefully managed under hospital supervision. The risks are carefully weighed with the patient's needs.

SELF-MANAGEMENT
Extremes of environment are best avoided and stressful situations may exacerbate the condition. Moisturizers are useful in reducing dryness and cracking. A dispersable bath oil and a moisturizing soap substitute are also helpful. Sunlight, with moderation, is often beneficial. Topical steroids are now available for anyone to buy over-the-counter, but do not use these in psoriasis without consulting your doctor.

SELF-HELP IN AN ATTACK
If psoriasis is red and angry all over and associated with shivering, you may be developing erythrodermic psoriasis. Keep warm, drink plenty of fluids and only use bland moisturizers. See your doctor quickly.

PATIENT'S EXPERIENCE
"I first developed psoriasis when I was eight, following a severe sore throat. It was a spotty, all-over, red rash, which went in about six weeks, with little treatment; my doctor actually gave me penicillin tablets for future sore throats. I didn't have any further trouble until I had another sore throat, which I didn't treat. This time the rash was treated with a coal tar cream and although it helped, it was difficult to use because there were so many small spots everywhere.

I had no further trouble with psoriasis until I was 17, when I had an accident; the rash developed in the healing scar. Soon after, the rash came up in my hair and on my knees. The knees were treated with a dithranol cream, which worked quite well – the brown marks soon cleared, but my bed linen was ruined with the stains. For my head, I was given a rather messy coal tar and salicyclic acid preparation, which was rubbed in at night and washed out in the morning with a coal tar shampoo. Once I had got used to the smell, it wasn't too bad.

On one occasion I got some psoriasis around my genitalia: unfortunately the dithranol was too strong, so the doctor gave me a mild topical steroid cream; occasional use of this kept the rash in the groin at bay.

This combination kept my psoriasis reasonably clear, but when I moved away from home I found it difficult to continue the treatment in rented accommodation. So my new doctor suggested I use a much stronger dithranol cream applied for only 15 minutes, then washed off. I can do this in the bathroom at night and it is much more convenient. My psoriasis tends to be quite variable; if I have a bad time at work it is worse, but on holiday it nearly clears up."

NAMES YOU WILL HEAR
Topical cytotoxic drug
Chemical name: 5-fluorouracil cream;
trade name: Efudix.

Sun screens
Chemical name: para-aminobenzoic
acid compounds; **trade name:**
Spectraban 4 and 15. **Chemical
name:** benzophenones; **trade name:**
Coppertone Supershade 15 (also
contains aminobenzoic acid). **Chemical
name:** cinnemates; **trade name:** Piz
Buin, available with various SPFs (also
contains benzophenone). **Chemical
name:** zinc oxide; **trade name:** ROC
factor 10 A+B Total Sunblock (also
contains cinnemate).

Caution: some sun screens can cause
staining of clothes, occasional allergic
reactions or even photosensitivity
reactions. Those with oil of bergamot
(which contains 5-methoxypsoralen)
have been implicated in causing skin
cancer, but this is not proved.

SKIN CHECK
Examine your skin ALL OVER once a
month, checking for patches, and
considering these seven points: **1** Is it
newly acquired? **2** Does it itch? **3** Is
its size increasing? **4** Has it changed
colour, or become variable in colour?
5 Is the border irregular in shape? **6**
Is there spontaneous bleeding or
ulceration? **7** Has it become nodular,
or does it extend into the underlying
skin? If you answer yes to one or
more of these, see your doctor.

WHAT IS SKIN CANCER?
– A growth on or in the skin which has the potential to
destroy tissue; some can spread to and damage other
sites. There are many different types, which vary considerably in local aggression and ability to spread.

The commonest cancer is the **basal cell carcinoma,**
alternatively known as a **rodent ulcer.** It varies in appearance, but is frequently a pearly-margined nodule,
which may or may not be ulcerated and form a deep
scab. The overlying skin often carries an increased
number of small, superficial blood vessels. These
nodules normally grow slowly and commonly occur on
sun-exposed sites, particularly the head and neck, but
can appear anywhere. Basal cell carcinomas are locally
destructive and will slowly enlarge, but do not normally
spread elsewhere.

Squamous cell carcinoma is the next commonest. It
usually presents as an unexplained ulcer or nodule on
the skin. It also occurs frequently on sun-exposed sites,
has the potential to spread. These tumours are uncommon, but there is real risk in neglecting them.

Malignant melanoma is one of the most aggressive skin
malignancies and, because of its ability to spread rapidly, always requires urgent treatment. These are usually,
but not always, dark brown or black in colour, and can
occur at any site, but again sun-exposed areas are the
commonest. They occasionally develop in pre-existing
moles. Some families seem more prone than others to
problems with moles, and should therefore be especially vigilant. See SELF-HELP.

Growths on the skin which have the potential, given
time, to turn into skin cancers, are known as **pre-
malignant skin conditions.** The commonest is the **solar
keratosis,** which occurs in middle age. It usually
manifests itself as a rough, darkened, scaly area of skin
in a sun-exposed area, frequently the head and neck, or
backs of the hands. Each patch of keratosis is small,
less than about $\frac{1}{2}$ in (1 cm) in diameter, and there are
often several of them. The risk of one of these lesions
developing into skin cancer is about one in a hundred
per year. They sometimes spontaneously resolve, but
can be treated as a preventative measure. If the lesion
becomes thickened, it is presumed to have become
malignant and needs treatment.

A similar condition, **Bowen's disease,** usually occurs as
a red-brown or orange scaly patch, which varies in size
and frequently occurs on sun-exposed sites.

With early diagnosis, most skin cancers are
treatable. However, recent studies show that deaths

from skin cancer are increasing, possibly because of the numbers of people taking holidays in the sun.

CAUSES The main factor is cumulative exposure to sunlight; whilst there is evidence that short intensive exposures can be harmful, it is the total exposure over the years that matters. In general, the fairer the skin, the greater the risk. Other factors are X-ray therapy, radiation exposure, ingestion of arsenic-containing tonics and certain types of immune suppressing drugs. A very few may be predisposed to skin cancer because in some cases it can run in families.

QUESTIONS TO ASK THE DOCTOR
■ Is my skin problem benign or malignant?
■ What are the risks?

TREATMENT
Basal and squamous cell carcinomas are, for preference, removed surgically; X-ray therapy is an alternative under certain circumstances. Occasionally other methods such as cryotherapy or lasers are used. Cryotherapy uses a freezing spray, usually liquid nitrogen. Malignant melanomas are always removed surgically as a matter of urgency. Solar keratoses are removed surgically, either by excision or by curretage – scraping off. Cryotherapy is an alternative, as is application of **5-fluorouracil cream** which destroys abnormal cells. Bowen's disease is treated in the same way as solar keratoses, but surgical removal may be preferred.

OVER-THE-COUNTER TREATMENTS
Sun screens have their role in limiting sun exposure, especially for those with fair skins. See **sunburn**, *page 278*. It is especially important to protect children.

SIDE EFFECTS
Some sun screens can cause staining of clothes, occasional allergic reactions or even photosensitivity reactions. Those with oil of bergamot (which contains 5-methoxypsoralen) have been implicated in causing skin cancer, but this is not proved.

SELF-HELP
Prevention is of course the key: follow the routine suggested in the opposite margin.

Limitation of, and protection from, sun exposure and other risk factors are especially important for those who burn easily. Use a high protection factor sunscreen.

PATIENTS' EXPERIENCE
"I lived overseas in a sunny climate until I was 20 years old. Like my father, I have a fair 'Celtic' skin. When he was in his forties, he noticed a small black mark on his back, but did nothing about it, as it didn't cause any trouble. Several years later it enlarged to form a nodule, which bled and seemed to leak a black colour into the surrounding skin. The doctors diagnosed a malignant melanoma and quickly arranged its removal, but it was too late: it had already spread to other parts of the body; Dad died a few months later. My mother, now in her fifties, has had several skin cancers develop on her face. Her doctor said that these were rodent ulcers and arranged for them to be removed. She hasn't had any more trouble, but the doctor keeps a check on her and freezes the occasional rough patch of skin on her face or the backs of her hands. Three years ago, I noticed a small dark brown mole appear on my leg. I was suspicious because I hadn't noticed it before and it seemed to be getting bigger. My doctor sent me to a dermatologist who thought it was a melanoma and arranged for it to be removed. Fortunately, it was still very thin, and I've been assured that there is every chance I won't have further trouble with it. The dermatologist told me that as a family we were prone to skin cancer because of our fair skin and degree of sun exposure abroad. Now in sunny weather, I wear a broad-rimmed hat and cool loose clothing that covers most of my body including arms and legs. On the exposed areas, I apply a factor 15 sun screen. Although I try not to be too neurotic about the sun, I avoid being out at midday and I no longer sunbathe. My dermatologist says this helps prevent further skin cancers, and also sun-induced ageing of the skin: reasonable advice for any woman in her 20s."

INDEX

Main references are in bold type.

A

abrasive preparations 274-7
abscess, corneal (eye) 269
ABVD combination 212
acebutolol 46, 56
ace inhibitors 54-5
acetazolamide 270-1
acetohexamide 158
acetylcysteine 70
acetylsalicylic acid 106, 238; see also aspirin
acne **274-7**
acquired immune deficiency syndrome (AIDS) **214-5**acromegaly 168
ACTH (adrenocorticotrophic hormone) 128, 168
acyclovir 140-1, 146-7, 210-1
additives, food 230
adenoma 168
ADH (antidiuretic hormone/vasopressin) 168
adrenalin 168, 184, 270-1, 288-9
adrenal insufficiency 168-9
aerosol medication 74-7
agonists 108
AIDS (acquired immune deficiency syndrome) **214-5**
alcohol 186-7
alcoholism **94-5**
alcuronium chloride 130
alexitol 22
ALG (antilymphocyte globulin) 226
alginic acid 22
alkaline gentian 90
ALL (acute lymphoblastic leukaemia) 210
allergent extract vaccine 260-1
allergy
    eczema 280-1
    food 230
    hay fever 260-1
    stings 288
allopurinol 246-7
almond oil 259
alopecia 207
aloxiprin 106
alphahydroxycholecal-ciferol 216
alprazolam 84
alprenolol 56
alum 260
aluminium acetate 258
aluminium hydroxide 22-3, 26, 184, 216
aluminium oxide 274
alverine citrate 32, 190
Alzheimer's disease **124-7**

amantadine 114-5
amenorrhoea 190, 220
amiloride 48, 50
amino acids 160
aminobenzoic acid 278, 292
aminocaproic acid 190
aminoglutethamide 206-7
aminophylline 70, 74
amiodarone 56-9
amitriptyline 109, 116-7, 124-5, 188, 220
amodiaquine 148-9
amoxycillin sodium 36, 68, 70, 78, 134, 138, 196, 262, 266, 288
amphetamines 103, **105**, 120
amphotericin B 264, 284
ampicillin 36, 70, 142, 144, 150, 256, 262-3
amylase 36
amyl dimethyl aminobenzoate 278
anaemia 34, 208, 210, **224-7**, 242, 264
anaerobic vaginosis 146
anaesthetics 34-5, 109, **130-1**, 185, 186, 266-7
analgesics 52-3, 78-9, 191-2, 203, 257, 266-7, 278-9, 288-9
    bones/muscles 234-7, 238-45, 248-9
    central nervous system 89, **98-9**, 100-01, **106-7**, 130
    children **196-9**
    infections 134-7, 140-1, 150-51
    pregnancy **184-7**
anaphylactic reactions 261
androgens (male hormones) 207; see also testosterone
angina **46-7**
anileridine 108
ankylosing spondylitis **248-9**
anorectic drugs; see appetite suppressants
anorexia nervosa **220-3**
antacids 22-3, 26-7, 89, 109, 184-7, with aspirin 106-7
antagonists 108-9
antazoline 260
anthralin 290
anti-arrhythmic drugs 52-3
anti-asthmatic preparations **74-7**, 185
antibiotics 28-9, 36-7, 99, 104, 109, 274, 288-9
    children 196-9
    ear/nose/eye 256, **258-9 262-9**
    infections **134-9**, **142-7**, **150-1**
    malignancy 203, 204, 209-1, 214-6

pregnancy 184-7
    respiratory 68-73, 78-81
anticholinergics 26-7, 32-3, 70-3, 74-7, 114-5
anticoagulants 64-5
anticonvulsant drugs 109, 110-3, 150-1
antidepressants 92-3, 99, **116-9**, 121, 124-7, 220-23
anti-diabetic preparations 156-61, 185
anti-diarrhoeal drugs **28-9**, 32-3, 38-9
antidiuretic hormone (ADH/vasopressin) 168
anti-emetics/anti-nausea drugs 22-3, **24-5**, 99, 138-9, 184-7, 202-7, 254-5
anti-epileptic drugs 99, **110-13**, 185, 186
antifibrinolytic drugs 190-92
antifungal preparations; see fungicides
antihistamines 25, 69, 92-3, 96-7, 136, 230-1
    ear/nose/throat **256-7**, **260-3**
    pregnancy 184-7
    skin **278-81**, **288-9**
antihypertensive drugs **48-51**, 172, 184-7, 216
anti-inflammatory drugs 106; see also NSAIDs
antilymphocyte globulin (ALG) 226
anti-nausea; see anti-emetic
anti-Parkinsonian drugs **114-5**, 120-3
antipsychotic drugs 120-3
antipyretics 134-7, 196-9; see also aspirin
antirheumatic drugs 242-5
antispasmodic drugs 32-3, 190-2
antithymocyte immunoglobulin (ATG) 226
anti-thyroid drugs 164-5
antitussives; see cough suppressants
anti-venoms 288-9
antiviral drugs 140-1, 146-7, 210, 214-5
anti-white cell; see immunosuppressive
anti-worm preparations 196-9
anxiety **84-7**
aplastic anaemia 226
appetite suppressants 154-5
arthritis 107, 236, **238-45**, 246
5-ASA 38-9
ascites 42
ascorbic acid 228
aspirin 42, 78-9, **106-7**, 190-2, 263, 266-7, 278, 288
    bones/muscles 234-8, 242-3, 246-8

cardiovascular 53, 60-1, 65
  central nervous system 98-101,
    109
  children 196-8
  infections 134-41, 149-51
  pregnancy 185-6
  see also analgesics
astemizole 230, 256, 260, 262
asthma **74-7**, 230-1
astringents 34-5, 258-9
atenolol 46, 56
ATG (antithymocyte immunoglobulin)
  226
atheroma 47, 52
atherosclerosis 172
athlete's foot 284
atrial fibrillation 54, **57**, 164
atracurium besylate 130
atrophy 158
atropine sulphate 130
azapropazone 106
azathioprine 42-3, 128, 129, 216

B

back pain **236-7**
baclofen 128-9
barbiturates 93; see also individual
  drugs
barrier creams 188-9
basal cell carcinoma 292
bath oils 280-1, 290-1
beclomethasone dipropionate 70, 260
beclomethasone propionate 74
bedwetting; see incontinence
bee-stings 288
bendrofluazide 48
benserazide 114
benzalkonium chloride-bromine 282
benzhexol 114, 120
benzoates 230; see also benzyl
  benzoate
benzocaine 266
benzodiazepines; see tranquillizers
benzoin 70
benzophenones 292
benzoyl peroxide 274-7
benztropine 120
benzydamine 106, 264
benzyl benzoate 286-7
benzylpenicillin 150, 288
bergamot, oil of 292
beta-blockers **46-7**; see also individual
  drugs
betahistine 24-5
betahistine dihydrochloride 96
betamethasone 34, 70, 258
betamethasone dipropionate 280

betamethasone esters 290
betamethasone sodium phosphate 260
betamethasone valerate 38, 70, 74,
  280
beta stimulants 74-7, 184-7
betaxolol 46, 270
bezafibrate 162-3
bicarbonates 68
bicarbonate of soda; see sodium
  bicarbonate
biquanides 157-9
biperiden 114
bisacodyl 30
bismuth 26-7
bismuth subgallate 34
bites **288-9**
bitters 90
bleomycin 212-3
blepharitis 268-9
blindness 270
blood
  circulation problems **62-3**
  clots **64-5**
blood pressure, high; see hypertension
boils (ear) 258
bones, 'thin' (osteoporosis) 36, 194-5
bowel problems 28-39
Bowen's disease 292
bradycardia 56
bran 30, 32-3
breast cancer **206-7**
breast-feeding 198-9
bromazepam 84
bromhexine hydrochloride 68, 78
bromocriptine 114-5, 168-9, 174,
  176-7
brompheniramine 256, 260, 262
bronchitis **70-73**
bronchodilators 68-9, 70-3, 78-9
bronchopneumonia 70, 78
budesonide 70, 260
bufexamac 106
buformin 158
bulimia **220-3**
bulking/bulk-forming agents 30-1,
  32-3, 154-5
bumetanide 52
bupivacaine hydrochloride 130
buprenorphine 108-9, 236
busulphan 208
butorphanol 108

C

caffeine **90-1**, 99, 191, 230-1
calamine 140-1, 279, 288-9
calciferol 250
calcitonium 109

calcium 37, 195
calcium blockers/antagonists 46-7,
  56-8
calcium carbonate 26
calcium gluconate 36, 250
cancer 108-9, **202-13**
  cervix 146
  secondary (metastasis) 206
  skin **292-3**
candida infection; see thrush
cannabis/dope/marijuana 102-5, 120
captoril 54
carbamazepine 99, 110-1, 113,
  128-9
carbaryl 286-7
carbenoxolone 26
carbidopa 114
carbimazole 164
carbocisteine 68, 70, 78
carboplatin 202
carcinoma; see cancer
carteolol 270
Castellani's Paint 284-5
catarrh 231
cefotaxime 216
cephalexin 256
cerebrovascular accident/stroke 60-1
chelated bismuth suspension 26
chemotherapy 206
chicken pox; see shingles
childbirth 184-7
children
  drugs **196-9**
  leukaemia **210-11**
chlamydia 144
chloral derivatives 92-3
chloral hydrate 92, 124-5
chlorambucil 208
chloramphenicol 150, 258, 268
chlordiazepoxide 84
chlorhexidine 264
chlormethiazole 92-3, 94
chlormezanone 236
chloroquine 148-9, 242, 244
chlorothiazide, 48, 278
chlorphenesin 284
chlorpheniramine 97, 256, 260-1,
  262, 278, 288
chlorpromazine 104, 120, 122
chlorpromazine hydrochloride 124
chlorpropamide 158
chlortetracycline 264
chlorthalidone 48
cholesterol 162
cholestyramine 162-3
choline salicylate 106
CHOP combination 212

chorionic gonadotrophin HCG 174, 176
chronic obstructive airways/pulmonary disease (COAD/COPD) 70-73
cigarettes; see nicotine
cimetidine 22-3, 26, 37, 216
cinchocaine 34
cinnamates 292
cinnarizine 24, 96, 254
circulation disorders **62-3**
cirrhosis **42-3**
chlorides 68
cisplatin 202
clemastine 256, 260, 262
clioquinol 258
clobazam 84, 110
clobetasol propionate 280
clobetasone butyrate 280
clofibrate 162-3
clomiphene 175
clomiphene citrate 174, 176-7
clonazepam 110
clopamide 48
clorazepate 84
clotrimazole 146, 258, 284
COAD/COPD (chronic obstructive airways/pulmonary disease) 70-3
coal tar 290-1
cocaine 90-1, 103, **105**
co-codamol 141
coconut oil 279
codeine 73, 98-9, **108-9**, ·278-9
codeine phosphate 28, 32, 38, 98, 103, 141, 266-7
  respiratory 68, 70, 78; see also codeine
co-dergocrine mesylate 124
coeliac disease 36-7
coffee 91
cola drinks 91
colaspase 210
colchicine 246-7
cold, common **134-7**
cold sores 146
colestipol 162-3
colic 197
conjunctivitis 145, **268**
constipation 28, **30-1**, 32-3
contraceptives **178-83**
  'pill' 169, 178-9, 190-1
converting enzyme inhibitors 49
convulsions
  epilepsy 110-3
  febrile 136, 137
  meningitis 150-1
COP combination 212
copper acetate 282

co-proxamol 140, 238
coronary thrombosis 52
corticosteroids 74-7, 274, 202-3; see also steroids
cortisol; see hydrocortisone
cortisone 109; see also steroids
cortisone acetate 178
co-trimoxazole **210-1**
cough **68-9**
cough linctus/mixture 68, 186-7
cough suppressants (anti-tussives) 68-9, 70-3, 78-9, 266-7
crabs (pubic lice) 286-7
cramp **250-1**
cretinism 166
Crohn's disease (regional enteritis) 36, 38
cromoglycate; see sodium cromoglycate
crotamiton 286
croup **266-7**
Cushing's disease 168
CVP 212
cyanocobalamin 224, 228
cyanosis 70
cyclandelate 62, 124, 250-1
cyclizine 24, 254
cyclofenil 174, 176-7
cyclopenthiazide 48
cyclophosphamide 128, 202, 206, 212
cyclosporin A 216
cystitis 88, **142-3**
cytarabine 208
cytotoxic drugs **202-15**, 290-3
  combinations 212-3

D

dacarbazine 212
danazol 190-1
D & C (dilatation and curettage) 191
dantrolene 128-9
dapsone 148
daunorubicin hydrochloride 208, 210
deafness 96, **254-5**
decongestants 68-9, 134-7, 256-7, 260-3
deep veinous thrombosis 64
dehydration/rehydration/fluid replacement 24-5, **28-9**, 151, 250-1
delirium tremens 94
delusions 120
depot injections 121
depression **116-20**
dequalinium chloride 266
dermatitis 258, 268; see also eczema

de-scaling preparations 290-1
desensitization/hyposensitization treatments 260-1
desferrioxamine mesylate 226-7
desipramine 116
desmopressin 168-9
desoxymethasone 280
dexamethasone 128, 202, 234
dexamphetamine 90, 104
dextromethorphan 70
dextromoramide 108
dextropropoxyphene 108, 141, 238
dextropropoxyphene hydrochloride 140
diabetes (diabetes melitus) 95, **156-61**, 172
diabetes insipidus 168-9
diamorphine 102, **108**; see also heroin
'Diane' pill 274-7
diarrhoea **28-9**, 32-3
diazepam 84, 96, 110, 113, 128-30, 150-1, 220, 236-7
dichloralphenazone 92
diclofenac 106, 248
dicyclomine hydrochloride 32
diethylproprion 102
diethylpropion hydrochloride 154-5
diet pills (abuse) 105; see also bulking agents
diflucortolone valerate 280
diflunisal 106, 248
digitoxin 54, 56
digoxin 54-5, 56, 59
dihydrocodeine 102, 108, 236
dilatation and curettage (D & C) 191
diltiazem hydrochloride 46
dioctyl sodium sulphosuccinate 258
diphenoxylate hydrochloride 28, 32, 38
dipipanone 102, 108
dipivefrin 270-1
disopyramide 52, 56-7, 59
disulfiram 94-5
dithranol 290-1
diuretics 42-3, 48-55, 189, 190-1
dizziness/vertigo **96-7**
docusate sodium 30, 254
dog bites 288-9
domperidone 22, 24, 202
dopamine 114
dopamine agonists 114-5
dope; see cannabis
dothiepin 116
doxorubicin 202, 206, 208, 212-3
doxycycline 144, 262, 274
droperidol 120
drostanolone propionate 206

drug misuse/abuse **102-5**, 186-7
duodenal ulcer **26-7**
dydrogesterone 190
dysmenorrhoea 190
dysrhythmias **56-9**

E

eardrops 254-5, 257, 258-9
ear problems **254-9**
eating disorders **220-3**
eclampsia (pre-eclampsia) 48
econazole 146, 284
eczema 231, 258, **280-1**
embolus/embolism 60, 64
emepronium 188-9
emepronium bromide 188
emphysema **70-3**
enalapril 54
endocrine preparations; see hormone
endocrine problems **154-69**
endometriosis 175, 190, 191
endorphins 107
enemas 31
enflurane 130
enteritis, regional (Crohn's disease) 36, 38
enuresis 188-9
enzyme deficiency 230
enzyme inhibitors 49
enzymes, pancreatic 36-7
eosin 230
ephedrine hydrochloride 134, 260, 262 epilepsy 60, **110-3**
epinephrine 270
epirubicin 206
ergometrine maleate 184, 186
ergotamine 100-1
erythema 278
erythromycin 28, 36, 70, 78, 185, 196, 274, 288
  ear/nose/throat 258, 262, 266
  infections 134, 144-5
ethacrynic acid 48, 52
ethambutol 80-1
ethamsylate 190
ethinyl oestradiol 168-9, 178, 190, 206
ethoheptazine 108
ethosuximide 110
etodolac 106
etoposide 202, 208, 214-5
etretinate 290-1
Evening Primrose Oil 162
exophthalmus 164
expectorants 68-9
eye drops 260, **268-9**, 270
eyes **268-71**

F

face washes 274-7
fatigue **90-1**
fecamfamin 90
fenbufen 106
fenfluramine 154-5
fenoprofen 106
fenoterol 70, 74
fentanyl citrate 130
ferrous fumarate 184, 224
ferrous gluconate 224
ferrous glucine sulphate 224
ferrous succinate 224
ferrous sulphate 36, 224
fibrillation/flutter 54, **57**, 164
fibrositis 234, 236
fish oils 162
fit; see epilepsy; convulsion
5-ASA 38-9
5-fluorouracil 292-3
fluclorolone acetonide 280
flucloxacillin 216, 258
flufenamic acid 106
fluid replacement; see dehydration
flunisolide 260
flunitrazepam 92
fluocinolone acetonide 280, 290
fluocinonide 280
fluocortolone 34
fluoride preparations 196-9
fluorouracil 206
5-fluorouracil 292-3
flupenthixol 104, 120
fluphenazine 32, 104, 120
flurandrenolone 280
flurazepam 92
flurbiprofen 106
folic acid 37, 184, 186, **224-7**, 228
follicle-stimulating hormone; see FSH
food
  additives 230
  allergies 230
  eating disorders **220-3**
  malabsorption **36-7**
  vitamin deficiency 228-9
food poisoning 28-9
formaldehyde 282-3
framycetin 258, 268
frusemide 42, 48, 50, 52, 216
FSH (follicle-stimulating hormone) 174, 176, 193
fungal infections **284-5**
fungicides (antifungal preparations) 146-7, 258-9, 264-5, **284-5**

G

galactorrhea 168-9
gamma benzene hexachloride (lindane) 286-7
gamma globulin 40-1
garlic 162
gastric ulcer **26-7**
gastroenteritis 28-9
gemfibrozil 162-3
genital warts **146-7**, 282-3
gentamicin 150, 216, 258-9, 268
gentian, alkaline 90
giardiasis 36
Gilbert's Syndrome 40
glaucoma **270-1**
glibenclamide 158
glibornuride 158
gliclazide 158
glipizide 158
gliquidone 158
glucagon 156-61
glucose-salt solutions 24-5, **28-9**
glutaraldehyde 282-3
glycerine 31, 259
glycerol 279
glyceryl trinitrate (GTN) 46
glycosides 56-8
glymidine 158
goitre 164-5, 166
gold 243-4
golfer's elbow 234
gonadotrophins 168, 174, 176
  FSH 174, 176, 193
  LH 176, 193
gonococcal conjunctivitis 145
gonorrhoea **144-5**
gout **246-7**
griseofulvin 284-5
GTN (glyceryl trinitrate) 46
guaiphenesin 250
guanethidine 270
guar 156-61
guar gum 158

H

haemorrhage, cerebral 60
haemorrhoids 30-1, **34-5**, 131
hair; see skin
halcinonide 280
hallucinations 94, 120
hallucinogenic drugs 102-5
haloperidol 104, 120
halothane 130
H2 antagonists 22-3, 26-7
hay fever **260-1**
headache **98-9**

heart, rhythm disorders of **56-9**
heart attack; *see myorcardial*
infarction
heartburn 22
heart failure **54-5**
heparin 64-5
hepatitis, viral 40-1
hernia, hiatus 22-3
heroin
  abused 102-3
  as analgesic *see morphine;*
  diamorphine
herpes
  herpes simplex **146-7**
  herpes zoster (shingles) 140
Herxheimer reaction 145
hiatus hernia **22-3**
histamines 260
HIV (human immunodeficiency virus)
  214-5
Hodgkin's disease/lymphoma 212
hormonal contraceptives ('pill') 169,
  178-80, 190-1
hormonal treatment/therapy 172-3,
  190-3, 206-7, 274-7
  hormone replacement therapy (HRT)
  166-9, 194-5;
  see also oestrogens
hormone suppression 168-9
housemaid's knee 235
housewife's hand 280
HPV (papillomavirus) 146, 282
HRT (hormone replacement therapy)
  166-9, 194-5
human immunodefiency virus (HIV)
  214-5
hydrochlorthiazide 48, 50
hydrocodone 108
hydrocortisone (HC)/cortisol **280**,
  290; *see also steroids*
hydrocortisone acetate 246-7, 278
hydrocortisone butyrate 280
hydroflumethiazide 48
hydrotalcite 22
hydroxocobalamin 224
hydroxyurea 208, 290-1
hyoscine 130
hyoscine butylbromide 32, 190
hyoscine hydrobromide 130
hypercholesterolaemia 162
hypertension **48-51**
hyperthyroidism **164-5**
hypertrophy 158
hyperuricaemia 246
hyperventilation 96
hynotic drugs/sleeping pills 92-3,
  102-3, 124-7, 131, 189

'hypo', diabetic (hypoglycaemia) 96,
  158, 161
hypoglycaemic drugs 156-61
hypoglycaemic drugs; *see 'hypo'*
hyposensitization/desensitization 260-1
hypotension, postural 96-7
hypothalamus 168
hyperthyroidism (thyroid deficiency)
  165, **166-7**, 168-9
hysterectomy 194

I

IB; *see irritable bowel syndrome*
ibuprofen **106**, 140-1, 185-6, 234,
  236-8, 242, 246, 248
idoxuridine 140-1
ifosfamide 202
imidazoles 146, 284-5
imipramine 116, 188-9
immune suppressors (immunosuppress
  ives) 128-9, 216-7, 226-7
immune system **212-7**
impotence, sexual 128, 168, **172-3**
incontinence, urinary 188-9
indapamide 48
indigestion **22-3**, 98
indomethacin **106-7**, 185, 234, 236,
  238, 242, 246-8
indoprofen 106
infertility 144, **174-7**
influenza **138-9**
  immunization/vaccine 138-9
inhalants 70-7, 263, 267
inosine pranobex 282-3
inositol nicotinate 62, 250-1
insect bites/stings 288
insomnia 90, **92-3**, 98, 116, 230
insomnia/sleep problems **92-3**
  tension 98
  depression 116
  caffeine 230
  fatigue 90
insulin **156-61**, 186
insulin zinc suspension 156
iodides 68
iodine 166, 186-7
  radioactive 164
ipecacuanha 68
ipratropium bromide 70-1, 74, 75
iritis 269
iron 37, 90, 184-7, 197, 216,
  224-7, 264-5
iron dextran 224
iron sorbitol 224
irritability 150
irritable bowel syndrome (IBS) **32-3**
isoetharine 70, 74

isoflurane 130
isoniazid 80-1
isophane insulin 156
isopropamide 32
isosorbide dinitrate 46
isosorbide mononitrate 46
isotretinoin 274-7
isoxsuprine 62
isoxsuprine hydrochloride 124
isphagula husk 30, 32-3
IVF (*in vitro* fertilization) 175, 176

J

jaundice **40-1**, 42
jealousy, delusional 120
joints **234-5**, **238-45**, 248-9

K

kaolin 28, 38
Kaposi's sarcoma 214-5
keloids 277
keratosis, solar 292
ketoconazole 146-7, 284-5
ketones 156
ketoprofen **106**, 238, 242, 246,
  248
kidney stones 246
kidney transplant 216-7

L

labetalol 48
labour
  analgesics 184-7
  induction 184
labyrinthitis 96-7
lactase 230
lactic acid 282-3
lactulose 30
lanatoside C 54-5
laryngitis 134, **266-7**
Lassar's Paste 290
laxatives **30-1**, 34, 109, 184-7, 220
L-dopa (levodopa) 114-5
lecithin 162
leukaemia
  adult **208-9**
  child **210-1**
levodopa (L-dopa) 114-5
levothyroxine (L-thyroxine) 166
levothyroxine sodium (USP) 168
LH (luteinizing hormone) 176, 193
lice **286-7**
lidocaine hydrochloride (lignocaine
  hydrochloride) 56, 130, 184-5, 288
lidoflavzin 46
ligament injury **234-5**, 236
lignocaine 34, 52; *see also lidocaine*

lignocaine hydrochloride (lidocaine hydrochloride) 56, 130, 184-5, **288**
lindane (gamma benzene hexachloride) 286-7
liothyronine 166
lipase 36
lipid disorders **162-3**
lipid-lowering drugs 162-3
liquorice 27
liquor picis carbonis 290
lithium 116-9
lithium carbonate 116
lithium citrate 116
liver, enlarged 42
loop diuretics 54-5
loperamide 28-9, 32, 38
lorazepam 84, 130
louse **286-7**
LSD (lysergic acid diethylamide) 104-5
L-thyroxine (levothyroxine) 166
L-thyroxine sodium (USP) 168
L-tri-iodothyronine 166
lubrican, bowel 30
lung cancer **202-5**
luteinizing hormone (LH) 176, 193
lymphatic system 212-3
lymphomas 212-3

M
magnesium 184
magnesium carbonate 26
magnesium hydroxide 22, 26, 30
magnesium trisilicate 22-3, 26, 216
malabsorption **36-7**
malaria **148-9**
malathion 286-7
malnutrition 220
manic depression 116
MAOIs (monoamine oxidase inhibitors) 116-8
maprotilene 116
marijuana; see cannabis
marine triglycerides 162
mast cells 260
mast cell stabilizers 74-7, 260
mastoiditis 256
mazindol 154
MCT (medium chain triglycerides) 37
mebendazole 196-8
mebeverine hydrochloride 32
mebhydrolin 256, 260, 262
meclozine 25, 185, 254
medigoxin 54-5
medroxyprogesterone acetate 168-9, 190, 206
mefenamic acid 98-9, 106, 190-2
mefloquine 148-9

mefruside 48
megestrol acetate 206
melanoma, malignant 292
Meniére's disease 24, 96
meningitis **150-1**
  tuberculous 80
menopause **194-5**
menorrhagia 190
menstrual problems 164, 166, 168, **190-3**, 220, 224, see also menopause
menthol 70
meperidine 108, 130; see also pethidine
meptazinol 108
mepyramine maleate 288
mercaptopurine 210
metaraminol 172
metastasis 206
metformin 158
methadone 102-3, 105, 108
methixene 114
methocarbamol 236
methohexitone sodium (sodium methohexital) 130
methotrexate 206, 210, 290-1
5-methoxypsoralen 292
methylcellulose 30, 154
methylclothiazide 48
methyldopa 172, 186
methyl prednisolone hemisuccinate 226-7
methyl salicylate 106
methylxanthines 71-3, 74-7
methysergide 100-1
metipranolol 270
metoclopramide 22, 24, 25, 100-1, 202
metolazone 48
metoprolol tartrate 46, 56
metronidazole 36-7, 146-7
mexiletine 56, 59
mianserin 116
miconazole 264, 284
midazolam 130
migraine 99, **100-1**, 231
minerals 36-7, 90
minocycline 274
mitomycin C 202
mitoxantrane 206, 208
moisturizers 279, 280-1, 290-1
moles 292
monoamine oxidase inhibitors (MAOIs) 116-8
monosodium glutamate 230
monosulfiram 286
MOPP combination 212

morazone 106
morphine 28, 38, 52, **108-9**
morphine sulphate 130
motion-sickness 24-5
mouth **264-5**
mouthwashes 264-5
MS (multiple sclerosis) **128-9**, 172
mucolytics 68-9, 70-3, 78-9
mucosal strengtheners 26-7
multiple sclerosis (MS) **128-9**, 172
muscle-relaxing drugs 109, 130, 236-7
muscles
  cramp 250
  injury **234-5**, 236
mushrooms, magic 104-5
MVPP combination 212
myasthenia gravis 90
myocardial infarction **52-3**
myxoedema 166

N
nadolol 46, 56, 270
naftidrofuryl 62
naftidrofuryl oxylate 124
nails 284, 290
nalbuphine 108
nalidixic acid 142
nandrolone 206
nappy rash 284
naproxen sodium **106**, 140-1, 234, 238, 242, 246, 248
narcolepsy 90-1
narcotic drugs/derivatives **108-9**, 236-7
nausea **24-5**
nebulizers 74-7
nefopam 106-7
neomycin 258-9, 268
neuralgia 98
nicardipine 46
nicotine/smoking 186-7
nicotinic acid 162-3, 250
nicoumalone 64
nifedipine 46, 62
night blindness 228
nitrates 46-7
nitrazepam 92
nitrofurantoin 142
nitrogen, liquid 283, 293
nitrogen mustard 212
nitrous oxide 130, 184-5
nits (head-louse eggs) 286-7
nystagmus 96
non-specific urethritis (NSU) **144-5**
non-steroid anti-inflammatory drugs (NSAIDs) **106-7**, 190, 234-49

INDEX

norethisterone 190
nortriptyline 32, 116
nose drops 134-7, 256-7, 260-3
NSAIDs (non-steroid anti-inflammatory
   drugs) **106-7**, 190, 234-49
NSU (non-specific urethritis) **144-5**
nystatin 146, 258, 264, 284-5

O

OA; *see osteoarthritis*
obesity **154-5**
oesophageal ulcer **26-7**
oesophagitis 22
oestradiol 190, 194
oestriol 190
oestrogens (female hormones) 169,
   175, 178, 190-5, 206-7, 276
olive oil 259
omega-3-marine triglycerides 162
opiates 102-5
opium 102, 108
orciprenaline 70, 74
orciprenaline sulphate 68
organ transplants **216-7**
orphenadrine 114, 120
orphenadrine citrate 236
osteoarthritis (OA) **238-41**
osteoporosis ('thin' bones) 36, 194-5
ovary/ovulation 193
ovulation inducers 174-7
oxerutin 250-1
oxpentifylline 62
oxphenbutazone 106-7
oxprenolol hydrochloride 46
oxycodone 108
oxygen administration 73, 78, 184-5
oxymetazoline 260, 262
oxymetholone 226-7
oxymorphone 108
oxytetracycline 144, 258, 274
oxytocics 184-7
oxytocin 184-7

P

pain **106-9**, 128, 231
   referred 236-7
painkilling drugs; *see analgesics,
   opiates, anaesthetics*
palpitations, heart 52, **56-8**, 84, 95,
   224, 230-1
pancreatic enzymes 36-7
pancreatitis 36-7, 95
pancuronium bromide 130
papaveretum 108, 130
papillomavirus (HPV) 146, 282
para-aminobenzoic acid 292
paracetamol 65, **78-9**, 191, 278, 288

bones/muscles 234-8, 242-5, 247,
   248
central nervous system **98-101**,
   106-7, 113
children 196-9
ear/nose/throat 257, 263, 266-7
infections 134-8, 140-1, 149-51
pregnancy 185-6
paraffin, liquid 30
paralysis 60
paranoia 120
parasites
   skin **286-7**
   worms **196-9**
Parkinsonism **114-5**
pelvic inflammatory disease
   (salpingitis) 175
penicillamine 242, 244
penicillins 144-5, 185
penicillin-V 262
pentaerythritol tetranitrate 46
pentazocine 52, 108
peppermint oil 32-3
peptic ulcer **26-7**
periods; *see menstrual problems*
peripheral vascular disease 62
pethidine 52, **108**, 130, 185-6
   abused 102
phenazocine 108
phenazone 106
phenazopyridine 106
phenelzine 116
phenindione 64
phenobarbitone 110, 113, 150-1,
   186
phenothiazines 96-7, 278
phenoxymethylpenicillin 256, 262
phentermine 154
phentolamine 172
phenylbutazone 106-7, 238, 248
phenylephrine hydrochloride 262
phenytoin 110-3, 150, 186
pholcodine 73
pholcodine tartrate 68, 70, 78,
   266-7
piles; *see hemorrhoids*
pilocarpine 270-1
pindolol 46, 56
piperazine 196-7
pirenzipine 26
piretamide 48
piroxicam 106, 248
pituitary gland **168-9**, 176, 193
pizitofen 100-1
placebo effect 90
plasmodia 148
pleurisy **78-9**

PMT/PMS; *see pre-menstrual tension*
pneumonia **78-9**, 134, 214
podophyllin 146-7, 282-3
polymyxin 259
polythiazide 48
POP (progestogen-only pill) 178-80
postural hypotension 96-7
post-viral syndrome 138-9
potassium 54
potassium citrate (pot. cit.) 142-3
pramoxine 34
prazosin 62
prednisolone 70, 74, 128, 226, 258,
   260
   bones/muscles 234, 242, 248
   gastrointestinal 34, 38, 42
   malignancy 202, 210, 212, 216
pre-eclampsia 48
pregnancy **184-7**, 197
premedication 130
pre-menstrual tension/syndrome
   (PMT/PMS) 190-1
prenylamine 46
primidone 110
probenecid 144, 246-7
probucol 162-3
procainamide 56, 59
procarbazine 212
prochlorperazine 24, 96-7, 254
prochlorperazine mesylate 202
procyclidine 114, 120
progesterone 169, 190-3
progestogens 175, 178-80, 194
proguanil 148-9
prolactin 168-9, 176, 193
prolintane 90
promethazine 24, 92, 96-7, 186,
   256, 278, 280, 288
promethazine theoclate 254
propranolol 46, 56, 88-9, 100-1,
   164 propantheline 32, 188-9
propantheline bromide 188
propylthiouracil 164
prostaglandins 106, 190
prostaglandin synthetase inhibitors
   190-2
protamine zinc insulin 156
protease 36
pseudoephedrine hydrochloride 68,
   134, 256-7, 262-3
psoriasis **290-1**
psychoses **120-3**
pulmonary embolism 64
pyelitis 142
pyrazinamide 80-1
pyridine 260
pyridoxine/pyridoxine hydrochloride;

see vitamin B6
pyrimethamine 148

Q

quinidine 56, 59
quinine 148-9, 251
quinine bisulphate 250-1

R

RA; see rheumatoid arthritis
rabies 288
rabies vaccine 288-9
ramitidine 22, 26, 37, 216
rash; see skin
Raynaud's phenomenon 63
regional enteritis (Crohn's disease) 36, 38
resorcinol 274
retin-A (tretinoin) 274
13-cis retinoic acid 274, 276
retinoids 290-1
Reye's syndrome 107, 136, 197
rheumatism 231
'soft tissue' 234
rheumatoid arthritis (RA) **242-5**
rhinitis, vasomotor 257, 263
riboflavine 228
'RICE' principle 235
rickets 228
rifampicin 80-1
ringworm 284
ritodrine 184
rubefacients 234-5, 237
rubella vaccine 184

S

salbutamol 68, 70-1, 74, 76-7, 78, 185
salicylic acid 274, 282-3, 290
saline nose drops 134-5
salmonella poisoning 28
salpingitis 175
salsalate 106
salt; see also sodium chloride
baths 34-5
tablets 250-1
water (saline) nose-drops 135;
scabies 286-7
schizophrenia **120-3**
sciatica 236
scurby 228
seborrhoea 276
seborrhoeic dermatitis 268
seborrhoeic eczema 81, 280
seizures, epileptic 110-3; see also convulsions
selegiline 114-5

selenium sulphide 284
senile dementia **124-7**
senna 30, 187
sex hormone deficiencies 168-9, 172-3
sexually transmitted diseases **144-7**
sexual problems/dysfunction 168, **172-3**; see also menopause
shampoo
medicated 268, 280
tar 290
shingles **140-1**
sickle cell anaemia 225, **226-7**
sickness; see nausea; vomiting
sight; see vision
sinusitis 134, **262-3**
skin **274**02-
bites/stings 288-9
'blotches' (Kaposi's sarcoma) 214
'blue' (cyanosed) 70
cancer 292-3
eczema 280-1
fungal infections 284-5
moles 292
parasites 286-7
psoriasis 290-1
'spots' 274-7, 282-3
sunburn 278-9
warts 282-3
sleeping pills/hypnotics 92-3, 102-3, 124-7, 131, 189
sleeplessness/insomnia 90, **92-3**, 98, 116, 230
SMO (superior mediastinal obstuction) 202-3
snake-bites 288
snake venom antiserum 288
soap, medicated 274-7, 290-1
sodium aurothiomalate 242, 243
sodium bicarbonate (bicarbonate of soda) 23, 143, 216, 259
sodium chloride 24, 28; see also salt
sodium cromoglycate 74, 230-1, 260-1 sodium fluoride 196
sodium methohexital (methohexitone sodium) 130
sodium salicylate 106
sodium valproate 110-2, 186
solar keratosis 292
sotolol hydrochloride 46, 56
spasticity 128-9
spermicide 180
SPF (sun protection factor) 278
spironolactone 42, 48, 50
sprains **234-5**
squamous cell carcinoma 292
squill 68

Stein-Leventhal syndrome (ovarian virilism) 177
sterculia 30, 32, 154
sterilization 182-3
steroids/corticosteroids **70-7**, 99, 109, 128-9, 175, 177, 202-5
bones/muscles 234-5, 242-5, 248-9
ear/nose/throat 258-61, 264-5
gastrointestinal 34-5, 38-9, 42-3
skin 274, **278-81**, **288-91**
stilboestrol 206
Still's disease 242
stimulant drugs 90-1, 102-5
stings **288-9**
strains **234-5**
streptomycin 80
stress 88-9
stridor 266
stroke/cerebrovascular accident **60-1**
strychnine 90
subfertility 174
sucralfate 26
sugar-free drugs 199
suicide 116
sulfadoxine 148
sulindac 106
sulphamethizole 142
sulphasalazine 38-9
sulphonamides 185-6, 278
sulphonylureas 157-9
sulphur 274
sulphur dioxide 230
sunburn **278-9**
sunscreens 278-9, 292-3
superior mediastinal obstruction (SMO) 202-3
suprofen 106
suxamethonium chloride 130
sympathomimetics 70-3, 270-1
syphilis **144-5**

T

tachycardia 56-9
tamoxifen 206-7
tardive dyskinesia 122, 123
tar preparations 280, 290-1
tartrazine 230
tea 91
tears, artificial 268-9
teeth 98, **197-9**, 220, 265
teething 197-9
temazepam 92
triazolam 92
temporal arteritis 98
tendon injury 234-5
tendonitis 234
tennis elbow 234-5

tenosynovitis 234
terbutaline 70, 74
terfenadine 230, 256-7, 260-3
terodiline 188-9
testosterone 172-3, 194
  esters 168-9
testosterone undecanoate 168
test tube babies 175, 176
tetanus 288
tetanus toxoid 288-9
tetracyclines 36, 78-9, 144-5, 185-6,
  258, 274, 278
thalassaemia **226-7**
theophylline 70-1, 74
theophylline hydrate 68, 70, 78
thiamine 228
thiazides 54-5
thioguanine 208
thiopental/thiopentone sodium 130
thioridazine 104, 120
13-cis retinoic acid 274, 276
thrombosis/thrombus 52, 60, **64**
thrush (yeast infection) 146-7, 258,
  264-5, 284
thymoxamine 62
thyroid gland disorders **164-7**, 168-9
thyrotoxicosis 164-5, 167
thyroxine (T4) 165, 166-7, 169
thyroxine sodium 168
tiaprofenic acid 106
timolol 270
timolol maleate 46, 56
tinnitus 96, 254-5
tiredness; *see fatigue*
tobramycin 268
tocainide 56
tolbutamide 158
tolmetin 106
tolnaftate 284
tonics 90-1
tonsillitis 134, **137**
tophi 246
tranexamic acid 190
tranquillizers/benzodiazepines 32-3,
  84-9, 92-6, 99, 124-7, 189,
  220-2
transient ischaemic attack 60-1
transplant surgery **216-7**
tranylcypromine 116
travellers' diarrhoea 28
travel-sickness (motion-sickness) 24-5
trazodone 116, 118
tretinoin (retin-A) 274
triamcinolone 234, 264
triamcinolone acetonide 280
triameterene 50
trichomonas (TV) 146-7

trifluoperazine 24, 32, 104, 120
triglycerides 37, **162**
tri-iodothyronine (T3) 166, 169
trimeprazine 92, 260, 278
trimeprazine tartrate 256, 262, 280
trimethoprim 68, 70
triprolidine 256, 260, 262
tuberculosis (TB) **80-1**
tuberculosis meningitis 80
tunnel vision 270
turpentine oil mixture 254
TV (trichomonas) 146-7

U

ulcer
  eye (corneal) 268
  genital 144
  leg 62, 280
  mouth 264-5
  peptic 26-7
  rodent 292
ulcerative colitis **38-9**
undecenoic acid 284
urethra **142-3**, 144, 194-5
  urethral syndrome 194
urine, incontinence of 188-9
urticaria 230-1
USP (levothyroxine sodium) 168

V

vaginal discharge 146-7
Valsalva Manoeuvre 57, **59**
varicose veins **62-3**, 280
vasectomy 182-3
vasodilators 49, 54-5, 62-3, 124-7,
  172-3
vasomotor rhinitis 257, 263
vasopressin (antidiuretic hormone/ADH)
  168
vecuronium 130
venereal disease; *see sexually
  transmitted diseases*
verapamil 52
verapamil hydrochloride 46, 56-7, 59
verrucae (plantar warts) 282-3
vertigo/dizziness **96-7**
vestibular sedatives 96-7
vincristine 202, 208, 215
vincristine sulphate 206, 210, 212-3,
  214
vindesine 202
viral hepatitis vaccine 40-1
vision, disturbed/impaired 60, 100,
  168, 269, **270**
  night blindness 228
vitamins 36-7, 90-1, 95, 216, **228-9**
  B6 (pyridoxine) 81, 190-1, 228

B12 224-7, 228
voice, 'loss' of 266
vomiting **24-5**

W

warfarin 60, 61, 64-5
wart-removers 282-3
warts **282-3**
  genital 146-7, 282-3
wasp stings 288
waterbrash 22
wax-softeners, ear 258-9
Whitfield's Ointment 284-5
worms **196-9**
writer's cramp 250

X

xipamide 48
xylometazoline 256, 262-3
xylometazoline hydrochloride 260

Y

yeast infections 146-7, 258, 264-5,
  284

Z

zinc 37
zinc oxide 279, 292
zinc oxide glycerol 288
zinc sulphate 36
zyclovucline 214-5

CONTRIBUTORS

Dr. D.N. Bateman, Consultant Physician, The Wolfson Unit, Newcastle upon Tyne (Parkinsonism); Dr. N.D.S. Bax, Consultant Honorary Physician, Royal Hallamshire Hospital, Sheffield (Migraine); Dr. P. Belchetz, Consultant Physician Endocrinologist, The General Infirmary at Leeds (disorders of the pituitary gland); Dr. Mary Belshaw, Liverpool (period problems, hay fever); Dr. M.J. Brodie, Consultant Physician and Clinical Pharmacologist, Gardiner Institute, Western Infirmary, Glasgow (epilepsy); Dr. M. Burke, Consultant Obstetrician and Gynaecologist, North Tyneside General Hospital (infertility); Dr. P. Campion, Senior Lecturer, Department of General Practice, University of Liverpool (indigestion, diarrhoea, constipation, haemorrhoids, obesity, middle and external ear infections, sinusitis); Dr. P. Carey, Consultant in Genito-Urinary Medicines, Royal Liverpool Hospital (sexually transmitted diseases, AIDS); Dr. I.S. Casson, Senior Registrar, General Medicine, Royal Liverpool Hospital (diabetes); Dr. Clare Connolly, general practitioner, Bradford (fungal infections, skin parasites); Dr. Jean Coope, General Practitioner, Bollingham, Cheshire (problems of menopause); Dr. Regina Curley, Senior Registrar in Dermatology, St. George's Hospital, Tooting (eczema); Dr. T.K. Daneshmend, Lecturer in Therapeutics, The University of Nottingham (jaundice, cirrhosis); Dr. J.M. Davies, Consultant Haematologist, Royal Liverpool Hospital (adult and childhood leukaemias, anaemia); Dr. Margaret Dodson, Consultant Anaesthetist, Royal Liverpool Hoaspital (anaesthetics); Dr. H. Elliot, Senior Lecturer in Clinical Pharmacology, Stobhill General Hospital, Glasgow (disorders of heart rhythm); Dr. Peter Elliot, General Practitioner, Denbigh (hyperthyroidism, hypothyroidism, strains and sprains, back pain); Dr. Christine Evans, Consultant Urologist, Royal Liverpool Hospital (impotence); Dr. Ronald Finn, Consultant Physician, Royal Liverpool Hospital (food intolerance); Dr. Katy Gardiner, General Practitioner, Liverpool (irritable bowel); Dr. Ian Gilmore, Consultant Gastroenterologist, Royal Liverpool Hospital (malabsorbtion, ulcerative colitis); Dr. R.M. Graham, Senior Registrar, Department of Dermatology, Royal Liverpool Hospital (viral warts, skin cancers, psoriasis); Dr. Susanna Graham-Jones, Lecturer, Department of General Practice, The University of Liverpool (stress, fatigue, dizziness, headache); Dr. John Green, Senior Lecturer in Medical Oncology, Clatterbridge Hospital, Wirral (lung cancer); Dr. G. Grennan, Hope Hospital, Salford (osteoarthritis); Dr. M. Grimmer, Senior Registrar, University of Liverpool (angina, heart failure); Dr. J.

Guillebaud and Dr. Gillian Robinson, The Margaret Pyke Centre, Soho Square, London (contracepion); Mr. S. Harding, Senior Registrar in Ophthalmology, St. Paul's Eye Hospital, Liverpool (chronic glaucoma, red eye/dry eye); Dr. P. Humphrey, Consultant Urologist, Walton Hospital, Liverpool (multiple sclerosis); Dr. D.H. Jones, Consultant Dermatologist, Raigmore Hospital, Inverness (acne); Dr. Denise Kitchener, family doctor, Liverpool (nausea and vomiting, pneumonia and pleurisy, cough, senile dementia, common cold, influenza, shingles, meningitis, drugs in pregnancy, urinary incontinence, drugs in children, disorders of eating, vitamin deficiencies, rheumatoid arthritis, ankylosing spondylitis, deafness, laryngitis, bites and stings); Mr. S. Leinster, Consultant Surgeon, Royal Liverpool Hospital (breast cancer); Dr. J.L. Maddocks, Reader in Clinical Pharmacology and Consultant Physician, Royal Hallamshire Hospital, Sheffield (lymphomas); Dr. J. Martin, Consultant Paediatrician, Alder Hey Children's Hospital, Liverpool (childhood leukaemias); Dr. J.P. Miller, Consultant Gastroenterologist, University Hospital of South Manchester (lipid disorders); Dr. M.E. Molyneux, Liverpool School of Tropical Medicine (malaria); Dr. A.I. Morris, Consultant Physician, Royal Liverpool Hospital (alcoholism); Professor Michael Orme, Reader in Pharmacology, University of Liverpool (introduction, myocardial infarction); Dr. Julia Parker, Senior Registrar in Psychiatry, Bristol and Western Health District (drug misuse, shizophrenia); Dr. David Roberts, Senior Registrar, University of Liverpool (hypertension); Dr. A. Scott, Senior Lecturer in Chemical Pharmacology, The University of Liverpool (problems of the circulation, blood clots); Mr. R. Sells, Consultant, Renal transplants, Royal Liverpool Hospital (organ transplants); Dr. M. Serlin, Consultant Physician, Southport General Infirmary (bronchitis and emphysema); Dr. E. Szabadi, Reader in Psychiatry, University of Manchester, and Honorary Consultant Psychiatrist, Withington Hospital (depression); Mr W.R. Tyldesley, Director of Dental Education, University of Liverpool (conditions of the mouth); Dr. C. Wells, Consultant in pain relief, Walton Hospital, Liverpool (pain); Dr. P. Winstanley, Senior Registrar, University of Liverpool (peptic ulcer, asthma); Dr. A.A.A. Zurek (cramp).

Acknowledgements

Editorial
Editorial Director	Andrew Duncan
Editorial assistance	Rosemary Dawe, Fiona Hardwick, Laura Harper
Index	Judy Batchelor

Susan Golombok's help in formulating the concept is acknowledged with thanks.

Design
Art director	Mel Petersen
Designer	Lyn Hector
Design assistants	Chris Foley, Gene Cornelius, Alastair Pether
Illustrations	Sandra Pond, Wil Giles, Andrew Popkiewicz, Paul Saunders, Tony Graham